Dialectically Integrated Psychotherapy

Dialectically Integrated Psychotherapy

A Unifying Approach to Theoretical Integration

Susan M Hingley

Editing, typesetting and publishing by UK Book Publishing
www.ukbookpublishing.com

ISBN: 978-1-914195-37-2

We shall not cease from exploration
And the end of all our exploring
Will be to arrive where we started
And know the place for the first time.

T. S. Eliot

Contents

List of Figures

About the Author

Sue Hingley is a clinical psychologist with over 30 years of experience in clinical and academic contexts. Most of her therapeutic work has been with adults in primary care, together with input into psychiatric rehabilitation and contributions to secondary care. She was a lecturer at Newcastle University from 1988 to 1998, and held an Honorary Visiting Lectureship with Teesside University from 2001 to 2018. Whilst at Newcastle University she was Academic Course Organiser for the Doctorate in Clinical Psychology focusing on curriculum development and teaching provision. She has extensive experience of teaching and supervising on the Newcastle and Teesside Doctorate courses. Her commitment to theoretically integrative therapy practice has been reflected in all of these contexts.

She lives in the North East of England, with her husband and their two cats.

www.dialecticallyintegratedpsychotherapy.com

Preface

I have always thought about psychotherapy in an integrative way, which has been influenced by my professional backgrounds and personal experiences.

Originally a biochemist, my introduction to psychotherapy took place in 1976, in my mid-twenties, with 16 sessions of therapy from a clinical psychologist in response to repeated experiences of depression. Within it I discovered the relief of talking to someone and feeling heard and understood for the first time; I discovered the tension reducing benefits of deep muscle relaxation; within my relationship with my therapist I experienced what I later discovered to be the psychodynamic concept of transference; and my sudden, spontaneous and totally unexpected connection with an anger I never knew existed reflected the concept of defence. I learnt a lot more as well, but these particular experiences stand out, because of their impact. They relate to three distinctly different theoretical approaches advised by different epistemologies. I discovered each of them by lived experience within the same therapy, and they were all valuable to me. Afterwards I never experienced depression in the same way again. I deliberately avoided reading about psychotherapy at the time, believing that it was better for it to unfold naturally. Afterwards, the books I found in my local university library told me about the concepts that my experiences related to, and made absolutely fascinating reading.

Three years later I had moved on from my rather stuck position of that time. I tried to follow through my childhood wish to become a doctor, was rejected by medical school, but accepted into the second year of a BA in psychology through a UCCA continuing application procedure; my biochemistry PhD giving me exemption from the first year. Summer was spent immersed in Hilgard, Atkinson & Atkinson's *Introduction to Psychology*, and making notes; and in the autumn of 1979 I started my psychology journey. I discovered that I loved the whole discipline of psychology; I had found my professional home.

I began my clinical psychology training in 1981 in Liverpool, where my evolving integrative perspective was supported by the broad-based functional analytic ethos of the training course, and input from a range of theoretical perspectives. My knowledge and commitment to client-centred and psychodynamic therapies inevitably influenced each other, alongside a valuing of cognitive and behavioural approaches. They were held together by the core principles of formulation: aetiology and antecedents, experiential triggers and current maintenance loops. Subsequent routine clinical work maintained those perspectives and my clinical psychology lectureship on the Newcastle Doctorate in Clinical Psychology from 1988 to1998, led me to think in more detail about theory and integrative practice. This was followed by a total of 12 years of clinical and supervisory work as an NHS consultant psychologist.

All of these professional experiences have contributed to this work, undertaken during the ten years since I left the NHS. It is the outcome of a much-loved professional life, and the product of many hours spent thinking and writing in my local university library and during lunch at Pret a Manger. It has been a fascinating and challenging journey, and I have learnt so much.

Sue Hingley, August 2020

Acknowledgements

I am indebted to all of the clients, trainees, supervisees, professional colleagues, supervisors and personal therapists who have contributed in untold ways to the meaningfulness of my professional life and to the knowledge and thinking reflected in this work. My gratitude goes to those of my clients who gave their consent for anonymised details of our work together to be used in published material, who at times thought of it as an opportunity for their painful experiences to be part of something constructive and hopefully helpful to others. All of their stories and our experiences together have contributed to the ways in which theory and practice have been thought about in this book, and aspects of one therapy are described in some detail.

The interest and support reflected in my regular meetings with Anna Jellema over the past six years have been invaluable. Her astute perceptions, our discussions of difference, the pleasure of shared understanding, and our experiences of mutual creative thinking have all been so very much appreciated.

To friends and family, your interest over the years has really mattered. To Steve for all the support, love and ups and downs of our daily lives, my love and gratitude always.

To Ruth Lunn and Jay Thompson of UK Book Publishing my sincere thanks for your interest, professionalism and hard work in support of this book.

As this work goes to press we are living through the loss, stress and uncertainty of the coronavirus pandemic. For all of us and the world as a whole, this is frightening, sad and uncharted territory. It has shaped the final months of my work on this book, and being involved in that work has helped to maintain my sense of self. My deepest gratitude goes to all the people who put themselves at risk to maintain our lives, and to give the best medical attention and human care to those who suffer and those who die.

Excerpt from "Little Gidding" from FOUR QUARTETS by T. S. Eliot. Copyright © 1942 by T. S. Eliot, renewed 1970 by Esme Valerie Eliot. Reprinted by permission of Houghton Mifflin Harcourt Publishing Company and Faber and Faber Ltd. All rights reserved.

Front cover image by the author.

Introduction

This book describes the work I have done in developing a unifying dialectically integrative rationale in relation to psychotherapy theory, Dialectically Integrated Psychotherapy. It is based on the five major theories that guide therapeutic understanding and practice: attachment, humanistic, psychodynamic, cognitive, and behavioural theories. It recognizes the theoretical depth of each of these approaches, and has two components: the Unifying Dialectical Model of human psychological functioning, the UDM; and the Dialectical Integration of Approaches to Psychotherapy, the DIAP meta-framework. Together they support the potential for any combination of these five approaches to be applied in a flexible theoretically integrated way on an individualized basis.

Within individual psychotherapy it is relatively rare for behavioural theory to be applied on its own, and both cognitive and behavioural theories are generally to be found within the integrative remit of cognitive behaviour therapy, CBT. So that equal status is given to both within this work, two theoretical sub-divisions within CBT have been created while still recognizing its overall integrative nature: cognitive and behavioural theory, in which theory relating to cognition takes the lead; and behavioural and cognitive theory, in which behavioural theory takes the lead.

In this chapter I will set the scene for this study of theoretical integration in psychotherapy, and describe the dialectical pathway I have followed. I will start by grounding us in the routine everyday world of practice, and the differing but also similar ideas that these approaches may offer us, by thinking about a single, but very meaningful therapy moment.

"So you've heard my story before."

These words were spoken by a client I will call 'Joan', who I worked with during my clinical psychology training and this therapy experience will become the starting point for our thinking about theoretical integration.

In a different place and a different way, I could imagine saying similar words to a potential reader. So much work has already been done by a wide range of therapists, researchers and academics in defining what psychotherapy integration is and exploring ways in which it may be achieved. There are many stories you may have read and valued already; will you decide to read my story too? Will it contain new messages and meaning, and is it worth your time and effort in joining with me to find out?

I heard Joan say these words right at the end of our second assessment session, after I had been describing ways in which cognitive behavioural theory helps us to understand and explain experiences of anxiety, and they taught me an important lesson about listening and making assumptions. I was feeling quite pleased at the time, the explanation fitted well with the anxiety symptoms she had talked about, and I assumed it would provide some degree of relief and reassurance that they could be understood. Her words might have indicated that was the case, might have reflected a sense of relief that her situation was known about, and she was not alone. But the tone of her voice told me otherwise. It was full of disappointment, and maybe some annoyance, and I sensed a feeling in her that I had dismissed and not listened to her story, and instead had offered a story of my own.

When we met the following week, we talked about it and I reflected her possible experience that I had not really listened to her. Yes, that was how she had felt. So, I listened properly. Later we did talk about ways of understanding anxiety reactions, but we thought about that understanding together in a way that integrated it with the personal and emotional context of her life and her experiences; everything about it was relevant to her in ways that could only happen because I had heard her, and we had connected with each other.

Thinking about Joan's reaction across our major theoretical perspectives might raise the following possibilities:

- From a primarily cognitive perspective we could think about her negative automatic thoughts, and wonder what had come into her head as she listened to me, and how did that make her feel. We might discover particular unhelpful and negative thoughts about herself, about me and about other people. We might further explore these negative thoughts, and identify unhelpful core beliefs about herself, and we may decide to challenge them in some way. We might also think that what happened between Joan and me might represent an unhelpful cognitive-interpersonal cycle that was relevant in the rest of her life, and related to underlying schemas about herself and others.

- From a primarily behavioural position we might think about operant conditioning and the principles of functional analysis, and wonder what she might have gained by responding as she did, what might have reinforced her behaviour? Since she experienced my behaviour as hurtful, it may have been rewarding in some respect to express her upset and disappointment, and positive reinforcement could be involved. In making this response she might also be pushing me away to avoid the risk of further hurt, in which case avoidance and negative reinforcement would be at play. My not listening could be understood as a discriminative stimulus for her experience of disappointment and hurt and her subsequent response, and all of these possibilities would be influenced by her learning history.

- From a humanistic, client-centred and experiential position we may think about the primary importance of empathic listening, unconditional acceptance and genuineness, and consider that this has failed in some respect, in the session and maybe in the past. We may also wonder whether her internalized conditions of worth are being reflected in some way.

- From attachment theory we may wonder about the security of her attachment relationships, and her need for the attuned relating associated with a secure base. Again we may consider that attunement has failed in this session, as may have been the case for her before, particularly within her childhood. This failure may be reflected in her internal working models of herself and other people.

- From a psychodynamic perspective we may wonder if she was not listened to or heard as a child, and whether other people still ignore her. Does she find it hard to speak up in relation to her own needs, wishes and opinions? We might think about ways in which early unhelpful experience might have affected her unconscious inner world of object relations, as well as her defence related processes, and wonder if an early problematic relational pattern was happening again in therapy. We might also think about the anger that her words might have been expressing towards me, what I had contributed to the process, and how important it was for her anger to be contained and understood.

These possibilities bear both similarity and difference in relation to each other. In the ways in which I have applied them, each of these theoretical contributions, except the cognitive perspective, recognizes essentially the same potential subjective experience for Joan: she has been hurt and has reacted to that hurt. This understanding is expressed in different ways, which may lead to differing options for intervention. From a cognitive perspective a more neutral position may be taken initially, and the nature of meaning and the experience of hurt may emerge as negative thoughts and beliefs about herself and others are explored, especially if cognitive-interpersonal cycles are taken into account. All interventions may end up being beneficial, depending on how they unfold. In addition some of those interventions might be combined with each other, to enhanced effect.

The strongest theoretical similarity here is between humanistic client-centred theory and attachment theory in terms of the importance of the attuned, empathic relationship and the consequences of its absence. The possibility of problematic early relationships is reflected within psychodynamic theory, attachment theory, and humanistic theory. Psychodynamic theory, attachment theory and cognitive theory refer to internal structures involving self and others that influence current relational experience, in terms of the inner world of object relations, internal working models and schemas respectively. Functional analysis focuses on the interaction between Joan and myself in terms of antecedents and consequences, generating ideas about its importance that are consistent with and potentially add to the other theoretical positions.

Contributions such as these from different theoretical perspectives add a greater richness and depth to the understanding and thinking that can be brought to bear within therapy, and can support each other in enhancing the therapeutic relationship. They have the potential to support a range of different interventions that may lead to positive change, and may actively complement each other. Where their understandings overlap, they provide us with greater confidence in the validity of our theoretical constructs, mechanisms and processes. This context of similarity and difference is at the heart of theoretical integration.

We will now look very briefly at the types of integration currently discussed within psychotherapy practice and research. A far more detailed overview of these approaches is provided by Norcross & Goldfried (2005).

Types of Psychotherapy Integration

Technical Integration or Technical Eclecticism: This refers to the use of therapeutic approaches on a largely pragmatic basis to address different aspects of a person's difficulties and to take the differing characteristics of individual clients into account. Approaches may be used as single-model therapies, or the techniques associated with several approaches may be applied within one therapy, but the integration is always on a pragmatic, technical basis rather than a theoretical one. Examples of technical integration are provided by Multimodal Therapy (Lazarus, 2005; Palmer, 2000), Systematic Treatment Selection and Prescriptive Psychotherapy (Beutler et al., 2005), and the incorporation of various techniques and strategies into CBT described by Harwood et al. (2010).

Theoretical Integration: This refers to therapies in which the mechanisms and processes associated with different models complement each other on a theoretical basis, and is often referred to as a synthesis of those approaches. Theoretically integrated approaches are often proposed as single-model therapies in their own right, with some key examples being provided by Transtheoretical Psychotherapy (Prochaska & DiClemente, 1983, 2005); Cyclical Psychodynamics and Integrative Relational Psychotherapy (Wachtel, 1977, 1997, 2014; Wachtel et al., 2005);

Assimilative Psychotherapy (Stricker, 2010; Stricker & Gold, 2002); and Cognitive Analytic Therapy (Ryle, 1995a; Ryle & Kerr, 2020).

Transtheoretical Psychotherapy addresses processes of change common to all therapies, and advocates the application of techniques associated with different theoretical approaches depending on the client's stage of change: whether they are at a pre-contemplation stage and unable to think about it; can start to contemplate change in themselves and their lives; are ready for the action involved in change; or need support to maintain change that has been achieved. Cyclical Psychodynamics recognizes the importance and value of overt behaviour in supporting the internal changes conventionally addressed by psychodynamic therapy, and the mutual cyclical relationship between the two. Active behavioural analysis and interventions are integrated into psychodynamic work on this basis. Assimilative Psychotherapy, primarily relating to psychodynamic theory, argues that useful aspects of a range of approaches can be assimilated into a main model of therapy, as long as they are defined within the theoretical terminology of that model. Cognitive Analytic Therapy has generated its own independent constructs based on psychodynamic and cognitive theoretical positions, which are used to guide largely overt interventions influencing ways of thinking, feeling, and behaving, particularly within relationships.

In other contexts, core processes of change are identified that can be influenced by interventions associated with a range of different theoretical approaches. Examples in this respect include the importance of the transformation of meaning as discussed by Power and Brewin (1997) and the disconfirmation of dysfunctional schemas considered by Safran and Ink (1995).

Common Factors Integration: A further approach to thinking about psychotherapy integration has been to assume that certain features that different approaches to therapy have in common are responsible for therapeutic change, and not their theoretically defined characteristics. In addition, the specifics of our theoretical approaches are deemed to be only those aspects that are unique to each of them. The common factors then tend to be referred to as non-specific or non-procedural factors, in effect detaching them from any theoretical understanding. The supportive nature of the therapeutic relationship, and the experience of hope are particularly identified as significant common factors responsible for change, with examples being provided by the work of Frank and Frank (1991, 2004) and the Contextual Model proposed by Wampold and Imel (2015).

My Approach to Theoretical Integration

In this work I am not looking to establish a theoretically integrated stand-alone model of psychotherapy. My aim is to articulate a model that supports the validity and constructive value of drawing on a range of theoretical approaches within any psychotherapeutic context.

Similarity and Difference: In thinking about what happened between Joan and myself from each of our major theoretical perspectives, important principles emerge that relate to this study of theoretical integration. Aspects of similarity and overlap support the validity of associated elements of theory; differences and unique understanding extend our theoretical awareness, and carry the possibility of interventions that might complement each other. The diagram in Figure 1 illustrates these principles, and portrays our major theoretical approaches as overlapping ellipses.

The extent of overlap varies between different approaches. The central area in which they all overlap implies that in some respect all of them will have something in common with each other. The areas of the ellipses that don't overlap represent

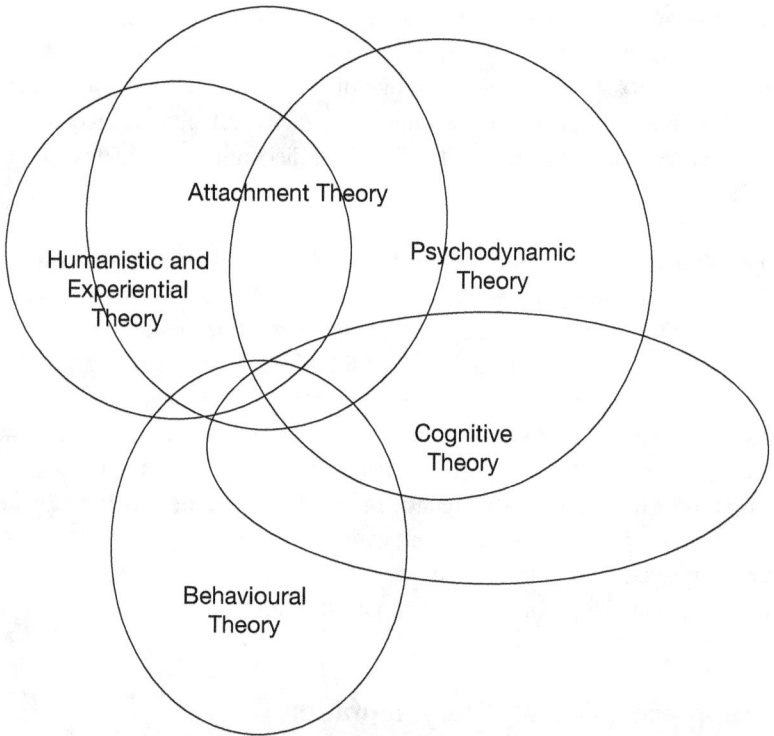

Figure 1 Overlapping and Unique Contributions of Theoretical Approaches to Psychotherapy

the unique contributions they each make to theoretical understanding and to therapy, differences that may powerfully complement each other within processes of change.

Our Human Mind: I now want to turn to some thoughts about the nature of our human mind, where the structures, mechanisms and processes of our theoretical perspectives will be at play. I will start by thinking about the experience of receiving psychotherapy, in order to reflect on what I believe to be a central and essential position in relation to theoretical integration.

If any of us were struggling with anxiety and depression, we might welcome the opportunity to see a cognitive behavioural, CBT therapist and gain really valuable benefits from a protocol-led Beckian approach. We might also find that to some extent although our anxiety levels were much more manageable, our depression not so disabling, we were still struggling with some source of unhappiness we could not quite understand or move on from. We might decide that an experience of psychodynamic therapy was worth a try and discover it was really helpful too. The process could just as well work out the other way around. After first benefiting from psychodynamic psychotherapy, we may find that our symptoms of anxiety linger on, and in spite of much else changing in our lives, our minds automatically take us to unhelpful positions at times. An experience of CBT could make all the difference.

In order to be helpful to us, the structures, mechanisms and processes associated with both of these therapy approaches must be present and active within our minds. We know that we do not have separate psychodynamic, cognitive or behavioural sections within our minds; they are whole, not fragmented entities. If that is the case, and if we truly believe that the mechanisms and processes of both psychodynamic therapy and CBT have validity, those mechanisms and processes must routinely exist together within our minds. Their differences have to be compatible with each other, and they all have to be able to co-exist. The same will apply to all of our validated theoretical approaches to psychotherapy.

My work reflects a basic belief in the theoretically unified functioning of our human mind. I do not believe that a fully defined and unified description of how that mind functions will ever be possible, or that we will ever be in a position to define a single, universally effective approach to psychotherapy on that basis. However, I do believe that all of our theoretical positions should be definable in ways that are not in conflict with each other, because their related processes and mechanisms must be functioning in harmony and seamless synchrony within the one human mind that we all possess. From a similar perspective Safran and Inck (1995) use the metaphor of different parts of the same elephant being addressed by our different theoretical approaches to psychotherapy. However, they come to the conclusion that although the same elephant is being referred to, theoretical integration in relation to these different parts is not possible. I very much disagree with this conclusion; if each theoretical approach has validity, and if we truly are examining the same elephant, ultimately theoretical integration must be possible.

I see the integrative consideration of psychological constructs on this basis as one of the most important tasks facing the study of human psychology. As long as we maintain a dissociative split across the different theoretical approaches that so obviously must be relating to the same human mind, we hold back our search for knowledge and understanding of ourselves, and the application of that knowledge.

This book is written from the position that theoretical integration and unification in relation to the psychological functioning of our human mind reflects its natural state of affairs. During our efforts to explore, understand and work with the amazingly complex phenomena that are our human psychological selves, our theories have become artificially segregated.

A Metaphor for Dialectical Theoretical Integration

Our current approaches to psychotherapy have been developed from, or at times, in opposition to earlier theoretical starting points, and each has set out to examine the psychological functioning of the same human mind from within its own frame of reference. Building on the theme of overlapping circles in Figure 1, we could imagine the elements of theory associated with each approach to be theatre spotlights, each casting a circle of light on the stage of human psychological functioning.

These spotlights are focused on the single stage of a theatre of study that researchers and therapists with allegiances to different schools of thought tend to visit on their own. They do not necessarily see the spotlights created by others. Sometimes the circles of light provided by different approaches would overlap with each other, if they were turned on together. They would maybe overlap virtually completely, or one may exist entirely within the sphere of another, but encompass only part of it, or it may be that only a limited area of some spotlights would cover the same ground as others. In the latter case the rest of the light from each spotlight would be shed on unique areas of the stage. None of this will be apparent unless the spotlights of the different theories are turned on and seen at the same time. Each of these relationships between the areas of light cast by our theoretical spotlights relates to ways in which the elements of our differing theoretical approaches relate to and connect with each other.

These connections and similarities may not be recognized at all within the writings and practices of the theoretical approaches concerned, and as readers and practitioners it will be for us to make our own judgements. At other times theoretical similarity, and/or the specific application of pre-existing concepts and understanding may be clearly acknowledged.

When the spotlights of our different theories do not demonstrate aspects of overlap, each will make their own unique contributions, complementing each other within an integrative, harmoniously functioning whole. This state of affairs requires theories to be compatible, and not in conflict with each other. The existence of one theoretical position must not logically wipe out the possibility that another one is functioning as well; they are able to co-exist and their spotlights can shine at the same time. If they are in logical conflict with each other they cannot co-exist, and their spotlights cannot shine in unison.

This context of incompatibility presents a particular challenge to psychotherapy integration. Only compatible constructs, mechanisms and processes may be drawn upon from an integrative perspective. If the premises associated with different theoretical approaches are incompatible with each other, they cannot be deemed to co-exist within our one human mind, and cannot be integrated. The only way to resolve this situation is for the premises of one or more of the approaches to be changed in a way that removes the incompatibility.

The Relationship Between Theory and Practice

As well as describing their individual perspectives on the nature of human psychological functioning, each theoretical approach to psychotherapy also defines its own principles regarding the practice and conduct of therapy. In this work I make a clear distinction between the two, and initially integration will be considered solely in relation to the psychological constructs, mechanisms and processes associated with human psychological functioning.

The principles adopted regarding therapy practice all relate to beliefs about what needs to take place in therapy, to enable beneficial changes in the particular constructs, mechanisms and processes that are the focus of each theoretical approach. In single-model therapy practice these beliefs are often stated as formal guidelines, supported by therapy protocols and definitions of therapist competencies. Significant aspects of routine practice that vary across different approaches to therapy include the style of therapist behaviour in relation to clients, the nature of the relationship between them, the nature of specific interventions, and the ways in which therapy is organized in terms of structure and content, across and within sessions. Principles of practice will also include judgments and criteria relating to the application of different therapies such as the nature of the problems it is best able to address, the characteristics of clients who are likely to benefit, and the nature of training needed for therapists to become competent. Compatible and incompatible differences in all of these respects will influence the feasibility of integrating our different major therapeutic approaches at the level of practice.

A Dialectical Study of Theoretical Integration

Before I overview the nature of the current work, a few more words need to be said about the context of our cognitive and behavioural theories. In terms of current approaches to therapy it is hard to separate them since they are both commonly applied as valuably integrated parts of cognitive behaviour therapy, CBT. This has become something of an umbrella term for a large group of integrative therapies all reflecting cognitive and behavioural principles and styles, which are often influenced by a range of other therapy-related theories as well. The boundaries between these individual, and sometimes very contrasting therapies, have not been maintained within what is often talked about as a single-model approach. In the midst of the 'cognitive revolution' unique core aspects of behavioural theory seem to have become somewhat eclipsed by cognition. As mentioned earlier, in order to reflect them as fully as possible within this work the theory underlying CBT has been separated into two parts: cognitive and behavioural theory, in which theory relating to cognition takes the lead; and behavioural and cognitive theory, in which behavioural theory takes the lead.

The current work adopts a comprehensive and transparent dialectical approach to the integration of psychotherapy theory across the five major theoretical perspectives. It initially addresses the theoretical nature of human psychological functioning on an integrative basis, and it is only after this work has reached its conclusion that therapy practice is brought into consideration. My intention is to explore ways in which the constructs, mechanisms and processes of these major theoretical approaches may all work together, and be involved in processes of change, within our one human mind. The work done to achieve this essentially constitutes a piece of informal qualitative research, in which the contents of our selected theoretical approaches are analysed, thought about and brought together on a dialectical basis that seeks to resolve incompatibility.

Philosophy and associated epistemology (the approach we take towards gaining knowledge) is very relevant to this analysis, because the position we take in relation to philosophy influences the range and nature of the knowledge that we work with and what we do with it. Some philosophical positions dramatically limit the nature of knowledge that may be taken into account. Within this work I have found Roy Bhaskar's critical realism particularly helpful, since it reflects ways I naturally think about knowledge of ourselves and the world around us, and is consistent with the nature of human psychology and psychotherapy. It allows for a range of epistemologies, and fundamentally supports dialectical process. Part 1, Chapters 2-4 will provide an overview of philosophical approaches and a discussion of the core principles of Bhaskar's critical realism.

In this work the spotlights of attachment, psychodynamic, humanistic, cognitive and behavioural, and behavioural and cognitive theories will all be turned on at the same time. Overlaps and similarities in their content will be identified, constructive use will be made of their compatible differences, and apparently incompatible differences will be explored in the context of their potential resolution. It is particularly this attention given to resolving incompatible or apparently incompatible differences that constitutes the dialectical strength of this work, and is consistent with Hegel's description of logic as following a dialectical pathway in which internal contradictions are transcended (Honderich,1995). The flow chart in Figure 2 illustrates the overall process of theory development.

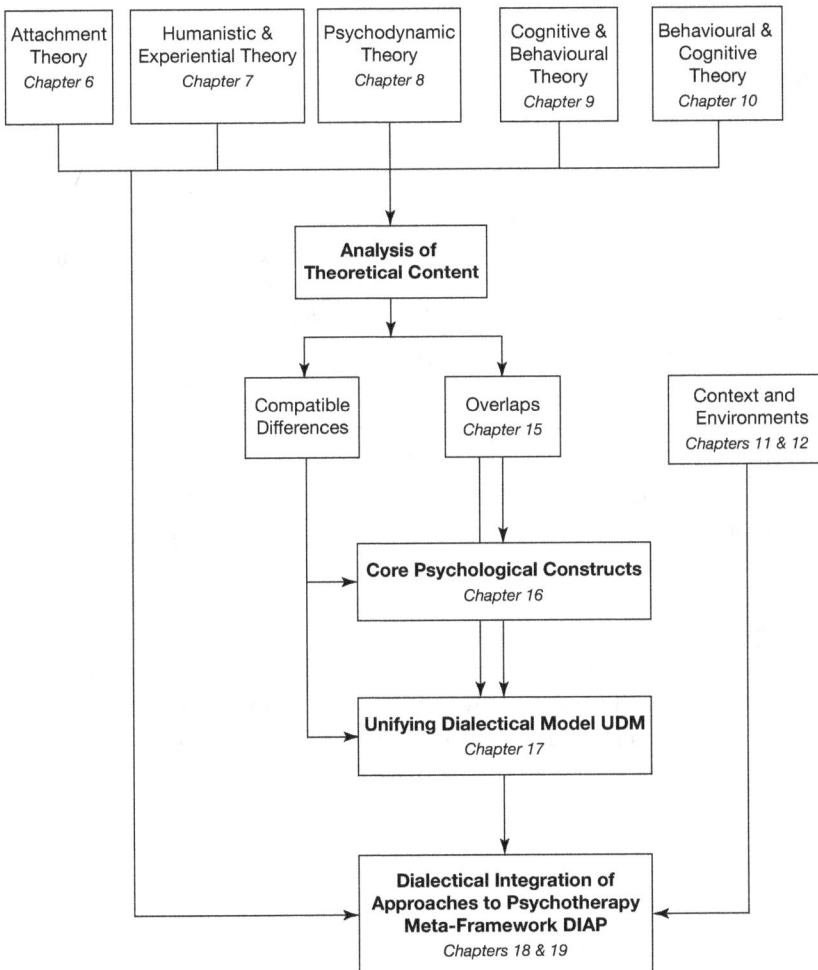

Figure 2 A Dialectical Study of Theoretical Integration

Part 2, Chapters 5-10, provides the theoretical detail on which this analysis of content across approaches will be based. We will look at attachment theory (Chapter 6), humanistic and experiential theory (Chapter 7); psychodynamic theory (Chapter 8); cognitive and behavioural theory (Chapter 9); and behavioural and cognitive theory (Chapter 10). In addition, Chapters 11 and 12 will address the theoretical importance of contexts and environments, looking at the nature of the world around us (Chapter 11), and our place in the lifespan (Chapter 12).

Part 3, Chapters 13-19, constitutes the core of this work in terms of the dialectical study of theoretical integration. In Chapter 14 I will further explore the importance and challenge of working with incompatible difference. In Chapter 15 I will discuss 11 significant theoretical overlaps between our five major approaches, identified by an analysis of theoretical content. These will include five core constructs, in which I judge our different approaches to be referring to the same psychological entity. In Chapter 16 differing aspects of compatible theory across the major approaches will be brought together to define each of these core constructs on a theoretically integrative basis. In Chapter 17 they will be used together with other aspects of significant overlap, to describe a coherent theoretically integrative model of human psychological functioning, the Unifying Dialectical Model, UDM. In Chapter 18 a meta-framework supporting theoretically integrative psychotherapy practice, the Dialectical Integration of Approaches to Psychotherapy, DIAP meta-framework will be discussed. This framework will illustrate the potential for each of our five major approaches to support constructive psychological change through their individual and mutual impacts on the processes of the Unifying Dialectical Model. Chapter 19 will discuss some of the practical implications and value of the UDM and the DIAP meta-framework. The Unifying Dialectical Model and the DIAP meta-framework together constitute Dialectically Integrated Psychotherapy.

Part 4 will explore a single experience of individualized integrative psychotherapy, and the different theoretical perspectives that have come together in support of practice within each session will be identified. Chapter 20 will analyse the proportions of different theoretical approaches used across the therapy, and summarize the therapy experience. Chapter 21 will then look at the nature of change in terms of the integrative understanding supported by the Unifying Dialectical Model and the DIAP meta-framework.

Part 5, Chapters 22-25, will discuss Dialectically Integrative Psychotherapy in the broader context of work addressing psychotherapy integration. Chapter 22 will look at its relation to the general aims and principles of integration, Chapter 23 will compare it with other approaches, and Chapter 24 will consider its implications in terms of theory development, the ways in which we conduct our research efforts, the practice of both integrative and single-model psychotherapies, and the nature of psychotherapy training. The final chapter will summarize the work done and reflect on the processes involved as it unfolded.

This book is designed to be read in sequence or approached on the basis of the parts and chapters that best fit the reader's existing knowledge and interests. Introductions are provided to Parts 1-3 and summaries are available at the end of chapters, to help readers decide where they want to start and to select those chapters they may most wish to read in detail.

Summary

This introductory chapter has defined the dialectical nature of my approach to theoretical integration in psychotherapy and overviewed the philosophical context of the work. It has described aspects of the qualitative analysis of the theoretical content of five major approaches that will lead to the development of the two components of Dialectically Integrated Psychotherapy: the Unifying Dialectical Model of human psychological functioning, the UDM, and the Dialectical Integration of Approaches to Psychotherapy, DIAP meta-framework. This material will be covered in Parts 1, 2 and 3 of the book. Part 4 will provide an example of integrative therapy practice that will be analysed in relation to the principles of Dialectically Integrated Psychotherapy. Finally, Part 5 will discuss this work in comparison with other approaches to integration, consider its practical implications, and reflect on key aspects of the work overall.

Part 1

The Crucial Importance of Philosophy

Introduction to Part 1:
Why Philosophy Matters

This book is about theory and how theory, in its various forms, may be applied within the practice of psychotherapy on an integrative and unifying basis.

Whenever we relate to our theoretical perspectives, we will be influenced in our thought processes by philosophy and by epistemology. Within any philosophical position associated epistemologies will guide the approach taken towards gaining knowledge, and will influence the nature of knowledge that we put our trust in. Each of us will be influenced by a range of factors in being pulled more towards some epistemologies than others, including our general education and professional training, our experiences of therapy with our clients, the therapy we may have had for ourselves, and the nature of the supervision we have received. Our own personalities will also play their part; we may just feel more comfortable with some epistemologies rather than others.

Sometimes we may consciously be aware that we are adopting a particular epistemology that guides our beliefs about the best ways to gain knowledge of the human mind and how to apply it. At other times, and maybe more routinely, we probably don't think about it consciously at all; we look for information, think and make decisions in relation to therapy theory and provision on an automatic basis. But we are still being guided at an unconscious level by our internalized beliefs regarding the nature and validity of related knowledge; our own individual epistemologies, outside of conscious awareness. In our routine professional practice I imagine it will be a rare occurrence for any of us to sit and think about the epistemological and philosophical assumptions that, moment-to-moment, lead us to consider one source of knowledge more meaningful, reliable and useful than another.

These processes will generally be automatic and implicit within our everyday practice. They may be restricted to a single epistemology, or involve more than one. Sometimes we may explicitly apply and adhere to one particular epistemology, but at the same time automatically and implicitly draw on others.

For each of us as individual practitioners and researchers, and for our profession as a whole, our overt and covert epistemologies will influence the ways we think about theory, and how we relate theory to practice. Some avenues of thinking will open up for us, and others may remain forever closed, however beneficial they may have turned out to be. In the end the way in which our understanding of the human mind develops, and the application of that understanding, depends on philosophy.

At institutional and societal/government levels we are significantly affected by the nature of philosophy and epistemology adopted at the higher levels of our professional and political systems, as is particularly evident in recent years with the evolution of single-model evidence-based practice. In addition, whilst by no means exclusively the case, psychology as an academic discipline is significantly influenced by the principles of logical positivism. In many respects it chooses to be seen more as a science rather than part of the arts or the humanities. Other psychotherapy contexts stand in more mixed positions in relation to philosophy and epistemology, depending on the nature and origins of their theoretical approaches, but in the context of public provision and therapies funded on an insurance basis, all approaches have had to consider the implications of the logical positivism that is associated with the requirements of evidence-based practice.

One of the major consequences of the push towards evidence-based practice is the powerfully restrictive impact that its formal implementation has had on the provision of integrative therapies, which cannot be allowed unless they can be branded and evaluated as single-model therapies. The benefit of drawing on more than one model in flexible ways that reflect the unfolding needs of individual clients, is totally denied within its ethos.

These influences of philosophy might be open to some degree of moderation if our epistemologies could be brought into the light of conscious thought, consideration and debate at institutional and individual levels. If it ever became possible for evidence-based practice to embrace a more pluralistic approach, its epistemological base would then be more in line with many of the therapies that it actually promotes, and would reflect the world of empirically supported psychotherapy that we actually live in. In support of this potential process, Part 1 of this book provides an opportunity to touch base in relation to philosophy and a range of epistemologies, and to consider the particular benefits that may be gained from drawing on the premises of Roy Bhaskar's critical realism.

Chapter 3 reviews the general nature of philosophy and epistemology, and considers the relevance of philosophy to the practice of psychotherapy. It provides brief definitions of some key epistemologies, giving particular attention to the characteristics of logical positivism, looking at the specifics of scientific method, the problem of induction, and the requirements of measurement associated with the role of statistics. The problems raised by its application to the study of human psychology and the practice of psychotherapy are summarized, and an overview is provided of the range of epistemologies reflected in our major approaches to psychotherapy. Finally, the need is argued for a philosophical approach that is consistent with the overall nature of human psychology and psychotherapy, and is supportive of theoretical integration.

Chapter 4 then introduces Roy Bhaskar's critical realism (Bhaskar, 2017), as discussed by Collier (1994). An overview of its core principles leads into a discussion of the ways in which its premises are consistent with the nature of the subject matter of human psychology and psychotherapy, conducive to theoretical integration, and supportive of the overall principle of theoretical unification within the human mind.

The Philosophical Context of Human Psychology and Psychotherapy

This chapter will be devoted to a discussion of the nature of philosophy, providing an overview of a range of traditional and currently popular epistemologies, a discussion of the fit between the subject matter of human psychology and psychotherapy and the principles of logical positivism, and a consideration of some current post-modern alternatives.

According to Rosenberg (2012) the noun 'philosophy' has its origin in words that mean 'love of wisdom'. In relation to the functioning of human society we might say that to have wisdom is to have awareness, knowledge and understanding that can be of reliable use or benefit in some way and therefore valued and trusted. Humans hold such knowledge in very high regard. In various ways the diverse outcomes of such wisdom help to enhance human well-being, they enable the development of the social and physical structures that support us, help to reduce existential anxiety, and satisfy our natural curiosity about ourselves and what we discover to exist around us. At other times, our assumptions about apparent wisdom that can be trusted prove to be ill-founded in some ways, and carry costs that we could not envisage, or did not wish to see.

Philosophy has as its subject matter the nature of the processes by which we come to have knowledge, and the processes that guide what we might do with it. Rosenberg (2012) defines four major sub-disciplines of philosophy: logic, ethics, epistemology and metaphysics. It is logic that we have come to rely on most strongly to give us a sense of security and trust in our human-based understanding of ourselves, and the space we live in within the universe. However, we often recognize and value the importance of meaning over logic within human existence, and meaning in some form is likely to influence the path of logic, whether we are aware of it or not. Ethics addresses our concerns about morality, right and wrong, good and evil, what is just and unjust, and therefore 'ought' to be the case within human society.

Epistemology refers to theory about human knowledge, exploring or defining the nature of that knowledge, the extent of it, and how it has been justified (Honderich, 1995). Any subject area could have its own epistemology that guides people in the processes they follow to establish its knowledge base. The same epistemology may be applied to other areas of knowledge and enquiry, or different epistemologies may be more appropriate.

Metaphysics is concerned with the features of ultimate reality, and has been described as the most abstract area of philosophy. Ontology is a branch of metaphysics, and relates to the nature of existence or being. It recognizes the existence of beings and entities, including both abstract and concrete entities, with the latter existing in the form of both substances and non-substances. In these respects, ontology recognizes that the nature of what exists in our world cannot be totally justified by empirical means within the natural sciences (Honderich,1995).

Epistemology is of central importance since without a secure theory underlying the acquisition of knowledge in any area of human understanding or endeavour, any further use to which that knowledge is put will be vulnerable to error or distortion. The nature of the epistemology guiding the acquisition and application of knowledge within human psychology and psychotherapy will influence the nature of knowledge that is accepted as valid and appropriate to guide day-to-day psychotherapy practice.

Since the nineteenth century it has been science and the use of observation and logic that has come to be the most highly valued approach to knowledge, particularly within western culture; a science that is now largely synonymous with logical positivism. To be recognized as a science has become associated with esteem, acceptance and influence, and this status has become a much sought after and defended prize for some disciplines. Gantt et al. (2016) provide an interesting discussion of this context in relation to social psychology. If a discipline is not a science it falls by default into the category of the arts or the humanities, although some may be defined as both a science and an art. We distinguish between natural science and social science, and between the pure and applied sciences, with pure science in relation to the natural world holding the highest status.

The political context of psychotherapy practice within the United Kingdom and the United States in relation to evidence-based practice and decisions made regarding financial support or remuneration for state and insurance-based psychotherapy provision, has raised the profile of philosophy and epistemology within psychotherapy practice and health care. In general, logical positivism has been adopted as the basis for decisions about the validity, effectiveness and availability of different psychotherapy approaches in these contexts. There has been no high-level governmental discussion in relation to this decision about philosophy, and the epistemology adopted seems to go unquestioned within the corridors of power.

On the positive side impetus has been given to encourage all psychotherapies to address issues of efficacy and effectiveness, and our research base has been much enhanced in this respect. However, serious issues in relation to the validity, reliability and generalizability of such research remain, as discussed by Roth and Fonagy (2006). In addition, the predominance of medical standard, randomized controlled trials (RCTs) in relation to psychotherapy outcomes, may have pushed research on underlying theoretical constructs into the back seat. Attention to underlying theory may be losing out to a pragmatic emphasis on practice and outcome, both in terms of research attention and as essential aspects of training in psychotherapy and the psychological therapies.

The following discussion hopes to take us back to basics in some ways, and overviews some key philosophical approaches and epistemologies that have relevance to human psychology and psychotherapy. It acknowledges the current debates between positivism and post-modern epistemologies, appreciating the value of using both alongside each other, as well as recognizing the polarized positions that may sometimes be adopted by practitioners and researchers.

The validity of research guiding important decisions about the public endorsement, application and availability of different approaches to psychotherapy is at stake here, as well as the crucial value of theory-led pure research. In the context of psychotherapy integration and theoretical integration in particular, we need to find a philosophical approach that supports the subject matter of our differing approaches, and allows for potential dialectical synthesis across areas of both similarity and difference. So perhaps a step across into the world of the philosopher may be helpful, in the belief that we are all guided at some level by philosophical and epistemological principles in carrying out our therapeutic work within the professional world of psychotherapy.

A brief review of some key epistemologies will be followed by a more detailed discussion of the requirements of logical positivism, looking at experimental method and the use of measurement and statistics in relation to psychological variables. Issues regarding the fit between the subject matter of human psychology and psychotherapy, and the principles of logical positivism and scientific method will be a central part of this discussion.

The post-modern position that has evolved within psychology to challenge the premises of empiricism and logical positivism will then be discussed, followed by an overview of the epistemologies reflected within psychotherapy theory and practice, and a look at the nature and relative status of theories compared with models.

A Brief Overview of Some Key Epistemologies

Stepping across into this world of philosophy is something of a challenge in itself, especially if we wish to gain a broad-based, critical and somewhat discerning perspective that is not simply influenced by current fashion and culture within psychology or psychotherapy. It also puts us in the position of considering the nature of both psychology and psychotherapy in relation to science: are they both sciences or not, or is one a science and the other not? If one or both are not sciences then how do we classify them, as an art or as one of the humanities, and how do we argue for the status and social value of their knowledge base?

How do we know that we know something? How do we judge that something exists or that some action is likely to produce a valued and beneficial outcome? The reason we want to answer these questions, particularly in the context of psychotherapy, is hopefully because we have a sense of responsibility towards others, and because we wish to function on an ethical basis.

Taking even a limited journey into the philosophical literature reveals considerable differences of perspective. It is one of those subject areas where it can seem hard to pin things down, where definitions vary from author to author, and where language can be esoteric and unfathomable. The following brief descriptions will overview some of the key epistemologies that illustrate the varied ways in which humans have considered the nature of the world around them. At this point we will look at ways in which realism, idealism, empiricism, positivism and logical positivism, hermeneutics, instrumentalism, relativism, phenomenology and post-modernism may be defined and some of their core characteristics (Honderich, 1995; Rosenberg, 2012).

Realism: This is the belief that the material world exists independently of our perceptions of it. However we might believe it to be, and whether we can perceive it or not, the material world has its own independent form and existence (Collier, 1994).

Idealism: In extreme form, called objective or absolute idealism, this is the view that what we perceive as the material world is created by the mind, and exists only if we have a thought about it. In a less extreme form it is the belief that our minds create the world as we perceive it by our senses imposing form on material things that are themselves unknowable; this view has been called subjective idealism. From this position idealism seems to somewhat overlap with realism in believing that an independent world does exist, even if it may be unknowable. More recently the term super-idealism has been used to refer to the belief that human beings can change themselves and the world they live in by changing how they perceive it, and how they convey this perception in discourse. In some respects the functional meaning of idealism and particularly super-idealism may seem to overlap with rationalism, which can be defined as the belief that it is possible to obtain knowledge of what exists in the world by reason alone, without empirical justification. (Collier, 1994; Flew, 1984; Rosenberg, 2012)

Empiricism: This is the position that all knowledge is based on experience, with the assumption that human beings have no innate knowledge, and only that which can be experienced through the senses can be known. In this respect it would be the opposite of idealism. John Locke saw the mind at birth as a 'white paper' that is provided with reliable sense experience by external objects which have their own independent reality. Empiricism importantly rejects the authority of received wisdom, custom and tradition, and emphasizes the importance of making judgments on the basis of observation and reason. In this respect it is seen as a significant part of the liberal philosophical positions developed during the European Enlightenment in the 17th century.

However, empiricism denies that the mind actively contributes anything to knowledge. It can reflect the belief that an accurate link exists between sense experience and the nature of material objects so that we know the world as it truly is, an actualistic perspective, or it may involve the belief that we cannot know the world as it truly is, but all that we can define as knowledge is what we know through sense experience. Knowledge is built up through repeated experiences of events and the relationships between them, and relies on the principle of induction, the belief that the regularities currently observed in nature will be reliably experienced in the future, and that what applies to finite sets of data will apply to a far broader, general set of data. In the 18th century David Hume questioned the principle of induction, believing that the regularity of nature cannot necessarily be relied on, and the future may not turn out to be the same as the present and the past. (Collier, 1994; Flew, 1984; Hartwig, 2007; Rosenberg, 2012)

Positivism: This involves the belief that all genuine human knowledge is obtained by the application of the systematic scientific study of phenomena, which provides evidence that has to be accepted as it has been found, and cannot be further explained. The epistemology was developed during the 19th century, building on the 17th and 18th century principles of empiricism, and was seen as carrying the optimistic potential of providing a reliable scientific basis for the reorganization of society to the benefit of humanity, in which fallibility and human bias have been removed. During the 20th century logical positivism sought to apply logic and the use of statistics to assess the probability that research outcomes supported the hypotheses being tested.

This was an approach designed to overcome the problem of induction, that the future may not be the same as the present, and requires phenomena to be measurable as well as observable. Positivism sees science as the only source of genuine knowledge, and if a question cannot be answered in this way it cannot be answered at all. (Flew, 1984; Rosenberg, 2012)

Phenomenology and Hermeneutics: Descriptions of phenomenology and hermeneutics relate closely to each other. Phenomenology is the study of conscious mind from a first-person point of view, looking at the nature of its processes and the ways in which it experiences objects in the outside world. Knowledge of the world is seen as existing within the experience of the human mind rather than in the fundamental nature of objects themselves. Phenomenology may also be described as the study and understanding of human cognition in the context of differing world experience and social/cultural contexts, and as such may explore the reasons a person may hold a particular belief. (Honderich,1995; Pietersma, 2000)

Hermeneutics sits within this overall phenomenological approach to knowledge, and places particular emphasis on investigating the individual meaning or interpretations that might be reflected in, or covertly underlie conscious human experience and behaviour. In their origins phenomenology and hermeneutics reflect the original thinking of Husserl and Heidegger respectively. (Gantt et al., 2016; Honderich, 1995)

Instrumentalism and Pragmatism: These perspectives view theories about the world as useful instruments for organizing our experience, rather than as literal claims that are either true or false. Theories and the evidence in support of them are accepted because they have functional value, not because they are deemed to be true. In a somewhat similar vein constructive empiricism refers to an empirically driven epistemology that withholds judgment regarding the truth or falsity of theories, as long as they enable us to predict and control phenomena and can therefore be considered adequate on those empirical grounds (Rosenberg, 2012). Pragmatism judges the truth of a theory by the effectiveness of actions guided by that theory, a position that risks putting the actual specifics of theory, their meaning and their inherent validity and reliability into the background (Honderich,1995), and reflects the prioritizing of usefulness that is central to instrumentalism.

Relativism: This is the belief that there are no absolute truths. It accepts the co-existence of alternative and conflicting views of the world, and believes that each has equal standing and is correct from its own epistemic perspective. Relativism would argue that there are no grounds for judgment between alternative theories, and in this respect it has also been referred to as judgmental relativism. It also recognizes the importance of the social environment and culture in determining the content of beliefs about the world, and the diversity of such environments. (Flew, 1984; Hartwig, 2007; Rosenberg, 2012)

Foundationalism: Some epistemologies argue their positions from a foundationalist perspective, believing that the knowledge gained through them is certain and will not be subject to error or change (Hartwig, 2007).

Important themes exist within this range of epistemologies regarding the possibility or not of gaining true knowledge of the world, the criteria by which the validity of knowledge should be judged, the fallibility or otherwise of that knowledge, and the limits that may be set on the nature and content of knowledge itself. These themes, and the different ways in which they are addressed, relate in some part to our human need for a felt sense of security and certainty.

Positions can become polarized, heightening perceptions of difference and reducing opportunities for the dialectical discovery of integrative possibilities. Within psychology and psychotherapy we may be particularly faced with this polarization at times in the divide between the principles of logical positivism and the premises of post-modern approaches. At other times practitioners and researchers may draw on them both, to complement each other, adding to the depth, richness, and hopefully the validity of our understanding.

As discussed earlier, all of our therapies and the associated study of human psychology exist within our prevailing Western culture, in which logical positivism, pragmatism and often a foundationalist perspective, hold a dominant place at societal and governmental levels, largely excluding the influence of other epistemologies from the processes of decision making. We will now look at the requirements of logical positivism in more detail and consider the problems of fit between the nature of human psychology and psychotherapy and those requirements in some depth.

The Requirements of Logical Positivism and the Problems of Fit with Human Psychology and Psychotherapy

The following discussion will relate primarily to the nature of experiments and their reliance on closed systems, the principle of induction and its associated problems, and the use of statistics and consequent need for observable entities to be measurable at the interval or ratio level. These are themes that typically emerge when psychotherapists, psychologists and others debate the limitations of logical positivism. O'Donohue (2013), Shean (2016) and Pilgrim (2018) provide recent examples of such debates.

Experiments, open versus closed systems, and the principle of induction: Experiments are established so that phenomena and mechanisms can be investigated under controlled conditions, in the belief that inferences and conclusions may be reached that are free from experimenter bias. This practice is deemed to enhance the empirical status of observations, and was much influenced by John Stuart Mill from a positivist philosophical perspective, during the 19th century. Experiments involve a relatively small number of instances of the phenomena to be studied, with the results being generalized according to the principle of induction. Core rules such as randomization, and the double-blind controlled studies of medical research were instigated by Mill to remove experimenter bias (Rosenberg, 2012).

Central to the nature of experiments is the context of the closed system, in which ideally one mechanism is isolated from the effects of others, to ascertain how that mechanism works on its own, and to test hypotheses about its relationship with other specific variables. In a closed system the mechanism should always produce the same result given the same stimulus, every time. The principle of induction, based on the belief that these outcomes will take place again under the same conditions in the future as they have in the past, then enables predictions about the future to be made.

Natural systems, however, are mostly very complex, multi-interactional open systems rather than closed ones. Some phenomena are much more suitable than others for investigation within a closed experimental system.

Collier (1994) warns that if we deprive a mechanism of its natural open system, we may significantly distort its functioning in misleading ways. In its natural state the human mind is a complex, multi-interactional open system, as is the practical, physical, social and cultural environment that each of us inhabits; in research terms the study of human psychology is dealing with at least two, and often multiple complex open systems in interaction with each other. In the contexts of experimental control it is impossible to truly isolate psychological variables of interest, and the natural environment in which they function becomes artificially distorted if we attempt to control independent variables and create a closed system for research purposes.

In the psychotherapy context the experience of therapy involves the interaction of at least four complex open systems, the two minds of the client and the therapist and the environments that influence both of them. The implementation of experimentally oriented research methodologies may distort the natural open systems of therapy and psychological change, and at the same time the uncontrollable multi-interactional open system of the client's world can influence the nature of client distress and the experience and outcome of psychotherapy, in helpful or unhelpful directions.

The problem of induction, the need for statistics and the implications for measurement: As mentioned earlier, the difficulty with the principle of induction is that we can never be sure that it will be valid, because we cannot observe the future. This situation became known as the problem of induction and was theoretically resolved by relying on statistics to demonstrate the probability of future occurrence. Limits were set in relation to the level of probability required for the problem of induction to be deemed to be resolved. The application of statistics requires that variables be measurable, and that measurement can be achieved in ways that enable statistical calculations of probability to be applied, which leads to the additional requirement of certain levels of measurement.

Measurement can be defined at different levels, nominal, ordinal, interval and ratio. At the nominal level an item is identified as being in a particular category of things, is named and allocated to that category. Statistics can look at the relationship between the numbers allocated to different categories. The ordinal level of measurement refers to the situation in which items can be placed in rank order, but there is no way of knowing the size or degree of difference between the items ordered. At the interval level of measurement items can be placed in rank order and it is known that there is an equal interval of measurement between each item on the scale. However, no absolute zero is possible, and any setting of zero is done on an arbitrary basis.

The interval level of measurement is the minimum required for the quantitative measurement of variables, and the application of statistical analyses in relation to hypotheses regarding quantitative relationships between them. At the ratio level of measurement there are equal intervals between items on a ratio scale and an absolute zero exists.

The nature of the statistics which can be used to assess probability depends on both the level of measurement of the variables and their mathematical distribution: traditionally parametric statistics have been used with the ratio level of measurement and with data that have a normal distribution with frequencies balanced around the mean, and non-parametric statistics for other levels of measurement and data with non-normal, unbalanced distribution around the mean.

In recent years there has been a greater emphasis on the relevance of statistical power, and the potential need for large research samples, which increases in importance as the anticipated effect size in any experimental situation decreases (Clark-Carter, 2007). In addition, parametric statistics have been developed for use with interval level measurements.

Observable and unobservable phenomena, and issues of measurement: The fundamental premise of logical positivism and science is that theoretical hypotheses should be tested and measured, in experimental conditions as discussed above. This requires phenomena to be accessible and amenable to direct observation and an appropriate level of measurement. Our variables of interest are often unobservable and very difficult, or impossible to measure.

Positivism will have its most straightforward and legitimate place when it is possible to isolate an observable human mechanism or variable, that can be assumed to function in a reasonably valid manner within a closed system, and that can be quantified with validity and reliability on a ratio or interval scale so that meaningful statistical analysis may be applied.

In some contexts the subject matter of human psychology may be ideally suited to these requirements, in others the fit between subject matter and logical positivism may be less straightforward, and in yet other contexts any valid fit between the two may be impossible to achieve.

Many of the phenomena of interest to us cannot be observed directly, particularly those related to our internal psychological functioning and to psychological distress. They are often measured by indirect measurement of their observable psychological or behavioural effects, or by measurement of other aspects of human experience that have been deemed to be theoretically and/or statistically associated with them.

Such measures are often composed of a list of such items, and at times there may be valid theoretical reasons to question how well and how comprehensively these items reflect the actual human experience of the phenomenon under study. Measures that are established in this way are often validated by a standardization process, demonstrating that the variable in question changes in size in relation to other variables as it would be expected to do, again on a statistical basis.

Some psychological test items are measured as the internal experiences of the individuals concerned, and then it is the individuals themselves who do the measuring, and in effect decide their own personal interval of measurement, often on a provided numerical scale.

Overall these considerations regarding measurement mean that the status of interval level measurement may be given to measurement processes that do not truly justify that status, or that only approximate to it, and may actually have a mathematical status somewhere in between the ordinal and interval level. Furthermore, we may not be truly sure that we are measuring what we believe we are measuring, and whether we are measuring all of it.

A Summary of Issues: The combined effects of the experimental alteration of natural open systems and associated tight control over the nature of research participants, the influence of variables and events that we are unable to predict or control and the above issues relating to measurement and statistics can markedly impact on research endeavours that aim to fulfil the requirements of logical positivism. They are likely to produce outcomes that are much harder to generalize, are open to far greater variation and are much harder to replicate than positivism would ever expect. They will also often fail to achieve the nature and level of measurement necessary for the statistics ideally needed to address to problem of induction.

In this situation we need to be open and accepting in relation to the limitations and fallibility of our research outcomes, rather than emphasizing any absolute authority.

The specific requirements of this epistemology limit our sources of knowledge to relatively simplified versions of psychological reality. Such simplified contexts may seldom exist in the real multi-faceted open systems of our human lives, and sometimes they will never exist, and may be totally spurious.

As part of the wish and maybe the political need for the discipline of psychology to be identified as a science, the danger exists that we distort our subject matter to make it compatible with the epistemology that we wish to apply, rather than feeling more free to choose from a range of epistemologies that may be more suited to aspects of the subject matter.

As practitioners interested in human psychology and psychotherapy we are not alone in struggling with these issues. The relevance of certainty versus fallibility, the prevalence of complex open systems, and the unobservable, unmeasurable nature of phenomena of interest are to be found elsewhere within the natural sciences, and are given clear attention by philosophers interested in the philosophy of science (Rosenberg, 2012).

As an example of an unobservable phenomenon that cannot be measured directly, Rosenberg discusses what we refer to as gravity, which does not fit the requirements of logical positivism: it cannot be observed, is completely undetectable except through its effects, can pass through a vacuum and has characteristics that we are completely unable to understand. It is, however, treated as something that is understood within the positivist world of science, and this is never questioned; to do so would be to question a theory that has enormous instrumental value and has become foundational to our human sense of security.

Within psychology, these problems in relation to logical positivism have led to a post-modern or post-positivist emphasis on the individual and social construction of knowledge, and the direct observation and recording of human functioning in natural open systems. Approaches such as these provide detailed descriptions of the complexities and subtleties of human experience and reduce the impact of research on natural processes.

Post-modern Psychology and Psychotherapy

This broad-based philosophical position within psychology encompasses a range of thinkers who take a critical approach towards empiricism and logical positivism, recognizing the complexity of the natural world and human existence, and challenging scientific orthodoxy. Within post-modernism a stance of deconstruction actively challenges positivist scientific theories of human functioning, re-writing them in alternative ways advised by a range of other epistemologies. These particularly include phenomenology, hermeneutics, and psychological constructivism. Associated methods of accessing and generating knowledge often involve the use of narrative and attention to discourse. In general, post-modernism seeks to recognize the complexities and ambiguities of our human existence within our social and cultural context, and gives a primary place to the role that our human minds play in constructing perceptions and understandings of ourselves and the outside world.

Constructivism within psychology is influenced by George Kelly's proposals in relation to Personal Construct Theory (Kelly, 1963) describing the capacity of our minds to actively generate our individual perceptions of ourselves, other people and the world around us in ways that are influenced by an unconscious internal construct system. This system is assumed to involve multiple clusters of bi-polar constructs, associated with each other, relating to characteristics that are particularly salient to us and have been influenced by our life experiences. The nature of our unique construct system influences how we each construe ourselves and other people, it affects how we think and feel about them, how we relate to them and how we live our lives.

Constructivism stands in direct contrast to empiricism's position that the mind does not actively contribute to the nature of our knowledge of the world. At times its proponents argue that all constructions of a particular reality are equally valid and true, no matter how different or incompatible they may be in their beliefs about their common subject matter, because each is based on its own different epistemology. This would allow multiple realities in relation to the same entity to exist at the same time. It is a position that denies the independent existence of the material world, and the existence of an absolute reality, and is reflective of radical relativism or anti-realism, and judgemental relativism.

In some contexts, constructivism and narrative/discourse- based approaches within psychology and psychotherapy may seem to reflect positions of super-idealism and rationalism, in which the nature of our thoughts and beliefs defines the actual nature of the world around us; changing how we think and how we define and describe the world within discourse is then deemed capable of changing the nature of the world we live in.

The epistemologies associated with post-modern psychology dispute the appropriateness of logical positivism and scientific method in the study of human psychology, and are reflected in qualitative research methodologies such as grounded theory and discourse analysis, where analysis of content aims to reveal important characteristics of human experience. In some respects, however, this work can become part of a somewhat polarized, oppositional position that can deny any value that logical positivism has to offer.

From a pragmatic perspective, post-modernism and logical positivism may be seen as offering complementary approaches to gaining knowledge through the use of both qualitative and quantitative methodologies to investigate the same aspects of human psychology, reflecting both positions within the overall research principle of triangulation.

Triangulation is an approach advocated within qualitative research methodology, which argues that we have greater reason to trust any knowledge we have gained if we obtain the same picture of our subject matter from different methodological perspectives. It is assumed to be of particular value when we are dealing with highly reactive phenomena in complex systems. Its philosophical background would seem to lie somewhere between logical positivism, realism and post-modernism, since its application reflects the belief that real characteristics of phenomena do exist but issues of observation and measurement and the open, complex systems they are part of makes it hard for us to study them.

We will now take a look at the range of epistemologies we may consider to be reflected within psychotherapy theory and practice across our major therapeutic approaches.

The Epistemologies Reflected in our Major Approaches to Psychotherapy

Our differing theoretical approaches to psychotherapy vary in the epistemologies that have guided theory development and are reflected in therapy theory and practice.

In general, our theories about human psychology and psychotherapy adopt a realist epistemology, assuming that phenomena have an existence independent of our human minds. Similarly, we rely on observation and hypotheses throughout our research and clinical practice, reflecting a broad-based empiricism, but vary in our adherence to the limits which empiricism places on the phenomena that may be considered to be real, and the extent to which we believe we can predict outcomes. In large part we very much reject empiricism's view that the human mind does not actively contribute to the nature of knowledge, rejecting an actualist perspective, and generally seeing our minds as influencing how we see ourselves and the world around us.

In a similar way logical positivism is reflected within all of our major therapeutic approaches in some way. All have been advanced to greater or lesser degrees by outcome-based research. Scientific method has been used to demonstrate the connection between the nature of the therapeutic relationship and therapy outcome, particularly within humanistic client-centred therapy. Insecure attachment relationships in childhood have been shown to be related to later psychological distress, and aspects of therapy process have been associated with evolving outcomes in psychotherapy process research. In addition, various constructs and mechanisms associated with our therapeutic theories have been supported and explored in ways that have been advised by positivistic scientific methodology.

Psychodynamic theory originated in the scientific medical paradigms of the nineteenth century and relies on broadly based empirical observations of human behaviour and narrative expression, together with indicators of internal emotional experience, to generate hypotheses about the nature of conscious and unconscious constructs, mechanisms and processes within the human mind. In these respects, whilst not explicitly guided by them, it also reflects the epistemological positions of phenomenology and hermeneutics. The importance of the direct experience of human relating within therapy, and associated subjective meaning is also consistent with these epistemologies.

Attachment theory uses scientific method, advised by the principles of logical positivism, in the form of the Strange Situation to study the nature of secure and insecure attachment relationships, and to categorize them. It also makes hypothetical assumptions about internal structures within the human mind, and developmental processes, and draws on relational emotion related connection and experience within therapy, reflecting the broad-based relevance of empiricism, as well as the principles of phenomenology and hermeneutics as discussed above.

The epistemological contexts of phenomenology and hermeneutics also particularly apply to humanistic client-centred and experiential therapies and theory, in their primary reliance on the directly experienced conscious nature of human relating, empathic connection and emotional awareness, whilst also making some assumptions about unobservable processes.

In general, behavioural, cognitive and cognitive-behavioural therapies have a close relationship with empiricism, logical positivism and scientific method, having their origins within those epistemological positions. Logical positivism is also reflected in the nature and structure of therapy. This position is at its strongest within radical behaviourism, early approaches to behaviour therapy and traditional approaches to cognitive behaviour therapy. Some approaches to cognitive therapy may also seem to reflect an epistemology equivalent to idealism, bordering on super-idealism at times, where it is assumed that the nature of the world we experience can be created and changed for the better solely by our own perceptions. In addition, traditional CBT also seemed to adopt something of this idealist position when it argued that it is only the way an adverse event is perceived that causes distress, and not the event itself. Overall, in these respects, any single approach within the cognitive behavioural therapies may be internally diverse and reflect multiple epistemologies.

Cognitive therapy's reliance on the assumed existence of unobservable schemas within latent unconscious mind, and its concern with individual interpretations and meaning is reflective of a hermeneutic epistemology, and is also inconsistent with logical positivism. This epistemological context is further extended when cognitive therapy incorporates more broadly-based influences, particularly those reflected in constructivist psychotherapy, where relevant epistemologies have moved more broadly in hermeneutic and phenomenological directions.

Any therapy context that pays attention to the listening, hearing and empathic relationship between therapist and client reflects a broad-based empiricism, an acceptance of the subjective first person experience of the client, and a valuing of meaning above logic that is generally reflective of more phenomenological and hermeneutic epistemologies.

In our overall valuing of effectiveness and its use to justify the nature of practice, and in our reliance on the utility of imaginative models we could also consider all of our major therapeutic approaches to reflect the principles of instrumentalism and pragmatism.

Overall, our major approaches to psychotherapy and their associated theories bear mixed and complex relationships to the epistemologies available to us; most reflect more than one, and some seem to be internally inconsistent regarding their main avowed epistemological position. Currently, it is primarily within psychology's post-modern position that such epistemological pluralism might be recognized and valued.

Theories and Models

Finally, we will touch on the rather thorny issue of the status of theory within human psychology. From a logical positivist and scientific perspective, Rosenberg (2012) refers to theories as sets of related hypotheses that work together to explain empirical regularities, and are backed up by strong empirical support in the form of studies of their observable consequences, which have been predicted by logic. He also sees theories as scientific hypotheses that are good candidates for becoming laws of nature.

Overall theories are deductive systems, and are developed by a hypothetico-deductive process. In these contexts, they are seen as having very strong empirical bases and as relating entirely to phenomena that can be subject to direct empirical observation, and to experimentation in closed systems. From a logical positivist perspective, the subject matter of theory also needs to be open to appropriate measurement and statistical analysis.

Within psychology we also frequently refer to models, often in rather the same way that we use the term theory, with these terms tending to be used interchangeably. Models are defined by Rosenberg (2012) as simplified theories that may leave out some variables and concentrate only on the important ones, whilst Collier (1994) sees them as potentially being entirely imaginative constructions that help to predict phenomena, or make them intelligible to us, but which cannot be directly empirically investigated.

From a logical positivist perspective we might consider that all of our theories could more appropriately be called models, since so many of our variables in human psychology can only have the status of imaginative constructs; we know them indirectly and by inference, they can never be directly observed. We also value the term model when we wish to give a sense of structure to the interactions between phenomena within the psychological systems we are imaginatively describing.

Within this work I have stayed with our conventional use of the term theory in relation to the bodies of understanding that constitute human psychology and the basis of our functioning as psychotherapists. I also use the terms theory and model on an interchangeable basis at times, and particularly refer to models when describing systems of interaction between psychological variables and structures.

A Philosophy Consistent with the Nature of Human Psychology and Psychotherapy and the Aims of Theoretical Integration

It is painfully evident that our nature as human beings, the nature of the complex social, cultural and demographic worlds we live in and the nature of our major approaches to psychotherapy (maybe with the exception of some tightly standardized and protocol-led cognitive behavioural approaches) are not consistent with the requirements and epistemological straitjacket of logical positivism when it is relied on as the sole or dominant epistemology.

In addition, logical positivism directs us towards categorization and the perception of difference, supporting either/or distinctions, rather than encouraging the discovery of similarity, compatibility and complementarity, and the potential for dialectical synthesis that are core elements of theoretical integration.

The alternatives available within the epistemologies of post-modern psychology avoid the problems with logical positivism, and offer us the very important concept of triangulation, but they may deny the validity of other valuable epistemologies within psychotherapy theory and practice, including logical positivism itself, as reflected on by Pilgrim (2018).

At this point it seems appropriate to say clearly that I believe in the independent existence of the material world, and in the existence of absolute reality, no matter how complex, incomprehensible or unknowable it may actually be. In this respect I reject the beliefs of absolute idealism, super-idealism, rationalism and judgmental relativism.

In all other respects I believe that we need a philosophical approach to human psychology and psychotherapy that is pluralistic in its attitude towards different epistemologies, seeing them as existing more on a continuum from strict logical positivism at one extreme to an absolute version of constructivism at the other, and that values the appropriate application of all of them. A philosophy that takes a critical approach to recognizing their individual strengths and limitations. A philosophy that believes an absolute reality does exist, but that we are limited in our human capacities to perceive, investigate and conceptualize that reality; accepts that our knowledge is fallible rather than certain, and that there actually is no absolute solution to the problem of induction.

We need a philosophy that will support us in using a range of epistemologies in complementary ways to study the subject matter of human psychology and psychotherapy the best we can, and in using well thought through criteria to help us make judgments about the knowledge we deem most appropriate at any one time to best support the practice of psychotherapy.

At present the philosophy that seems to me to best fit these requirements is the critical realism of British philosopher Roy Bhaskar. I first came across his philosophy in 2011 whilst exploring American university psychology and philosophy curriculum materials online. Recently, Alderson (2021) has endorsed its benefits within health and illness research; support for its value within systemic psychotherapy has been provided by Pocock (2015); and Pilgrim (2019) recommends it as an appropriate general philosophy for psychologists. Chapter 4 will describe the core principles of Bhaskar's critical realism and discuss its value as a philosophy that is consistent with the subject matter of human psychology and psychotherapy, is able to take complex open systems into account, allows for hard to measure and unobservable phenomena, and accepts the validity of a range of epistemologies. A philosophy that is naturally supportive of theoretical integration.

Summary

Chapter 3 has touched base in relation to some core aspects of philosophy, overviewed a range of epistemologies that can guide us in gaining knowledge of ourselves and the world around us, and looked in particular at logical positivism in its role as the lead epistemology guiding us within the philosophy of science. We have discussed the problems of fit between logical positivism and the study of human psychology, and acknowledged the wide range of epistemologies reflected within our major theoretical approaches to psychotherapy. Finally, it has been argued that a philosophical approach is needed that is consistent with the nature of human psychology and psychotherapy, and is supportive of theoretical integration.

The Principles of Critical Realism and its Value to Human Psychology and Psychotherapy

4

Critical realism as developed in Britain by Roy Bhaskar (Bhaskar, 2015, 2016, 2017) and comprehensively discussed by Collier (1994), takes an approach to philosophy that seems particularly consistent with the complexity of human psychological phenomena. This chapter will provide an overview of core characteristics of Bhaskar's critical realism, and argue for its value as an appropriate philosophy to support our search for knowledge in relation to psychotherapy and its practice.

Critical realism in general is a philosophy that believes the phenomena in the world around us have an absolute reality, which is independent of our knowledge of them and of our thoughts about them, and recognizes that there can be problems and limits in our human capacity to gain knowledge of them (Flew, 1984). British philosopher Roy Bhaskar has developed a particularly discerning version of critical realism that addresses complex issues involved in the study of both the natural and human, psychological and social worlds.

Bhaskar's critical realism is seen by Collier (1994) as existing in the space between relativism and idealism on the one hand, which both deny the absolute reality of the material world, and logical positivism on the other, which believes in that reality, sets very narrow limits on what can be known and always assumes direct correspondence between what can be observed and what actually exists. Critical realism accepts the value of reason and logic, and is fully committed to a thorough, objective and discerning approach to the study of the natural and human social worlds (Collier, 1994; Hartwig, 2007).

The following brief summary of core principles within Bhaskar's critical realism is advised by Andrew Collier's book *Critical Realism. An Introduction to Roy Bhaskar's Philosophy* (Collier, 1994), Roy Bhaskar's transcribed lectures *The Order of Natural Necessity: A Kind of Introduction to Critical Realism*, edited by Gary

Hawke (Bhaskar, 2017), and the *Dictionary of Critical Realism* (Hartwig, 2007).

Roy Bhaskar's Critical Realism

Core principles:

- *Realism and objectivity:* The material world in all its forms has an absolute reality, and exists independently of our knowledge of it, our thoughts about it and the scientific methods that we use to study it. It can exist and be real even if we are not able to observe it at all.
- *Fallibility:* All theories and the data that have led to them are fallible, and may subsequently be shown to be wrong, and the scientific beliefs of any given time may prove to be mistaken. The nature of every subject of study will go beyond the data that we are able to observe.
- *The transitive nature of theories in relation to the intransitive absolute reality of the ontological world:* Scientific theories represent our current best approximations to truths about ourselves and the world around us. They are transitive objects, always in transition towards a potential full and accurate knowledge of intransitive absolute reality, a reality that we may never actually come to know. The intransitive world exists independent of our knowledge about it, and involves the entirety of existence, being or ontology of ourselves and the world around us.
- *Transphenomenality:* An object of study may have both an observable surface structure and an underlying deeper structure which is not directly observable. It may be possible to investigate and gain knowledge of underlying structures. These structures may also be more enduring than the observable characteristics of surface indicators, which they may be responsible for creating.
- *Counterphenomenality:* The knowledge that may be gained about deeper structures may contradict and not appear to be consistent with the knowledge that has been gained about the surface structure of the same object of study.

Critical realism sees our knowledge as transitive, continually moving forward towards a better picture of entities as they exist in their intransitive state. In some instances we may be able to come to a full and accurate knowledge of the intransitive object, in others we may never be able to do so. It also recognizes the full importance of the entire world around us, our total existence, whether the entities within that world can be subject to scientific study or not, all of the ontology or 'being' of our world matters, and has an absolute intransitive nature of being, at any one time.

Fundamentally, it puts human beings in a relatively unknowing place, it recognizes the fallibility of our capacities to perceive and conceptualize, as well as the value and benefits of our current best approximations to the truth about the world. In this respect it clearly rejects the foundationalist certainty of epistemologies such as logical positivism. It does not accept that all theoretical beliefs are equally valid as judgmental relativism does, but does believe that they are socially produced, transient and fallible. These core characteristics of critical realism lead it to be seen as a depth realism in contrast to the shallow realism or actualism of empiricism and especially logical positivism, which denies the existence of underlying structure and sees automatic direct and infallible equivalence between what is observed and what exists in absolute reality.

In addition to these core characteristics of critical realism, Bhaskar has given particular attention to the prevalence of complex open systems in nature, the value of imaginative models within science, and the dialectical relationship between different epistemologies. Each of these themes will be discussed before turning our attention to the value of critical realism in relation to human psychology and psychotherapy.

The recognition of natural open systems: Critical realism asserts that natural systems always exist as open multi-interactional systems. Collier (1994) discusses the ways in which the unnatural experimental creation of a closed system may distort the functioning of phenomena and generative mechanisms and possibly lead to misleading results.

This position leads to the conclusion that the capacity of a generative mechanism to produce a particular outcome within an experimental closed system should be referred to as a tendency. This is an important position to hold, since it accepts that the generative mechanism under study can produce the outcome that has been observed in the closed experimental system; however, it also recognizes that in a natural complex open system the situation may be different. The generative mechanism under study may produce the outcome that it has a tendency to produce, or it may produce a different outcome depending on the functioning of the other generative mechanisms it is interacting with as part of that system. It will not necessarily always be triggered and the observable outcome of it being triggered may not always be exactly the same. Empirical evidence has demonstrated that generative mechanisms function in unpredictable ways in complex open systems, and Collier (1994) sees this as an empirical truth as much as any other.

Crucially, the principles of critical realism challenge the expectation that the practice of science will necessarily lead to prediction and certainty. Collier (1994) specifically argues that sciences which address mechanisms that only function in complex open systems can achieve high explanatory power without making predictions, and that the inability to make predictions should not be seen as a failure. He supports the mutual value of studying both closed and open systems.

Unnatural experimental closed systems can valuably demonstrate the existence of generative mechanisms and explore their possible tendencies, which may then be looked for at work in natural open systems.

Unobservable phenomena and the value of imaginative models: The belief in the transitive nature of human knowledge, and the concepts of both transphenomenality and counterphenomenality within critical realism provide a secure epistemological home for the value of imaginative models of understanding. The existence of both observable phenomena and the underlying unobservable entities that influence them is a clearly accepted reality within critical realism.

Collier (1994) sees imaginative constructions as helping to make unobservable entities clearer to us, and as supporting us in making predictions about how those entities or phenomena might behave. We are then able to investigate the potentially observable consequences of their functioning, although they themselves cannot be directly investigated because they are not that kind of a thing. As transitive knowledge develops over time, what were previously proposed as imaginative models, may be discovered to exist as real structures underlying those phenomena.

A dialectical philosophy: A core characteristic of Bhaskar's critical realism has been defined as its dialectical nature, and at times it has been referred to as dialectical realism (Collier, 1994). Since the way the term dialectic is used within philosophy may vary, it may be helpful to start by clarifying its meaning. Flew (1984) refers to Hegel's classical use of the term, using it to describe the logical pattern that productive and creative thought processes need to follow. Ideas need to be brought together that have been judged to be contradictory to each other, sometimes referred to as thesis and antithesis. These two will often be kept separate because they have been assumed to be incommensurable and cannot be brought together. However, progress is made from a dialectical perspective if contradictions can be resolved in some creative way and a synthesis achieved that moves both thesis and antithesis to different positions. It is this process that Hegel defines as dialectic.

In this context the nature of incommensurability becomes quite crucial. Collier (1994) gives particular attention to this issue, and points out that thesis and antithesis always have something in common because they represent different transitive knowledge about the same intransitive phenomenon. Two theories cannot clash with each other if they have no shared meanings; they can only clash about something. As an example, Collier reminds us of Lavoisier and Priestly whose theories clashed about the gas that one called oxygen and the other called de-phlogisticated air. This something is the start of a possible dialectic process, in which apparently incommensurable theories may learn from and support each other, moving in new dialectically integrative directions.

The dialectical approach within critical realism would look at what apparently incommensurable theories have in common as well as recognising their differences. It would also seek to examine those differences and consider ways in which they might be resolved, potentially prompting creative dialectical thinking.

As with Priestley and Lavoisier different scientific communities may see no overlap of sense in their differing theories, and may be unaware that they are actually referring to the same intransitive thing. Connections and degrees of potential synthesis may be possible across a range of different epistemologies and associated theoretical positions. Critical realism's support for the mutual relevance of a range of epistemologies and its belief in the potential for dialectic synthesis between apparently incommensurable positions sits at the heart of its relevance to theoretical integration.

Critical realism also takes the position that we can apply reason and logic to choose the aspects of theories that best represent the state of transitive knowledge at any given time. It encourages us to keep an open mind; to stand back from the perspectives, paradigms and epistemologies available to us and be as objective as possible in thinking about the constructive contribution that different approaches to knowledge and different theoretical positions may have to offer; to look for similarities and common ground as well as recognizing differences; to base criticism and judgment on in-depth understanding; to avoid the lure of fashion; and in general to adopt a process of theory development that speaks more of discerning evolution than dramatic revolution.

Doing so would inevitably mean that we would no longer raise particular theoreticians to the status of idols or heroes, since theoretical perspectives would be valued alongside each other rather than exist in status-driven competition.

The Value of Critical Realism to Research, Theory and Practice in Human Psychology and Psychotherapy

The importance of unobservable phenomena: As discussed above critical realism is totally accepting of the existence and importance of unobservable phenomena. It would support our reliance on them within therapeutic theory and practice, and our efforts to study them.

This is an extremely important benefit for human psychology and psychotherapy. When dealing with the internal subjective experiences of the human mind and the potential generative mechanisms and processes that may underlie them, we are largely dealing with phenomena that cannot be known directly and are hypothesized to exist on the basis of observable surface phenomena such as the verbal and non-verbal expression of thoughts and feelings, and the overt behaviours we engage in.

We give material terms to elements of human experience and functioning that we judge to have consistent enough characteristics to justify their status as entities with a name, such as self-esteem, locus of control, aggression, love, guilt, depression, and anxiety and we develop imaginative models involving generative mechanisms that logic and reason lead us to consider may underlie these human experiences and the relationships between them.

Our imaginative psychological structures and processes include schemas, transference, defence mechanisms, positive and negative reinforcement, reciprocal inhibition, procedural memory and many, many more. To the extent that we have evidence in support of their potential existence, all of these mechanisms and processes whatever theoretical perspective they are associated with, are part of the functioning of our human minds and will have as their substrates our human brains, our nervous system and the rest of our human bodies. The intransitive absolute reality of our human functioning will underlie all of our currently diverse transitive theoretical perspectives and associated psychological constructs.

In addition, critical realism thinks about the relationship between observable surface structures and deeper unobservable ones related to them. In observing the observable cognitions, emotions, and behaviours that we consider to be the surface outcomes produced by underlying deeper structures, we are drawing on the principle that critical realism refers to as transphenomenality. When we recognize the possibility that a phenomenon such as emotion may exist in one form on the observable surface and in a different form at a deeper level, for example anger on the surface, and fear at a deeper level, we are reflecting critical realism's principle of counterphenomenality.

Issues of experimental control and open versus closed systems: The natural everyday context of open systems is totally accepted within critical realism, but at the same time the value of studying entities within more controlled closed systems is not at all excluded. It is the interpretation of research outcomes that are changed, to now reflect tendencies and possibilities. Phenomena can be studied and explored within both open and closed systems with equal validity, with uncertainty and fallibility being seen as the norm in both contexts.

Issues in relation to measurement and statistics: Within critical realism measurement and associated statistics are not essential. As with experimental control they will be used and valued when appropriate to the phenomena under question, and the epistemology that is best suited to their study: all levels of measurement will be allowed.

The existence of multiple epistemologies: Critical realism is accepting of the epistemological pluralism that is characteristic of psychotherapy theory and practice overall, and it is accepting of the need for research epistemologies to fit the nature of the phenomena under study, rather than impose procedures and practices that are incompatible with them.

From this position critical realism would not deny a place to methods of study derived from logical positivism, but would not adhere to the belief that the outcomes of such studies provided infallible answers to the questions we were asking, or that positivist science was the only source of knowledge. Positivist methods would be seen as making fallible contributions to a wider picture alongside other approaches to gaining knowledge, and all would be seen as contributing transitive understanding that might gradually move closer to intransitive reality.

From a critical realist perspective we would always say that something could be the case, that a certain therapeutic approach can be effective, and we would never say that we could predict, but would be content to say that current evidence pointed towards the possibility of certain outcomes.

Implications for theoretical integration: It is particularly in the context of theoretical integration that critical realism comes to the fore, in supporting us in crossing the boundaries that may otherwise be assumed to separate the knowledge associated with our different epistemologies. It dissolves the need for forced categorization, the emphasis on what is different between approaches, and the need for direct observation and measurement imposed by logical positivism. At the same time it avoids the relativist and idealist pitfalls of post-modern psychology. It gives us permission and encouragement to look at the knowledge available to us across theoretical perspectives on a neutral basis. To feel free to identify and acknowledge the similarities between different theories, and to explore both their commensurable and currently incommensurable differences, whatever their epistemological background. The similarity of constructs identified by different approaches may support the existence of the same intransitive entity, and through their related compatible differences, they may contribute unique aspects of transitive knowledge about that entity, from their particular perspective.

That similarities may logically point towards the same phenomenon having been recognized independently from the basis of different epistemologies, echoes the principle of triangulation that is valued within qualitative research, and provides us with instances of theoretical triangulation. In addition, we will be encouraged to consider the creative possibilities of dialectical synthesis between differences that can logically be argued to relate to the same phenomenon. Critical realism supports us in doing this, even if the theoretical perspectives themselves do not acknowledge that particular constructs may have a common identity, just as was the case between de-phlogisticated air and oxygen.

We are also supported in trying to work towards the resolution of incommensurable and apparently incompatible differences. If that cannot be achieved in any theoretical context that is deemed to be referring to the same intransitive phenomenon, then critical realism advises us to accept that theory in some respect has got it wrong. It does not accept the possibility of more than one reality, or the co-existence of multiple incompatible constructions of the world around or within us. It is from this position that critical realism supports the overall principle of theoretical unification in relation to any single intransitive phenomenon. If we see our human mind as having an absolute reality, as ultimately being an intransitive entity, then in the final analysis all of the mechanisms and processes associated with our different theoretical perspectives have to be functioning effectively within it. If this cannot be argued to be the case, if some are simply not compatible with others, then somewhere along the line theory is wrong, and it is our job to resolve the incompatibility.

Finally, in recognizing the importance of ontology, the overall real, complex life experience of being, critical realism supports us in taking all aspects of human life into account within the practice of psychotherapy, and in giving full, legitimate and equal place to the contexts and environments within which we live, the complex open systems of our experienced worlds.

Conclusion: Overall human psychology and psychotherapy sit comfortably with Bhaskar's critical realism. From this perspective our current theories about human psychology and psychotherapy all represent fallible and transitive, best current approximations to aspects of what are ultimately intransitive realities. Accepting this could remove the motivation for competition in having claim to the right answer. We would no longer have the option of certainty, and having let go of that, accept that none of our theoretical positions can provide the comfort and reassurance of knowing anything exactly, completely and for sure. We might open ourselves up to greater collaboration in exploring the ways in which different epistemologies and theoretical perspectives may complement each other and help us come to a better understanding of our human selves and the world we live in.

I believe that critical realism as developed by Roy Bhaskar and discussed by Collier (1994) is in a good position to provide a secure philosophical ground for existing and future theoretical approaches to psychotherapy, where the complex and often unobservable nature of their subject matter can be fully appreciated and taken into account, where epistemological pluralism can be supported and where the value and fundamental validity of theoretical integration, and the principle of unification can be recognized and developed.

Summary

In Chapter 4 we have looked at the philosophical basis of Roy Bhaskar's critical realism, considering its core characteristics and discussing the ways in which its principles are consistent with the nature of human psychology and psychotherapy and supportive of research, theory and practice. It avoids the problems raised by logical positivism, and supports the use of multiple epistemologies including logical positivism, which can then be matched to the nature of the phenomena under study. It supports the study of phenomena that function within complex open systems and is primarily dialectical in its approach to knowledge. It is also thoroughly consistent with and directly supportive of the principles of theoretical integration.

Bhaskar's critical realism is consistent with my belief in the absolute reality of our one human mind, and in the unified functioning of the constructs, mechanisms and processes associated with our different theoretical approaches to psychotherapy within that mind, as discussed in Chapter 1. Discovering his philosophy early on in this work provided invaluable formal support to my position, and fed into the ways in which the work unfolded.

Summary

Part 2

The Major Theoretical Approaches to Psychotherapy

Introduction to Part 2: The Major Theoretical Approaches

Having explored the philosophical context of this work in Part 1, and identified the foundational support provided by Roy Bhaskar's critical realism, Part 2 will now look at the five major theoretical approaches that form the basis of this study. A chapter each is allocated to core elements of attachment, humanistic, and psychodynamic theories, and two chapters are given to cognitive and behavioural theories. Alongside this focus on psychotherapy theory, we will also look at the importance of our social and demographic environments, and the significance of our place in the lifespan. In each chapter my intention is to present theory solely from the perspective of the approach being discussed, and to avoid making cross-theoretical comments or connections at this point.

A substantial amount of theoretical detail and depth will be provided, but not so much that the potential process of theoretical integration risks being overwhelmed. In all instances the constructs, mechanisms and processes of theory are the main focus of attention. Aspects of practice come more to the fore when they are needed to convey important elements of theory. Content aims to provide introductory level material as well as summaries of core principles that reflect more advanced levels of knowledge. None of the chapters do anywhere near full justice to the approaches they represent; they do, however, provide considerable substance in relation to these perspectives, and details of practice that help to illuminate them. It is often within the detail of our different positions that the potential for theoretical integration is best explored. If we rely on overly brief summaries of approaches, we may be vulnerable to integrating what amounts to simplified caricatures. Such simplifications may emphasize difference and reduce the opportunity for similarities between perspectives to be appreciated. As we delve into detail more complex pictures emerge for all of our approaches, aspects of similarity become increasingly apparent, and valuable aspects of difference become clearer and more available to integrative consideration.

I have decided to maintain a distinct boundary between psychodynamic and attachment theories. Within psychotherapeutic practice this boundary can become blurred at times. Psychodynamic therapists often see themselves as incorporating attachment principles into their work, and see the essence of the attachment relationship as a core aspect of psychodynamic theory, particularly supported by object relations and self-psychology perspectives. Somewhat similarly, therapists working from an attachment perspective may implicitly see attachment theory as including much that could be defined as aspects of analytic and psychodynamic theory and practice. In this sense the boundaries can become blurred both ways round, and this context is usefully discussed by Fonagy et al. (2008).

Whilst having its origins partly within psychodynamic theory, attachment theory defines its own independent concepts, draws on a range of other theoretical positions, and includes a very strong research component that adds support to various aspects of theory and to the part played by insecure attachment in the evolution of psychological distress. Much that is discussed from an attachment perspective stands on its own ground, particularly outside the context of psychotherapy, and its boundary of separateness is maintained within this work.

The order of these chapters reflects my support for the primary importance of secure and nurturing close relationships, within our individual developmental experiences, our adult relationships and the experience of psychotherapy.

Chapter 6 overviews attachment theory as developed by John Bowlby, Mary Ainsworth and many others, looking at its core specifics and associated research base. It will highlight the real-world relevance of parents' behaviour towards their children, the complex nature of the attuned relating at the heart of attachment security, the developmentally important consequences of that security and the long-term negative impacts of insecure and disorganized attachment. The contributions that attachment theory makes to the practice of psychotherapy will be discussed, particularly the attuned, emotionally connected and containing relational experience it can provide. The chapter will also consider the related observational work of Daniel Stern and Colwyn Trevarthen, looking at the moment-to-moment realities of connection and communication between infants and parents, their contribution to the development of a sense of self, and the development of subjectivity and inter-subjectivity. Finally, it will consider the neurobiological underpinnings of emotional, non-verbal early experiences and associated developmental processes; and will look at the role of secure attachment in supporting our capacity to mentalize: to see our own mind as separate from the minds of others and to consider the perspectives of other people when they are different from our own.

Chapter 7 on humanistic and experiential theory connects us with the fundamental belief that each person has their own natural potential to grow and develop, and that a relationship characterized by genuineness, acceptance and empathy, can support that natural developmental path. The theoretical and practical principles developed by Carl Rogers and others will be reviewed, including the concepts of organismic valuing and conditions of worth; material that at its heart speaks of the challenges and essential value of empathic attuned human relating, and of the importance of experiential self-awareness and human connection.

Chapter 8 on psychodynamic theory focuses on the specifics of key psychological constructs and processes associated with psychodynamic and analytic theory, rather than on the detail of particular schools of thought. The content reflects my own understanding of their nature, value and usefulness, and their place within typical processes of psychological change and development. Whilst the work of some key figures in theory development, particularly Sigmund Freud and Donald Winnicott, will be acknowledged, I will generally refer to literature that provides broader based theoretical overviews, or looks in some depth at particular psychological constructs. We will discuss a range of unconscious processes, the crucial roles played by early as well as later relationships, the significance of emotion, the concept of unconscious conflict, and the nature of some psychodynamic approaches to psychological development. We will also look at the importance of the therapeutic relationship and the nature of analytic listening. The chapter will end with a simplified psychodynamic rationale for change.

As discussed in Chapter 1, I have created two sub-divisions within the CBT umbrella therapies, recognizing those that are led by cognitive theory as a separate group from those led by behavioural theory. Within both these groups the nature and range of theoretical constructs, mechanisms and processes is best appreciated by looking at the pragmatics of therapy practice; detail in relation to specific interventions will therefore be much more evident in these chapters compared with other approaches.

Chapter 9 addresses cognitive and behavioural theory, and considers the impact of Aaron Beck and the 'cognitive revolution', looking at traditional cognitive therapy, the associated application of behaviour therapy methods, plus a broader range of more integrative approaches including Schema Therapy, Constructivist Psychotherapy, Mindfulness Based Cognitive Therapy, and Compassion Focused Therapy. Aspects of theory related practice will be overviewed which reflect attention given to increased awareness of conscious thoughts and beliefs, access to cognitions that are not routinely available to conscious awareness, the appraisal and challenge of unhelpful thoughts and beliefs, as well as interventions aimed at influencing the nature of schemas of self and others, and the processes of interpersonal relating.

Chapter 10 considers behavioural and cognitive theory. It is here that the theoretical premises of behaviourism will be discussed in more detail, reflecting the classic contributions of key figures such as Ivan Pavlov, Joseph Wolpe, and

B F Skinner. We will look at methodological behaviourism, radical behaviourism and applied behaviour analysis, and the recent application of radical behaviourism to cognitive functioning and related verbal and non-verbal behaviour reflected in relational frame theory. In discussing the integration between behavioural and cognitive approaches, specific attention will be given to stage of 1 Dialectical Behavior Therapy, Acceptance and Commitment Therapy, Behavioral Activation and Functional Analytic Psychotherapy. In some instances, a broader basis of theoretical integration will also be evident.

Chapter 11 looks at the theoretical importance of the world around us and discusses the relevance of the social, demographic and cultural contexts of our lives, recognizing the crucial interaction between ourselves and the environments in which we live. In many ways this theme is most clearly reflected in therapy when we take the relational environment into account, both in the context of early development and the nature of current relationships. The psychosocial literature reflects and adds to these understandings, and provides empirical support for many of the premises of our theoretical approaches to psychotherapy. A wide range of evidence in relation to adverse aspects of childhood experience will be considered, and the enduring vulnerability associated with their long-term consequences. The interactive impact of adverse adult life contexts and life events will be discussed, including the powerful impact of loss in its many forms, plus the benefit of supportive relationships and factors associated with resilience. In addition, particular attention will be given to the psychosocial context of gender and sexual orientation, and to contexts of difference and discrimination.

Finally, Chapter 12 will discuss our place in the lifespan, recognizing the continuing processes of development that take place during our adult lives, the changing nature of our psychosocial and demographic environments and the accompanying experiences of transition and adaptation. All of these factors may raise issues that are important for us to consider as therapists at every point in our clients' lives. Models of lifespan development will be discussed, focusing on themes and issues deemed to be particularly supportive of therapeutic practice. The strengths and limitations of traditional stage-based models will be recognized, including the risk of conveying unhelpful cultural influences, especially in relation to older age. Erikson's classic work on psychosocial development will be given particular attention, reflecting its enduring relevance to psychotherapy practice, and will be followed by an overview of the ways in which lifespan perspectives may be drawn upon in psychotherapy. The chapter will end with a discussion of the particular context of older adulthood and the experience of approaching the end of life at that time.

Attachment Theory   **6**

The power of attachment theory lies in its capacity to convey the lived realities of our human need for sensitive love and care within close intimate relationships throughout the lifespan, and the problematic and damaging consequences we may live with if those needs are not fulfilled, especially during infancy and childhood. We are brought face to face with descriptions of real-life ways in which parents behave in relationship with their babies and young children, and the nature of helpful or problematic internal processes, thoughts, beliefs and behaviours in relation to self and others that are likely to develop in those children as a consequence, and that can endure for a lifetime. In addition to its connections with clinically based observations, it is a picture of human psychological development and functioning that has been directly and longitudinally observed and investigated by researchers grounded in developmental psychological theory and in the study of adult relationships over the past sixty years. It is through attachment theory research that we have the strongest evidence that psychological and relationship problems in adulthood can be linked to problematic experiences in relationships with parents or other primary care givers, in childhood. A truth that at times seems to be hard for society and individuals to accept: it really does matter how we relate to our children.

Attachment theory does not constitute a separate model of therapy, but seeks to be a theoretical approach that can advise and influence particularly psychodynamic and analytic therapies. It also has an extensive base within purely academic and research circles. It has strong implications for the practice of psychotherapy overall, and clearly supports the tenets of other therapy related theories, particularly those that pay attention to early life experiences and the nature of human relating. It was influenced by object relations theory and Freudian theory, with other powerful influences lying within evolutionary theory, biology, psychology and cognitive science and the ethology of Konrad Lorenz.

Attachment theory grew in John Bowlby's mind at least in part, as a reaction to Melanie Klein's perceived rejection of the importance of the child's actual interactions with real people during the 1930s to 1950s, and was markedly influenced by his own direct observations of the psychological impact on children of separation, and emotional deprivation and loss, in his professional psychiatric roles with London's Child Guidance Centre, the World Health Organization, and the Tavistock Clinic. He believed that what happened in the relationships between children and their parents was of great importance psychologically and emotionally, in ways that were primary in themselves, rather than being driven by the need for food, by orality or by an infantile, childish dependence that would disappear when maturity was achieved (Bowlby, 1988; Holmes, 1993, 1996, 2001; Holmes & Slade, 2018; Wallin, 2007). In the early 1930s the analyst Ian Suttie had come to similar conclusions about the significance of love, the child's primal attachment to mother, and the basic fear of losing that love, with later social attitudes depending on the nature of that early relationship (Brown, 1961; Clarke, 2006; Suttie, 1935/1988;). This position was fundamentally echoed in Fairbairn's emphasis on the absolute primacy of relationships in infancy and later childhood in his work on ego development and structure of mind (Clarke, 2006; Fairbairn, 1940/1952).

Attachment theory and its associated research tells us about parental capacities and ways of relating and responding that support sound and secure infant and child psychological development. Availability, sensitivity, instinctive attunement, and responsiveness from a position of personal psychological security characterize those parents who are best able to support healthy and resilient psychological development in their babies and children.

Wallin (2007) brings these capacities alive for us as he describes the sort of mother reflected in Ainsworth's research (Ainsworth et al., 1978). He tells us of a mother who is sensitive and does not delay in picking up her infant when she cries, but quickly and calmly holds her with tenderness and care, and only for as long as her baby wishes to be held. She can sense the meaning of her child's responses, and reciprocates in ways that enmesh with her own rhythms and with those of her baby, without imposing her own pace or her own agenda. There is sensitivity rather than mis-attunement, acceptance rather than rejection, cooperation rather than control, and emotional availability rather than remoteness.

Ainsworth's early intensive observational research of mothers in interaction with their infants supports the existence of the close and specific psychological and emotional bond, the attachment relationship between mother and infant that Bowlby argued for. As well as being associated with a sense of safety and the security to play, the attachment relationship plays an important part in supporting the infant's capacity to explore his or her immediate environment, and to interact with it in ways that facilitate the processes of learning. A pattern of repeated exploration and return is observed, particularly if the infant is surprised or upset by an experience during exploration, a return that can settle the child and enable further exploration; mothers are seen as functioning as a secure base for their babies. Ainsworth developed the structured laboratory experience of the Strange Situation to prompt these attachment related behaviours under controlled conditions, enabling observation of the nature of the play relationship between mother and infant, the infant's reaction to the presence of a stranger, to their mother briefly leaving the room, and to the reunion with her when she returns. This procedure has become a research marker for the importance of the attachment relationship between parents and their children, for its association with the psychological development of the child, and with their psychological health as they grow into adulthood. Within the Strange Situation, as at home with their mothers, it is the infants of the sensitive, attuned mothers who are relaxed and engaged in play and exploration in her presence, are distressed by her leaving, and unresponsive to the efforts of the stranger to comfort them, but soothed and comforted by their mother when she returns, regaining their capacity to play and to explore. Wallin (2007) describes secure babies as having equal access to their impulses to explore when they feel safe and to seek solace when they do not. A profound sense of comfort, emotional and physical safety and security can be associated with a good attachment relationship, and a powerful, maybe desperate need to be reunited and close again if separation takes that person and sense of security away.

The concepts of secure and insecure attachment emerged from Ainsworth's studies of the attachment relationship between infant and mother. As family observation and video data accumulated, she and her colleagues started to identify different patterns of infant behaviour. As well as the pattern of security described above, they also observed infants who showed very different behaviours, such as very little capacity to explore, being constantly anxious about where their mother was, being very passive, or rocking themselves, who cried greatly in their mother's absence, and were anxious to find her but did not seem to enjoy contact when they were with her again. It is these patterns of behaviour that have come to be defined as indicating insecure attachment in infancy and childhood, with distinction being made between two types of insecurity: ambivalent or anxious resistant attachment, and dismissive or avoidant attachment.

Ainsworth sees the prime marker of attachment security as the infant's capacity to be reassured by reunion with the mother, and to be able to resume play, however distressed he or she had been at separation. Infants are observed who seem constantly preoccupied with their mother's whereabouts, unable to explore freely, and intensely distressed when their mother leaves the room. Reunion with their mothers does not end their distress or resolve their preoccupation with where she was; some try to make connection, only to then express rejection, and others are passive and unresponsive. It is these infants who are considered to show the ambivalent or anxious resistant type of insecure attachment. Ainsworth's observational studies in the home show that the mothers of these infants are unpredictable in their sensitive attunement towards their babies. Sometimes they are able to respond in helpful, accurately attuned ways and at other times they are mis-attuned and/or unresponsive; at the same time they are discouraging of their infants' autonomy (Wallin, 2007). In addition, Bowlby (1988) associates ambivalent attachment with clinical evidence of separations, and with threats of abandonment being used as a means of control.

A further contrasting pattern led to the definition of dismissive or avoidant attachment. Some infants show no apparent distress during the Strange Situation procedure, and little overt attachment behaviour in relation to their mother. This external calm is associated with increased heart rate and greater increases in the stress related hormone cortisol compared with secure infants, and is understood as a defence related state. In such contexts, mothers tend to actively rebuff their infants' efforts to connect with them, withdraw when their babies appear sad, be uncomfortable with physical contact, and be generally inhibited in their expressions of emotion. Infants on the receiving end of these experiences on a daily basis can be left with no expectation of, or confidence in, true emotional connection with their mother, or the experience of care that connects with the emotions they hold within themselves. Emotions and needs become hidden to protect the self, and apparently self-contained distance becomes the solution for psychological survival.

Later, in looking through 200 research videos of the Strange Situation where the behaviour patterns of the infants had seemed to fit neither secure, or insecure categories, Main and Solomon realized that 90% of these included a pattern of strange, inexplicable, contradictory or bizarre responses from the infants, which often lasted only a few seconds and were dispersed amongst behaviours which otherwise could be defined within the existing categories (Main & Solomon, 1990; Wallin, 2007). This was defined as disorganized attachment, associated with the attachment figure being experienced as a source of fear and danger. This fear or sense of danger can be part of an otherwise safe haven of security, or exist within a relationship characterized by insecure attachment. In research samples it is particularly identified in infants maltreated or abused by their parents, and may be evident in those whose parents suffer from mental health problems, or live with the consequences of their own abuse or socially related stress. This disorganized pattern of infant responding seems likely to reflect internal processes of dissociation, resulting from traumatic experiences inconsistent with other aspects of relating, experienced as overwhelming and impossible to integrate.

Main has also been amongst the researchers interested in the context of attachment in adult life. A key aspect of Bowlby's theory lies in the importance of secure attachment relationships throughout the life span, and the central role that our attachment patterns play in influencing the nature of adult relationships.

Whilst there is no direct equivalent of the Strange Situation that is feasible to directly assess adult attachment security, several researchers have developed questionnaires to assess the relational patterns that adults are consciously aware of, using the responses to differentiate between secure and insecure adult attachment (Bartholomew & Horowitz, 1991; Hazan & Shaver, 1987; West & Sheldon, 1988). Main, on the other hand, developed the Adult Attachment Interview, AAI (Main et al., 1985) to prompt verbal and behavioural responses from adults that would reflect their inner psychological processes in relation to personally significant attachment material, particularly in their childhood. Differentiation between secure attachment and types of insecure attachment on the AAI relies on characteristics of the narrative emerging during the interview, revealing the nature of early attachment experiences, and the ways in which they can be remembered, connected with, felt and talked about in the present.

Current secure attachment on this basis is deemed to be associated with the capacity to remember past experiences, both good and problematic, to be aware of feelings associated with those experiences and to talk about them in a coherent narrative, demonstrating the absence of problematic defence related processes, the capacity to deal with and contain associated meaning and emotion, and the capacity to reflect on and think about the nature and consequences of those experiences. Insecure attachment is categorized as either preoccupied (equivalent to the ambivalent/anxious resistant attachment category in the Strange Situation) or dismissing (equivalent to the dismissive/avoidant attachment category in the Strange Situation). A category of unresolved/disorganized attachment is similarly seen as equivalent to disorganized attachment in the Strange Situation.

Whilst the questionnaire-based approaches to adult attachment assess the overt nature and quality of current close relationships, the AAI connects with unconscious processes that are part of the Internal Working Model (IWM) that Bowlby assumes results from the internalization of early attachment experiences, and that influences the nature of future intimate relationships throughout life. The IWM is assumed to encompass representations of self, others, patterns of relationship and associated unconscious processes. Holmes (1996) summarizes the IWM in secure attachment as including an internal model of a loving reliable other and a loved self, with an absence of defensive exclusion. Insecure attachment that has involved living with the internal dilemma of maintaining attachment in childhood with a care-giver who is unpredictable or rejecting was seen as including an internal model of an unreliable, and/or uncaring other and an unloved self, with the potential defensive exclusion of one's own needs and of emotions such as anger.

The importance of parental attachment status in relation to the attachment security of their children is particularly evident, especially in relation to parents' states of mind in relation to attachment as indicated by the AAI. Overall, research shows that the AAI classification of the parent predicts the Strange Situation classification of the child with 75% accuracy in regard to security versus insecurity (Wallin, 2007), and the trans-generational transmission of attachment security has been demonstrated by Hautamaki et al. (2010).

Used in combination in correlational and longitudinal research studies, indicators of attachment status in infancy, childhood, adolescence and adulthood, support Bowlby's assertion that attachment security or insecurity in childhood relates to the quality of parental care, and becomes an enduring aspect of personality from then onwards, with consequences during adulthood in terms of individual well-being and the quality of intimate relationships. Waters et al. (2000) discuss the stability of attachment security from infancy to early adulthood, and McConell and Moss (2011) review studies addressing stability and change in attachment status across the lifespan, looking at factors that relate to both. In terms of psychological well-being, the connections between attachment insecurity and disorganized attachment, and a wide range of psychological problems in childhood, adolescence and adulthood are discussed by various authors including Deklyen and Greenberg (2016); Green and Goldwyn (2002); Holmes (1993); Sheftall et al. (2014) and Stovall-McClough and Dozier (2016).

Importantly, and as Bowlby believed, as well as being an enduring aspect of who we are, our attachment status, and our internal working models can change in positive directions over time if our lives provide us with the good attachment relationships that we need. Research using the AAI has provided evidence that what has come to be termed earned security, can be achieved in adulthood. In spite of damaging early childhood experiences some adults are able to function psychologically in ways consistent with attachment security, and it is this capacity that is most strongly associated with attachment security in their children (Wallin, 2007).

Within recent approaches to attachment the implicit aspects of communication and meaning within attachment relationships has received particular attention. In relation to the early development of secure attachment between infant and care-giver, it is particularly non-verbal communication that has been emphasized since this must be the major basis for the development of secure attachment in the earliest months of life before the capacity for language has developed. It has also been argued that non-verbal behaviour then remains the most powerful attachment related communication throughout the life span, without denying the importance of words and their meaning (Wallin, 2007).

These positions of attachment theory in relation to early infant development are heavily supported and illustrated by the independent work of Colwyn Trevarthen and Daniel Stern, (Trevarthen, 2005; Trevarthen & Aitken, 2001; Smidt, 2018; Stern, 1984/2018) who discuss the moment-to-moment realities of connection and communication between infants and parents, their contribution to the development of a sense of self, and the development of subjectivity and inter-subjectivity.

Trevarthen's research involving the video recording of infants as young as a few hours old interacting with their parents, demonstrates the innate capacity for human connection and dialogue, and the need for that connection from the early moments after birth onwards. The vital role fulfilled by parents and primary care givers who can respond with attuned sensitivity is evidenced within those recordings. Within minutes of birth, babies are able to engage in two-way dialogues of imitation involving interest and effort. They experience emotion in response to interactions with others, and feel and express pleasure or sadness and distress depending on how people respond to them. Babies need to feel content and alert for these exchanges to take place, and they need to be with adults who wish to communicate with them, who are aware of and sensitive to the process that may unfold between them, can be in tune with the ways in which babies can respond and who will be prepared to let the baby take the lead. It is sensitive and attuned care by adults that provides the social environment in which infants can experience the reciprocal human connectedness that they need.

In his seminal work *The Interpersonal World of the Infant*, originally published in 1985, Stern (1985/2018) explores the ways in which physical, non-verbal and verbal communication between mother/parents and infants influences the development of a baby's sense of self from birth to 18 months of age, addressing pre-linguistic relational interactions and the early stages of language acquisition. In looking at the development of an emergent sense of self from birth to 2 months of age, Stern refers to the importance of the nature of communication that exists within primary care givers' movements, non-verbal and paralinguistic aspects of behaviour while carrying out the routine aspects of essential physical care, and the abstract social dance that can unfold between a mother and her very young baby. It is these aspects of communication and relationship that are crucial to the infant's developing sense of an emergent self. This work is consistent with Trevarthen's research and deepens our sense of the importance of the security and quality of the attachment relationship in early infancy.

Stern defines the subsequent developmental categories of a sense of self as the core self (from 2 to 6 months), the subjective self (from 7 to 15 months) and the inter-subjective and verbal selves (from 15 to 18 months) with the reality-based nature of the attachment relationship playing a crucial part in the secure evolution of each of these. The core self is considered to involve the sense of being a separate, cohesive, bounded physical unit, that can experience agency, affectivity, and continuity in time (Stern, 1984/2018). Its development is influenced by the repeated experience of coherence and consistency within the physical and sensory experiences of the infant's own body, his or her own actions and their consequences, and the reactions and behaviours of others. The infant's relationship with primary care givers, the nature of their responsiveness, the emotions they evoke and those they help to contain and regulate, and the intimacy, holding and security of their love and care, all make crucial contributions to the infant's development of a sense of core self. A self that is differentiated and boundaried, with its own capacities to feel and to act, and exists in interaction with others.

Stern describes the development of the subjective self as the infant's discovery of its own mind and the discovery that others have separate minds, and sees this as involving a theory or working sense of separate minds. The evolving potential to communicate and share subject matter between those separate minds then moves towards the capacity for inter-subjectivity; sensitive, meaningful and mutual exchanges with parents and others can now increase in quality and quantity. Good and secure parental responses in these respects, are seen by Stern as fundamentally enabling the baby to experience psychic human membership rather than psychic isolation; a capacity described as a basic psychological need. It is essential that parents are able to read their infant's feeling state and infants are able to read their parents' responses.

By the time infants have reached 18 months of age Stern describes them as knowing they are objects that can be experienced by others, and as able to imagine others' subjective states and to experience empathy. As it develops, verbal communication is seen as enabling the overt negotiation of meaning between the child and others, providing new ways of creating relatedness, opening up the possibility of mixed and contradictory verbal and non-verbal messages, and playing a central part in crucial issues of attachment regarding autonomy, separation and intimacy. All categories of the sense of self are now available to be further supported or limited and distorted by the nature of the continuing attachment relationship between children and their parents.

In the adult context an emphasis on communication sits alongside a recognition that individuals need to conceptualize other people's minds as being separate from and different to their own, as described by Stern in relation to the developmental category of the subjective self. They need to be able to develop sufficiently accurate models of those other minds to take them into account when relating to other people; to think about how those other minds work and to empathize with them. Bowlby sees this capacity as essential for a harmonious relationship between any two people (Bowlby, 1988).

Subsequently these abilities have been referred to as the capacity to mentalize, supported by an unconscious theory of mind, a personal theory about how the different, separate minds encountered in human relationships may be working, echoing Stern and Bowlby's earlier work (Fonagy & Bateman, 2007; Fonagy & Target, 1996, 2006). A theory of mind is seen as enabling us to develop the reflective capacity to step back from the immediate impact of interpersonal experience, understand it better, and take contextual factors into account. Overall, such capacities lie at the heart of the ability for sensitive and empathic attunement so essential to the secure attachment relationship between child and parent, and at the heart of true mutual understanding and emotional connection between people of any age.

Moving on further or maybe deeper into human functioning, Schore (2012) reviews his own and other research addressing the neurobiological context of the attachment relationship, making connections between brain development and the nature of interpersonal relatedness from early infancy onwards. This research and discussion of ideas related to attachment and brain development has also involved a particular emphasis on the infant's early pre-verbal experience of empathic attunement and emotional containment. Uncontained and unregulated emotion resulting from a failure of non-verbal empathic attunement influencing the right brain at this time is deemed to have a particularly detrimental effect on brain development, because it occurs at the same time as the brain is experiencing a surge in overall neuronal growth and proliferation. In somewhat similar vein, Dana (2018) discusses the neurobiological basis of fundamental human connection, soothing and emotional regulation in the context of polyvagal theory (Porges, 2011).

Whilst attachment theory has been developed and applied in a wide range of academic and social contexts, it was first developed in the context of psychoanalytic psychotherapy and other approaches to clinical work in support of children who experienced deprived and damaging environments. In particular, Bowlby sought to develop a broader theoretical basis for psychoanalytic therapy practice that took the real world into account and paid attention to theory and evidence from other disciplines with important things to say about human development and psychological functioning. It was not designed to become a new and different therapy, but to be a theory that would support and maybe transform existing therapeutic approaches and practice.

Bowlby (1988) and many others, including in particular Holmes (1996, 2001), Holmes and Slade (2018) and Wallin (2007), have defined and discussed the ways in which psychotherapy practice can be advised, and led by attachment theory, seeing the therapeutic relationship in many ways as a parallel of the good, secure attachment relationship. Bowlby sees this as the context in which amidst a potentially emotionally dependent and intense anxious attachment to the therapist, clients may be able to recover an emotional life that was lost to them in childhood. Similarly, Wallin (2007) discusses the potential for us to be given a second chance, when new relationships within adult life may enable us to think, feel and love more freely, from within the security and safety afforded by the experience of secure attachment. When it unfolds well, psychotherapy may be able to provide this healing relationship.

Patterns of thinking, feeling and behaving in relation to ourselves and others may now have the chance to change, as our internal working models of attachment become open to modification. Bowlby (1988) refers to the following five therapeutic tasks to help guide analytic psychotherapy from an attachment perspective:

- The provision of a secure base enabling exploration of the painful past and present
- The exploration of the nature of current relating to significant others, and associated unconscious biases
- The encouragement to explore the relationship with the therapist and what it can reveal of clients' internal working models of relationship with an attachment figure
- The consideration of links between current ways of being in relationships and those experienced in the past; accessing ideas and feelings about parents that may have been felt unimaginable or unthinkable, with the possibility of strong emotions
- The possibility of recognizing that images of self and others derived from a painful past may not be appropriate to the present or the future, and may have never been justified at all; freeing people from old unconscious stereotypes and enabling them to feel, think and behave in new ways.

The attentive, attuned and empathic relationship provided by the therapist is central to this experience of a secure attachment relationship, and secure base to support thinking, feeling and being. Bowlby emphasizes the importance of clients taking the lead, being given the opportunity to discover experience and understanding for themselves, whilst acknowledging the need for supportive challenge at times, particularly in the face of defensive avoidance. He believed in the innate human capacity for growth and recovery, with the psychotherapist's job being to provide the conditions in which self-healing can best take place.

It is the emotional communication between therapist and client that is seen as enabling changes within the internal working models of the client. Aspects of client past and current experience of insecure attachment may be thought about, relived and enacted within the therapeutic relationship, in the context of an empathic and emotionally containing, but not intrusive, warmth and acceptance. Previously unmanageable feelings may now be experienced by clients, as their therapists become people who are able to receive and respond to their projections of intensely painful emotion (Holmes, 1993; Wallin, 2007). In Wallin's terms, a connection and relationship is provided that is experienced as valid, real and personal, and creates a developmental crucible for the client.

The more recent work of Schore (2012) and other researchers from a neurobiological perspective has involved increased attention to the non-verbal expression of emotion that may represent defensively hidden experience within clients relating back to their earliest pre-verbal relational contexts. The importance of non-verbal experience between therapists and clients within the therapeutic attachment relationship has now been brought to the fore from a perspective that sees it as representing a fundamental level of psychological and emotional relating. Wallin and Schore argue that the holistic and emotion focused right side of our brain as therapists matters in a particularly special way, because its activity in relation to our clients can connect with the consequences of very early pre-linguistic experience within the infant. These consequences are deemed to be especially significant to all future functioning, since pre-linguistic relational experience is likely to have been taking place during the very intensive period of infant neurobiological brain development, and is seen as having constituted the core of the early developing self. Any adverse experience that became defensively excluded at this stage of development could only ever exist in a non-verbal form, and would only be accessible in the therapeutic relationship through emotional attunement to non-verbal aspects of being within the client and the therapist.

Loss and separation are intimately embedded within attachment theory. It was through a recognition of the impact of loss and separation that the importance of secure attachment was identified, in everyday life and on a research basis through Ainsworth's Strange Situation. Separation and loss are unavoidable human experiences. They present in many forms, and can engender difficult, painful emotions such as sadness, anger, fear and despair. The ways in which we are or have been treated by the other person involved in a loss or separation will have significant effect on how it is experienced, and the impact of the loss will be influenced by our internal working models and underlying attachment security. Attachment theory can help therapists to consider both the importance of loss within clients' lives, past and present, as well as the separations and losses experienced within the therapeutic relationship.

The way in which the categories of attachment are used within clinical practice is often very different when compared to their use in research contexts. With a focus on the uniqueness and complexity of individual people rather than group-based data, therapy involves recognizing the variations and overlaps of behaviours and categories that empirical research cannot take into account. Therapists find it useful to think more broadly, in terms of overall secure versus insecure attachment status. The discrete categories of attachment may be used on a dimensional rather than categorical basis, and used to help therapists generate ideas about the possible nature of attachment related thoughts, feelings, defences and behaviours experienced by their clients within their intimate relationships (Holmes, 1993).

Crucially the reality of external experience is accepted within attachment theory, particularly the impact of environmental and relational trauma. Bowlby clearly argues that client reports of their real worlds are to be accepted as reasonable and acceptable approximations to the truth; they should be believed, unless clear indications existed to the contrary, and not to do so is damaging (Bowlby, 1988). Alongside the realities of the external world the realities of the child's (and adult's) internal world, their own agency and potential resilience are also recognized: both external and internal worlds play their part (Holmes,1993).

Having evolved as a result of this interaction between internal and external worlds, internal working models then have their own potential to play a part in maintaining problems. Therapy involves a real and genuine attachment relationship, co-created by therapist and client, in which honesty and openness may prevail and helpful changes within internal models may take place.

Summary

In Chapter 6 we have looked at the main principles of attachment theory, reviewed its associated research base, recognized the crucial developmental importance of the attachment relationship, and made connection with other closely related observational studies of infant development. We have thought about the real-world nature of relationship and attunement associated with secure attachment, its importance throughout the life span, the ways in which attachment theory may help us understand the nature of psychological distress, and the role it may play within the experience of psychotherapy.

Humanistic and Experiential Theory   **7**

Person-centred therapy and related theory enshrine the core principle that it is the person who has decided to come for therapy who should take the lead in making decisions about the nature of his or her life, the ways in which that life might be changed and how any changes may be brought about. The motivation behind such change within people is seen by Carl Rogers as lying in the natural human capacity for, and tendency to move towards, growth and development, towards becoming more fully and more freely the unique person that all of us naturally have the underlying capacity to be. Therapeutic principles argue against any goal directed interventions on the part of the therapist, and any therapist led decisions about the desirable nature of change. In these respects, it is a therapy that is very conscious of issues of power within the therapeutic relationship, explicitly arguing that the power to make choices and to take the lead should lie with clients. Their empowerment sits at the heart of person-centred practice, plus the fundamental belief that all people have within them the potential for constructive psychological and emotional growth and development. It is these characteristics that define it as a humanistic approach (Mearns & Thorne, 2013; Nelson-Jones, 1982; Rogers, 1957, 1961/1967, 1980, 1951/2003; Thorne, 2003; Tolan, 2003; Wilkins, 2016).

The nature of the therapeutic relationship is seen as the origin of the therapist's capacity to help people grow and change, to help them become the people they might be. Roger's belief in the power of the therapeutic relationship in combination with the clients' natural propensity to growth evolved in the context of his early work with children and families. His colleagues such as Jessie Taft worked from a relationship therapy perspective and were influenced by Otto Rank's work including his concept of 'will' (Barrett-Lennard, 1998; deCarvalho, 1999; Taft, 1933). The essence of Rank's position seems at times to have become lost in translation, with will being interpreted as active, almost forced, conscious intention, rather than reflecting Rank's belief in naturally unfolding processes of constructive self-direction and creativity, capacities that could be freed to function by the experience of psychotherapy. If that underlying capacity is affirmed and supported rather than negated and denied, Rank believed that our life instinct would naturally lead us towards a happiness founded within those capacities for creation and being, and our acceptance of our lives as they are lived (Rank, 1936/1978).

Rogers first experienced the facilitative role that therapy may play and the power of listening rather than providing his own interpretations, in his work with the mother of one of his young clients. Following his subsequent belief that there could exist a common set of relational characteristics that might be identified within all effective therapies, he then pursued a thoughtful analysis of his own therapeutic work and undertook numerous research projects, exploring the connection between such assumed characteristics and therapy outcomes (Thorne, 2003).

Through Carl Rogers' work we are placed as close as is professionally possible to our human psychological nakedness as therapists within our professional place, as one person relating to another. We are asked to lay aside status, certainty, and decision making, preconceptions, assumptions and stereotypes, and as truly as possible to meet and to hear the other person. It is this person-to-person human encounter and connectedness that Rogers identifies as being of primary importance within person-centred therapy, and for him the therapeutic relationship is fundamentally a deeply egalitarian one.

An essential tension may at times seem to exist between the experience of a natural and genuine human connection within the therapeutic relationship and the academic, professional and ethical need to develop a sound and comprehensive theory and to describe the ways in which good and helpful therapy may be provided. Defining theoretical concepts and processes, and developing techniques to be used in therapy, may run the risk that the opportunity to share a genuine personally meaningful and unique human connection may be lost in the process. Much of the writing on person-centred therapy reflects on and describes the personal experience of therapists within themselves and between themselves and their clients, with theory being quite broadly based and using a terminology that differs somewhat from the more conventional and scientific language of other therapy approaches. This may reflect something of the need to protect the personal relationship that lies at the heart of therapy.

The human capacity to grow and develop into the person that we have the potential to be is referred to as the actualizing tendency, and the positive unconscious motivation to develop the self that we can naturally become is referred to as organismic valuing. The self that evolves and that is experienced as self by the child and later adult is termed the self-concept or self-structure. The childhood development of the self may become disrupted by unhelpful judgemental parental attitudes and behaviours. When such disruption occurs and parents treat their children in ways that are not valuing of the person they are naturally becoming, and focus their valuing instead on how they want and need their child to be, they are seen as generating conditions of worth, which are internalized by the child. Depending on the nature of relationship between children and parents, the self-concept may be consistent with a developmental path influenced by organismic valuing or it may be more or less heavily influenced by parentally induced conditions of worth, following a path that is shaped more by parental values, wishes and needs. People are defined as congruent or incongruent, depending on how much the naturally unfolding path of the self-concept has been distorted by conditions of worth. Incongruence involves internal tensions that result in the defensive exclusion of aspects of self-experience that are at odds with the distorted self-concept, in an attempt to achieve a state of apparent congruence. If defensive exclusion fails, overt incongruence results in anxiety and other symptoms of psychological distress. If defences are well maintained, they limit the extent to which reality in relation to self and others is accurately perceived, and distortions in perception are likely to create problems in different aspects of life and relationships. Those parents who are able to accept their child as the person they may naturally become will raise children who are minimally affected by conditions of worth as adults, are able to be accepting of themselves and who they naturally are, and who will be more likely in turn to be accepting of their own children (Nelson-Jones, 1982).

Whilst Rogers' concepts were developed in the context of humanistic psychology, it is important to define the differences between his use of the term actualizing tendency and Maslow's definition of actualization (Maslow, 1943). Bohart (2007) discusses this context, making it clear that Rogers is referring to the human motivation to maintain, enhance and develop the self, the tendency to grow and adapt to function better within the environment in which we find ourselves. Rogers' actualizing tendency would not necessarily result in personal characteristics that might be judged as morally and socially positive. Maslow, on the other hand, explicitly defines morally and ethically positive attributes as qualities that identify the fully actualized person. For Rogers the fully functioning person is someone who is open to their experience of themselves and others, is not overly impeded by defensive exclusion, and is therefore able to adapt and learn from experience.

Bozarth and Motomasa (2005) summarize the six conditions that Rogers (1957) identifies as related to effective therapy, seeing their value as relevant across all therapies of all theoretical orientations, and judging them to be both necessary and sufficient for beneficial personality change to take place:

- clients and therapists need to be in psychological contact, which involves both having the capacity to be affected by their experience of the other

- clients are defined as needing to be in state of incongruence, that can no longer be held at bay by defensive exclusion of experience
- therapists need to be congruent within their relationship with their clients, having undefended access to their perceptions of all that their clients bring to them, and to their own capacities to understand the other person; it is only from this undefended place that therapists may experience truly genuine, authentic ways of relating
- therapists need to be in a personal position to experience unconditional positive regard towards their clients, involving a basic respect, valuing and acceptance of the person as they are, that is not conditional on whether they do things that please and gratify the therapist
- from these positions within themselves therapists need to be able to experience empathic attunement with their clients' inner worlds, however different these may be from their own, to connect with where clients may be within their lives, in relation to their past and current experiences, and imagine the possible meanings, thoughts, feelings, wishes and motivations, from within the clients' frame of reference
- clients need to be able to receive and perceive these responses from their therapists, to connect with them and feel the impact of genuineness, acceptance and empathic connection, within their own minds.

Implicit alongside these six conditions lies the therapist's belief in the humanistic basis of person-centred therapy, a belief and a trust in the actualizing tendency (Bozarth, 1998). Rogers believes that given these necessary psychological conditions, the actualizing tendency will naturally result in clients discovering what they need to do in order to change in positive and constructive ways: that people will become freed for normal growth and development (Rogers, 1942). Similarly, if one or more of the conditions is absent, he believes that constructive personality change will not be possible (Rogers, 1957). Rogers also referred to three of these six conditions: empathy, unconditional positive regard/prizing of the client, and being a real person, as the facilitative conditions provided by therapists that make such change most likely to take place, giving rise to the commonly used term of the therapeutic triad.

During infancy and childhood it is parents' capacities for genuineness, acceptance, unconditional positive regard and empathic attunement that provide an environment in which the actualizing tendency may foster healthy personality/ self-development, free from the unhelpful impact of conditions of worth. Being valued and experiencing a sense of love from other people are essential to human well-being from earliest childhood onwards, and they are the essence of what Rogers refers to as positive regard. When conditions of worth have distorted the development of the self, incongruence is survived with the help of defensive exclusion, and a price is paid within personal relationships and the capacity to live and to thrive; finding these conditions within a therapy relationship may provide a second chance. Therapist acceptance and unconditional positive regard may foster self-acceptance and positive self-regard, conditions of worth may be reduced and the actualizing tendency may result in growth and development starting to follow a path that is congruent with the client's organismically valued self, naturally reducing the functioning of defences and moving them towards being the person they have the potential to be.

Rogers brings us to a very personal place in thinking about the nature of empathy and the challenge it may present for us at times. It involves us at an essentially personal level within a clearly professional relationship. He refers to entering the private perceptual world of the other in a way that enables us to become familiar and at home with its characteristics and nuances, comfortable with who this other person is from the inside, with all their range of experiences, emotions, meanings and expression, but maintaining our separate psychological place at all times as well, sensing the client's private world as if it were our own, but without losing the 'as if' quality (Rogers, 1980).

In allowing ourselves to become closer to the inner, often hidden experiences of another human being, some aspects of experience may be easier for us to connect with than others. It can be disturbing to feel touched by another person's fear, anger or pain and our own defences may naturally pull us back from that connection. Our task is to accept the disturbing discomfort, feel the impact of anger or pain, but also contain and manage it within ourselves. If something in our face conveys that we have been able to truly hear that distress, and if our words are felt to have recognized and understood their experience, clients' emotions may then emerge with greater clarity, fullness and meaning. However, we may pull back from empathic connection precisely because we know that this can happen, and fear of that expression of emotion may stop us from empathizing in the first place. Balance and care are also needed, however, so that we avoid the risk of unhelpfully prompting deeper and deeper emotions, when this could actually be damaging and even destructive.

We are challenged to find connection across a wide and varying range of meaning, thought and feeling, recognizing love, tenderness, warmth and humour alongside the darkness of fear, anger and confusion and sometimes the terrible consequences of trauma and abuse, finding our own way to live with their impact within ourselves. At times we may come to understand some aspect of human experience in a new and completely different way because we have empathized with it, and now know it differently for the first time: in some way we may be changed, and never be quite the same again (Rogers, 1961/1967); Welch (2003) considers empathy to be "a matter of risk, a matter of courage" (p.137).

The six factors described by Rogers (1957) as necessary and sufficient, elaborate on the prerequisites for empathic connection between therapist and client. No empathy can exist if therapist and client are not in psychological contact with each other, each sensing and being affected by the other; it cannot exist if the meaning and feeling are only experienced in the therapist's mind and do not resonate, echo and find they have a home in the mind of the client; it cannot be trusted and is meaningless if it is not felt to come from someone who is truly being genuine in whatever they do and say, and who is accepting and valuing of who we are. The defences that may normally maintain apparent congruence within the client, also need to have lost enough of their strength for underlying incongruence to assert itself in the form of distress.

Therapists are hampered in listening and in finding emotional resonance within themselves for the personal, often painful experiences of their clients if their own psychological needs and defences associated with incongruence, get in the way. As well as being crucially important in relation to conditions of worth, the fundamental respect, acceptance and valuing of the client that constitute unconditional positive regard are also essential to empathic understanding. The two go hand in hand; an emotion, a wish, a belief, a thought, a behaviour has to be accepted as it is before it can be empathized with. Any judgemental positions, either positive or negative, will impede the experience of empathy, interfering with therapists' capacities to become psychologically connected with the meaning and feeling that may lie within the client. Acceptance is essential to empathy and empathy communicates acceptance, care and understanding: it is a connection that ends psychological isolation.

Empathy is personally precious; and, as clients if it has not happened to us in the same way before, it may mean that finally we are no longer on our own. It lets us know that someone understands us with validity, because they could not have realized our thoughts and feelings had they not truly understood. We are not mad or bad for thinking and feeling the way we do. Another human being has been able and willing to hold who we are in their own mind, and care enough to think and find their own words to express what they have come to know, understand and accept of us. The sense of relief may be palpable. It may become safer then, for difficult unacceptable or painful feelings to come into consciousness, when we had barely known they were there. If another person has not needed to hide away from those thoughts and feelings, then it becomes safer for us to feel them. They grow stronger, and we discover the hurt or the anger or the despair, in the presence of another who can bear and accept them. Our unhelpful defences start to change and may fall away as they are no longer needed.

We may also discover our particular abilities, strengths and interests as they are also recognized and empathized with, and as the defences associated with all that has gone before start to ease. The sense of rapport and closeness between ourselves and our therapist deepens and we naturally talk more openly, freely and deeply about ourselves and our lives. A freedom may develop in which we become able to imagine possibilities within our daily lives that could not come to mind before. In small and maybe not so small ways, aspects of our lives may start to change as we make some decisions to try out doing things differently.

Rogers recognizes the paradox of people accepting who they are, including the aspects of themselves and their lives that they wish could be different. It seems on the face of it a potentially counter-productive thing to do, to accept that difficult or distressing things about ourselves are as they are, since acceptance could be thought to imply that things either do not need to change or cannot change. Rogers talked about this paradox, reflecting on his own experience that valuable change could take place spontaneously, once he had truly accepted that things just were as they were. The nature of the self-acceptance that Rogers is talking about is not an acceptance that reflects despair and giving up, but an acceptance that reflects a willingness to face the truth just as it exists now. This truth may include associated feelings of sadness, guilt, shame, and grief and despair, but all are known and accepted. It may also sometimes include the recognition and reality that aspects of our behaviour are detrimental and damaging to others. Change may be hindered by internal unhelpful processes associated with non-acceptance, such as self-blame, criticism, denial, the wish that the awful experience would just go away, maybe a wish for miracles; self-acceptance can help relieve their counterproductive and undermining power.

As self-understanding, valuing and acceptance evolve, people become more free to live in their own spontaneous and maybe creative ways, with their evaluation of what they do coming to lie more within themselves rather than being overly influenced by conditions of worth and defined by the real or imagined judgments of others. They may then sometimes experience a different kind of disappointment in themselves, if they come to realize they have been betraying their own personal values rather than failing by not meeting someone else's expectations, wishes or demands (Mearns & Thorne, 2013). For Rogers, self-acceptance is equally important for both therapists and clients.

More recent developments in person-centred theory have recognized that the developmental drive of the actualizing process needs to be balanced and moderated by a process of social mediation that takes into account the needs of others and the society we live in (Mearns & Thorne, 2000, 2013). This involves a valuable acceptance that the outcomes of the actualizing tendency with its goal of survival and development in whatever circumstances people find themselves, may not always be positive from a wider social perspective, and that 'healthy social restraint' has an appropriate place in developmental experiences. This has led to the valuable recognition that setting limits can also be an important part of person-centred theory and therapy.

This may be of particular relevance in the context of early childhood deprivation and trauma. The consequences of very damaging developmental environments, including the routine absence of parental empathic understanding have been recognized as resulting in what can be referred to as fragile process, in which adults experience very low or very high intensity emotions when faced with personally meaningful experience, and a difficulty in appreciating the perspectives of other people while high emotion is activated (Warner, 2000).

Taking their inspiration from Rogers' work, various practitioners, including Nelson-Jones (1982), Tolan (2003) and Welch (2003), have developed structured approaches towards the development of the therapeutic skills involved in listening and relating to clients from a person-centred perspective. Other work such as Egan's classic text (Egan, 2017) define Rogers' style of working as active listening, specifying and describing the skills involved, and supporting their active development in therapists, hopefully without spoiling the unique human connection between them and their clients. Rogers sees empathy as a way of being, and Mearns and Thorne (2013) describe it as a process rather than a technique. The concern has long been expressed that skills training on a technique basis will destroy the spontaneous human connection that empathy involves. However, structured practice may always be needed for new therapists to start putting a potential understanding of another person's private world into words that may carry meaning, and with practice and familiarity, technique may become part of the therapist's natural and authentic way of being. The capacity for human emotional connection may need to be learnt, but the learning process need not invalidate the power of that connection.

Person-centred therapy is now seen as part of a family of experiential therapies (Sanders, 2013). This family includes the non-directive approach fulfilling the criteria that Rogers defined, but also allows for a broader range of therapies that fulfil some of these conditions but not others. All of them give a central place to therapists' empathically attuned connection with their clients and the importance of clients' awareness of their own internal experiences and processes.

Some members of the family put particular emphasis on the accessing, processing and management of emotional experience as discussed by Westwell (2016) and illustrated by Focusing-Oriented Therapy (Gendlin, 1996). Others recognize the cognitive processing needed for therapeutic change, especially in trauma related contexts (Murphy & Joseph, 2016). The process-experiential therapies, including Emotion-Focused Therapy (Elliott & Greenberg, 2007; Greenberg, 2004, 2011), involve active collaborative tasks oriented towards explicit goals for change. Similarly, Gestalt therapy includes active approaches towards enhancing experiential awareness of different aspects of self, and in support of changes within the nature of experience (Clarkson & Cavicchia, 2013). The two-chair technique is a good example in this respect: having become experientially connected with disparate and often hidden aspects of self, clients are encouraged to take the role of both aspects, in dialogue with each other, in the hope that through doing so awareness and understanding of both positions within the self will be enhanced, and greater internal integration may be achieved. All therapies within the experiential family hold the therapeutic relationship to be of core importance, and within that the therapists' empathic understanding, acceptance and valuing of their clients.

Overall, a wide range of therapies have found their home within the humanistic and experiential family. The most powerful and enduring legacy of Carl Rogers' work, however, may be the universal recognition of the importance of empathic connection between therapist and client within counselling and psychotherapy as a whole, whether his work is formally acknowledged or not.

Summary

In Chapter 7 we have thought about the powerful and universally important positions held by Carl Rogers and others regarding the experience of genuine and accepting empathic connection and valuing, that can enable people to develop and change, so that each may move closer to the person that they have the potential to be. In doing so, we have discussed core principles of client-centred theory and specifics of therapeutic relating that can enable constructive change to take place. We have also recognized the wider range of experiential therapies that draw on, and add to, these principles.

Psychodynamic Theory   8

Psychodynamic theory sees our unconscious minds as playing a very important part in our psychological and interpersonal lives, in constant interaction with experience that lies within conscious awareness. It gives a central role to the importance of emotion, and sees our ongoing relationships with others as being crucially influenced by accumulated unconscious complex representations of past relational experience. It is also at its heart a developmental theory, paying deep and intricate attention to the nature of early and subsequent relationships and the ways in which they may influence the developing self. It is a process-oriented theory which believes in the complexity of the human mind, and recognizes the contribution which multiple factors, both conscious and unconscious in the past and the present can make towards our current states of mind and personal and interpersonal difficulties.

Theory takes the view that changes in important aspects of unconscious functioning within therapy will influence the ways in which conscious experience and behaviour unfold, that time is needed for this to happen, and that the ways in which it happens will be unique to each individual and cannot be known in advance. In these respects, psychodynamic theory supports a facilitative approach to therapeutic change and personal development, and sees the relationship between therapist and client as central to the processes of change.

Important core theoretical concepts reviewed here will include unconscious conflict and related psychological defences, identification, internalization, projection, projective identification, transference, countertransference and the inner world of object relations, emotional containment, corrective emotional experience and re-enactments, and parallel process. This chapter will discuss these concepts and look at further aspects of theory and practice including analytic listening, processes of psychological development, and the significance of intra-psychic and interpersonal boundaries.

The discussion of psychological development will include the core concepts of basic trust, the basic fault, early primitive/immature and later more mature defences, the contrast between true self and false self, the nature of early symbiotic closeness and subsequent separation, rapprochement, and individuation, and the concepts of self-objects, empathic mirroring, optimal frustration, and developmental arrest. The chapter will end with discussions relating to the therapeutic relationship and therapeutic frame, and a simplified psychodynamic rationale for change.

Throughout this chapter my writing is primarily advised by my personal understanding of this range of concepts and processes, reflecting my therapy practice, teaching, training and supervisory roles. It supports a post-Freudian position that recognizes the topographical distinction between conscious and unconscious mind, rather than Freud's structural model of ego, id and super-ego. It is reflective of positions such as Fairbairn's in which self is synonymous with ego, which is vulnerable to fragmentation under the influence of damaging developmental experiences (Clarke, 2006; Fairbairn, 1940/1952).

The material overall is supported by the following texts: Bateman et al. (2010); Brown (1961); Casement (1985/2014); DeYoung (2015); Freud (1895-1926/1979, 1911-1940/1984); Jacobs (1995, 2004); Kahn (1997); Leiper and Maltby (2004); Lemma et al. (2011); Malan (1995); Segal (1973/2018); Siegel (1996); and Symington and Symington (1996).

Unconscious Conflict and Defence: Unconscious or intra-psychic conflict and defence play a constant part, together with transference and countertransference, in the unfolding nature of our emotional lives and our relationships with other people. Unconscious conflict refers to the conflict between our feelings (wishes, impulses, emotions, needs or drives) and the anticipated negative consequences of experiencing and acting on them. This conflict leads to what Freud refers to as signal anxiety which triggers the functioning of psychological defences. These in turn disguise, distort or in other ways hide the feelings that have triggered the anxiety. In the case of our emotions, the pain associated with the conscious experience of an emotion may lead directly to unconscious conflict and related signal anxiety. The painful, maybe unbearable emotion may remain unconscious, and others may take its place within conscious experience.

An important distinction is made between primitive/immature developmentally early defences which can have particularly powerful capacities to distort reality, and mature defences. As adults we each function with our own unique mix of both mature and immature defences. Theory defines a range of defence mechanisms at both conscious and unconscious levels. The most notable mature defences are suppression, the holding back of a feeling that is consciously known to exist, and repression where a feeling is deemed to exist at an unconscious level, unavailable to conscious awareness. Immature defences include the splitting of emotional experience into polar extremes with no grey areas in between; projection of one's own emotions onto others with the consequent perception of them as belonging to those others rather than to ourselves; and the delusional denial of reality.

Defences are often constructive processes, helping to maintain effective emotional and interpersonal living, but at times they may be unhelpful to us. If they have been influenced by earlier problematic experiences, especially in childhood, they are likely to have played an important part in our psychological survival at the time. However, they may no longer be needed, and their persistence will distort our experience of ourselves and others, and prove damaging to our current abilities to lead less painful, happier and more fulfilling lives.

Other unconscious processes play key roles within psychodynamic theory's understanding of the human mind. Central among these are internalization, identification, projection and projective identification.

Internalization, Identification, Projection and Projective Identification: Internalization refers to the ways in which aspects of other people and/or the ways in which they have related to us, can be taken into our own unconscious minds and become part of who we are. This may be associated with a process of identification as we consciously or unconsciously see a connection and similarity between who the other person is in certain ways, and who we are or may become; we identify with them. When we project an aspect of who we are, we may perceive someone else as having a characteristic that we are loath to recognize within ourselves. Projection in this respect may then be functioning as a defence. Alternatively, we may assume that others have the same acceptable qualities as we do, when actually that may not be the case. We may also behave in a way that prompts others to feel an emotion that originates in ourselves, and in this way project emotions into others. This may particularly happen when an emotion feels hard for us to experience and to bear.

Projective identification involves complex interpersonal processes, which maintain and potentially intensify a psychological state of affairs involving two or more people that may be beneficial or unhelpful. Within psychotherapy we most often focus on this process in the context of unhelpful consequences. It is one of those processes that is not easy to put into words, and since I believe it to be very significant within therapy and supervision, and within all our relationships, I will describe it here in some detail by giving an anonymised example involving myself and a trainee.

My trainee and I have just finalized his contract for the first placement of the three-year training course, and as I shut the door to my room I feel pleased, and somewhat relieved, that it has been completed. I feel secure in my judgement that we have struck an appropriate balance between enough learning opportunities and a quality/quantity of work that could risk being unhelpfully challenging at his stage of training. Minutes later, however, there is a knock on the door; my trainee has returned. He says that he really feels he wants to work with a client with alcohol-related problems as part of his goals for placement. I find myself feeling uncertain and somewhat anxious - should I have dealt with the contract differently? We go to the filing cabinets; I look and find a possible client for him and I add this goal to his contract.

Back in my room I am unsettled. This does not feel right, but can I take back my decision and face his disappointment? After some time of thinking I decide, yes that is what I need to do. I tell him that I think we were right in the first place, we have a sufficient range of therapeutic work planned already, and there is no need to extend it; in fact, to do so could be unhelpful. He is disappointed but accepts and does seem to understand. Returning to my room, my sense of uncertainty is markedly eased. The placement unfolds well, my trainee makes good and sound progress, and he works successfully with clients with alcohol-related problems later on in his training.

In terms of projective identification, I imagine my trainee experiencing anxieties about not being good enough when he comes back and knocks on my door. I identify with that and feel anxious too - am I good enough? We could say his anxiety is projected into me, which only happens if we identify with each other, share a similar underlying anxiety, and I become anxious as well. I respond to my anxiety, sort out another client, and our mutual anxieties are initially reduced, but lurking in the background is more uncertainty and the risk that this solution will actually cause more problems. We are at the start of a process of unhelpful projective identification that could result in a cycle of increasing anxiety if it is not identified and ended. Doing so is often not comfortable - processes of defence are in there fuelling our mutual responses to the anxiety of not being good enough, and helping us avoid personal and interpersonal discomfort. This process does nothing to actually resolve our self-esteem related concerns, and if anything might risk intensifying them. Facing my trainee's disappointment and living through it, taking us both back to the more secure ground of our original contract was actually the only way to break that vicious cycle, to reduce anxiety and to affirm that we were both good enough already.

Transference, Countertransference and the Inner World of Object Relations: Transference refers to the internalized experience of our relationships with significant other people, particularly those who have been most important to us while we were growing up. The patterns of those relationships, how others behaved towards us, and how we also felt and responded, live on within us and colour our perception of other people and our behaviour towards them, in our current lives, especially if something of the role relationship of the early experience is reflected within the present. The situation is more powerful the more the person in the present behaves in ways that are similar to the person in the past.

People in this theoretical context are referred to as objects, because it is believed that it is not necessarily the nature of whole people that are reflected in internal memory, but also separate parts of them that have had particular emotional impact on us. Within our minds our experiences of others and our relationships with them may be unconsciously remembered and held together in terms of whole and part-objects, whole people and aspects of people, parts of who we experienced them as being. Such memory structures exist as part of an unconscious inner world of object relations. They may relate to specific people, as well as to more generalized types/categories of people and the roles that others played in relation to ourselves. Within this internal world, our self is also an object which can exist as a whole as well as a number of part-objects. These processes of transference are fuelled by relationships with people who are significant to us in the present as well as in the past.

Our inner world of object relations influences the ways in which we perceive and make sense of ourselves, other people and our relationships with them, and how we behave in relation to ourselves and others. It holds within it the depth and complexity of the conscious and unconscious experiences and processes associated with the nature of our self, of others and of our relationships; incorporating our emotional reactions, our processes of defence, the ways in which we behaved, how others behaved towards us, plus the many unconscious processes that may have been involved in them all. This unconscious inner world constantly influences the ways in which we experience ourselves, and the ways in which we think, feel and behave in relation to ourselves and others in our current everyday world. It may also be referred to as reflecting a dynamic unconscious, and its influences may be prompted by experiences that are symbolic of, rather than directly replicating, other relational contexts. Our inner world of object relations will influence us, our lives and our relationships in positive, neutral or unhelpful ways, and will make a major contribution to the nature of our dreams.

Within therapy the nature of the therapeutic context is likely to enhance the role that transference plays in the emotional significance of the therapist for the client, in both positive and negative ways.

The term countertransference refers to the reactions that a person's behaviour elicits in other people, and is generally used to refer to thoughts and feelings that therapists experience in relation to their clients, providing that they are not primarily due to the therapist's own transference. These reactions may be understood in several ways. They may be thought of as examples of the way other people may feel in the clients' everyday lives, when clients behave in certain ways. They can also be understood as a form of unconscious communication from clients, in which aspects of their own hidden feelings are generated in their therapist.

Emotional Containment: How therapists deal with the thoughts and feelings that they experience, and how they respond to their clients is crucial to the process of effective therapy, and in this context the concept of emotional containment is paramount. Psychodynamic therapy provides a place in which it hopefully becomes safe enough for clients to experience hidden painful emotions within themselves, and safe enough for patterns of relating to emerge between themselves and their therapists that may reflect problematic relationship dynamics of the past. In all of these situations, it is important that therapists retain a place within themselves where they can feel, think and reflect on what they are experiencing. A place where difficult feelings are held, processed and understood in relation to the client's psychological context and needs, avoiding automatic responses that may risk putting unhelpful emotions back into the client.

Therapists need to be able to live with, rather than defensively avoid, whatever fear, pain, guilt, anxiety, or anger has come to them before giving back something more containable to the client. We will experience many emotions as therapists in relation to the story of each client's life, as reactions to the emotions they express or those that are hidden, and in relation to the ways they respond to us and who we appear to be for them. Crucial to the capacity of therapists to effectively contain and work with emotion is their own ability to experience a wide range of feelings, to reflect on the origins of those feelings within themselves, to experience empathic connection with others, and to retain the capacity to think, so that the context of their own and the client's experience may be contained by being heard and by being understood. This can apply to intense positive emotions as well as painful ones. Bion believed that the containment of powerful emotions, and the associated reduction of anxiety and arousal was essential to the capacity to think, to link thoughts and ideas within the mind, for them to grow and develop, and for connections to be made between different minds (Bion, 1984).

Corrective Emotional Experience and Re-enactments: Within the developing secure relationship, its unfolding matrices of transference and countertransference, the evolving capacity of clients to speak of themselves and their lives, and the empathic and containing capacity of the therapist, lies the potential for aspects of corrective emotional experience: new and different relational outcomes to echoes of the painful past which have been relived in the present relationship. This may take many forms, but all involve clients experiencing an accepting and developmentally helpful response when a negative, damaging one had been anticipated. It is a corrective emotional experience for a client to find that what they have only known in the past to elicit criticism or dismissal from others, is received with acceptance, care and understanding by their therapist.

Within the sometimes-complex dynamics of the therapeutic relationship particularly significant corrective emotional experiences may be part of a re-enactment of a relational experience. Processes of transference and countertransference may result in the re-living of a significant problematic relational pattern within the therapeutic relationship, with both client and therapist playing their part (Maroda, 1998). For example, the client may respond to their therapist in ways typical of their early responses to a parent, and initially the therapist may respond back in unhelpful ways that are evocative of the parents' responses in that distant past, which will be received by and responded to by the client accordingly. A potentially damaging repeat of the past is underway, but this time in the therapy environment, it is possible for therapists to have the capacity to step back within their own minds and examine what is unfolding. This means that the damaging process may be brought to an end, may be empathically understood, and be thought about in the context of the client's current life and relationships. Containment and understanding may replace damage and shame.

Such enactments bring important aspects of clients' inner worlds of object relations to life within current relational experience, and are most likely to involve the processes of defence, identification, projection and projective identification, transference and countertransference discussed above. Therapists' conscious understanding of what may be happening can be crucial to their capacity to enable such experiences to be resolved in beneficial ways, helping them to curtail potentially damaging processes, put their understanding into words, and acknowledge their own potential contribution. Emotional containment is essential in this context, and when a difficult re-enactment is lived through in a constructive way it may result in a particularly valuable corrective emotional experience.

Parallel Process: Parallel process is a psychodynamic concept that is particularly thought about in the context of the supervisory relationship; a process by which the therapeutic relationship and its associated issues start to influence and be reflected within the supervisory one. This experience may primarily reflect an aspect of the clients' problems, or the therapist's own issues; and it may be influenced by the therapist's identification with the client. It may also involve therapists unconsciously putting their supervisors in the same position in relation to them, as they experience in relation to their clients. Whichever way it evolves, therapy related issues become evident within supervision, with the therapist/supervisee functioning as the connection between the two.

This process may vary in its complexity. It may reflect a relatively straightforward situation in which the supervisor is a neutral observer of some change within the supervisee, a change that comes to be understood as stemming from the supervisee's own issues and/or the nature of their clients' problems. Alternatively, the supervisor may become a mutual part of the process, with both professionals being influenced at an unconscious level by the therapy-related material. In this context the changes within the supervisory relationship may also stem from the supervisors' issues and the potential effects the client has on them at an unconscious level. He or she can be a fully equal participant in the parallel dynamics emerging within supervision. Both relationship dyads may influence each other, potentially to detrimental effect within both of them, until one party, usually within the supervisory dyad, and most often the supervisor becomes consciously aware of what might be happening. When conscious minds become able to appreciate the processes underway, and they can be talked about and understood, significant progress may be made within the supervision and the therapy. Frawley O'Dea and Sarnat (2001) and Morrissey and Tribe (2001) provide discerning perspectives on parallel process.

Analytic Listening: A capacity for analytic listening is crucial to the application of psychodynamic theory within therapy. In order to appreciate the nature of client experience in ways that can be advised by this perspective, it is essential that the process of therapy allows clients to access material in their minds that may not usually be available to conscious awareness. It is also essential that therapists can connect with, think about and respond to that material in empathic, sensitive and meaningful ways. Doing so requires a capacity for attuned connection and imagination, that is able to travel into the realm of the individual, unique and sometimes unwished for possibilities that may be the distressing reality for the client.

We need to be able to listen for both overt and symbolic, unconscious or latent content, relating particularly to the contexts of intra-psychic conflict, defence and transference. Frederickson (1999) provides a particularly accessible and well-structured account of specific aspects of psychodynamic understanding, the nature of listening that will help us to connect with client processes, and ways in which we may respond. Interpretations are offered not imposed; for Frederickson this involves mutual confirmation, rather than an authoritative assumption of validity on the part of the therapist.

Psychological Development: Psychodynamic theory pays considerable attention to processes of psychological development, being particularly addressed from post-Freudian positions by object relations and self-psychology theorists. It is the self in the context of nurturing relationships that lies at the heart of development, rather than the drive-related and psychosexual processes of traditional Freudian theory. The nature and quality of early relationships with primary care givers are thought about in depth, from birth onwards, in terms of their influence on the development of self. The crucial importance of early relationships characterized by sensitive attunement, responsiveness to infants' ways of being and their emotional and physical needs, containment of anxiety and powerful feeling, and the optimal experience of difference and limits, are reflected in the work of theorists such as Donald Winnicott within the object relations school (Winnicott, 1971/1974,

1986, 1965/1990) and Heinz Kohut (Kohut, 1977, 1984) from a self-psychology standpoint.

Secure development of a self that can be sure of its existence, survive in the world of emotions, be psychologically separate from other selves, and carry forward into later childhood and adulthood a secure sense of intrinsic worth, is deemed to depend on such a relationship. Similarly, from a life span development perspective Erikson (1980) describes the importance of gaining a psychological foundation of basic trust from an emotionally and physically secure environment in the early months of life.

Winnicott uses the term true self to refer to that self we naturally have the potential to become, as opposed to the false self, a distortion of that potential, which could evolve as a defensive protection, enabling us to survive childhood experiences that failed to provide a good enough maturational environment (Winnicott, 1986). Some difference of emphasis exists between Klein and other object relations theorists regarding the importance of innate factors within the infant rather than the nature and quality of care. For example, Klein considers the experience of intense anger and rage within the infant to be ubiquitous and of genetic origin, rather than the possible result of problematic experience within the infant-parent relationship.

The path of psychological development over time from infancy onwards is also reflected in several further fundamental respects: the development of defences from early immature/primitive defences to later mature defences, as discussed by Vaillant (1971); the path from early infant symbiotic closeness with a primary care giver, to the parallel pathways of psychological separation and individuation as elaborated by Mahler et al. (1975); and the pathway through stages of psychological development across the life span from infancy to old age described by Erikson (1980).

The overall outcome of development is reflected in the concept of ego strength. The secure, integrated and cohesive development of the self leads to high ego strength: a range of adult personality characteristics that includes the capacity to develop and maintain constructive relationships with others in intimate, social and work contexts and to cope with strongly felt emotions. Developmental experiences that have failed to meet the needs of the infant and child and may also have been characterized by trauma and abuse, will result in varying degrees of low ego strength, involving problematic relationships and difficulty coping with intense emotion. In discussing these consequences of early developmental failures, Balint elaborates on his concept of the basic fault (Balint, 1968), which in essence describes the damaging consequences of an environment that has not enabled Erikson's concept of basic trust to become established.

Balint and Erikson both attribute great importance to very early attuned relating, and the consequences of its fundament failure, which results in damage to the core basis of self on which all further psychological development is founded. For Winnicott early empathic connection and mirroring is also fundamentally important in conferring a core essence of secure existence, and is conveyed in his very simple but powerful words, "when I look I am seen, so I exist" (Winnicott, 1971/1974, p.134).

Kohut (1977, 1984) also recognizes the central importance of empathic mirroring, associating it within the overall capacity for care-givers to act as primary selfobjects for their infants and children, those people who accept, love, see, hear, validate, joyously celebrate, and emotionally contain them. He gives an absolutely core developmental place to the self-selfobject relationship, and recognizes its importance throughout the lifespan. Overall, Kohut sees adverse experiences in childhood as resulting in developmental arrest which carries with it the positive potential that having become arrested, development may later be given the opportunity to resume a more constructive path. This relates to Freud's original belief that individuals could become stuck or fixated as a result of difficult experiences at different stages of development.

In addition to recognizing the importance of mirroring, Kohut also emphasizes the essential experience of optimal frustration in which a child's need or wish is not responded to immediately or perfectly, but with some delay or disappointing imperfection. Frustration needs to be significant and felt, but not traumatic and damaging. Its experience conveys the separateness between the child and its caregiver, and the difference between an inner wish and the existence of external reality. It also enables the development of realistic rather than idealized self and selfobject representations. These processes are necessary to the development of a secure and boundaried sense of self as separate from others, and of a mind that is separate from others' minds; they all relate to Freud's original concept of the reality principle.

In understanding the origins of parents' difficulties in providing loving emotionally-attuned care, and in containing their children's anxieties and powerful emotions, psychodynamic theory recognizes that parents may not have received developmentally needed love and care themselves. The emotional and psychological needs of childhood will still live on within them as adults, and they may struggle to provide what their own children need, as damage carries from one generation to another: a theme so powerfully echoed in Philip Larkin's poem *This Be The Verse,* Larkin (1974).

Intra-psychic and Interpersonal Boundaries: Boundaries define where one thing stops and another starts, crucially marking the existence of separateness. They also hold matter in place, retaining structure and preventing chaos. An example from the physical world illustrates this - if the boundary provided by the glass containing water becomes broken, it goes all over the place. This is a very simple metaphor, but one that may quite graphically describe the psychological consequences when intra-psychic and interpersonal boundaries become compromised. One of the defining characteristics of psychodynamic theory and practice is the attention it pays to boundary-related issues. It is particularly the intra-psychic psychological boundary between self and other that concerns psychodynamic theory. This boundary is seen as playing a crucial part in the security of the self, needing a balance between strength and permeability, so that our own minds may function without undue influence by the minds of others, yet be able to connect with experiences other than our own.

Thought is given throughout theory to the developmental experiences and therapy practices that may weaken or strengthen such boundaries, and to potential ways of understanding the complex processes that may evolve when boundaries between ourselves and others become weakened. The experience of problematic aspects of countertransference for therapists, difficulties in relation to emotional containment, and difficulties with the practical boundaries of time and place may in part relate to and also influence the nature of the intra-psychic boundary between self and other within the therapeutic relationship. The maintenance of needed and appropriate interpersonal boundaries in our relationships with others, including the therapeutic relationship, may well be harder to maintain when the intra-psychic boundary of self is compromised. The two relate crucially to each other.

The Therapeutic Relationship: In many ways the therapeutic relationship sits at the heart of psychodynamic theory and therapy, and this has been increasingly the case with the more recent evolution of relational models of psychodynamic work (DeYoung, 2015). It is a relationship that always reflects a subtle mix of managed structure and interaction alongside the human reality of two people relating to each other. To the extent that it is a managed relationship, it is managed and structured in ways that relate to theory. Whatever unfolds within that relationship is then available to be thought about and understood between therapist and client, and may lead to greater awareness of clients' everyday psychological functioning, to their experience of a growth promoting psychological and emotional environment, and to their capacity to change. Managing the therapeutic relationship in psychodynamic work relates strongly to the issues of boundaries, in terms of time, place and nature of relationship. The existence of boundaries and limits within our everyday world is powerfully represented by the time boundary of the therapy session, which tends to be firmly held within psychodynamic therapy, and given serious thought if it is not. The psychological impact of this boundary is then available for unique understanding, and may automatically contribute to the development of a more secure and separate self.

The Therapeutic Frame: Within psychodynamic theory the general term therapeutic frame refers to aspects of practical and relational structure that influence and frame the environment within which the therapeutic relationship develops and change processes evolve.

The practical and emotional security of the therapeutic space is recognized as crucially important to psychodynamic therapy process, and is addressed in structural terms by attention to the nature of the furniture and fittings of the therapy room, as far as these can be controlled, and particularly to the security and reliability of time, place, privacy and confidentiality.

Other aspects of the therapeutic frame relate to the nature of relationship between therapist and client, and the limits and boundaries between what is talked about within this relationship and what is not. The belief that the therapist should, or could ever be a blank screen reflecting the inner workings of their clients' minds which have simply been projected onto it, with no contribution made by the nature of the relationship, has largely been abandoned. However, the principle of relative neutrality still remains important and central to psychodynamic therapy practice. Therapists remain relatively unknown to clients regarding their personal lives, and in the extent to which they may choose to explain their thoughts and actions.

This ensures a middle ground, a space for the therapist to think and reflect on what may be happening in the client's mind, and what may be happening between the two of them. Here understanding may be formulated that sheds light on the inner life and everyday experiences of the client, in the context of their past and present, that may support growth and the processes of change. A clear distinction is made between the professional role of the therapist in relation to the client, and any other types of relating. The understanding and empathy that the therapist may bring to these encounters, the limits of relationship and the reliability of time, place and environment may all contribute to enough safety and security on both sides for the most difficult and distressing aspects of client psychological and emotional experience to emerge between them. As discussed above, this can involve re-enactments of the dynamics of past interpersonal contexts, and the essence of relational psychodynamic therapy lies in the therapist being able to allow themselves to become part of such re-enactment, but also able to then sit outside of that process, understand what may have been happening, and to share and develop that understanding with their client.

A Simplified Psychodynamic Rationale for Change: The diagrams in Figures 3 and 4 provide flow charts of the consequences of problematic experiences in childhood, and the potential change processes within therapy that constitute a simplified and generalized psychodynamic rationale for change. The evolution of psychological problems will commonly involve far greater individual complexity than can be represented here, and the changes that may take place during therapy will be influenced by the unique nature of each client's childhood experience, the complexity of the problems that have developed, the evolving therapeutic relationship, and the intensity, depth and duration of therapy. The choices therapists make in relation to their therapy approach, and the schools of psychodynamic and analytic theory that advise their work, will influence the nature of the therapeutic relationship, the processes of therapy and the nature of change within clients at conscious and unconscious levels. The overall experience of therapy will also be affected by the frequency of sessions and whether it is brief and time limited, or long term and maybe open ended.

From a psychodynamic perspective, childhood experiences crucially influence the development of the psychological self and the ways in which our minds function at conscious and unconscious levels, affecting our emotional reactions, thoughts and feelings, our defences, our unconscious inner worlds of object relations,

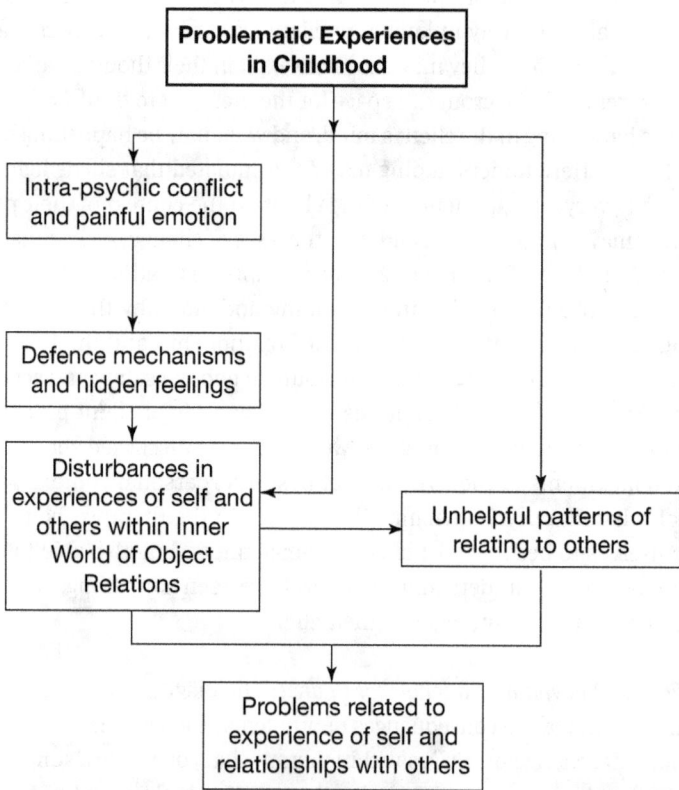

Figure 3 A Simplified Psychodynamic Rationale for Change: The Origin of Psychological Difficulties

and the ways in which we relate to ourselves and others. Within the attuned relationship, emotional security, containment, exploration and understanding that therapy may provide, aspects of our self-experience may become more known to us and have the opportunity to develop and grow.

The intra-psychic conflicts underlying our defences may become apparent, be survived and their power diffused; the unhelpful relational patterns that unfold between ourselves and others may be recognized and understood, and our inner world of object relations may change for the better. Our thoughts, feelings and behaviours in relation to ourselves and others may be enabled to change, helping us to live our lives more easily, with greater fulfilment, and with less discord and greater satisfaction in our relationships with others.

The therapeutic relationship sits at the heart of all the above processes, and for Kohut (1977, 1984) it provides the essential component that moves us

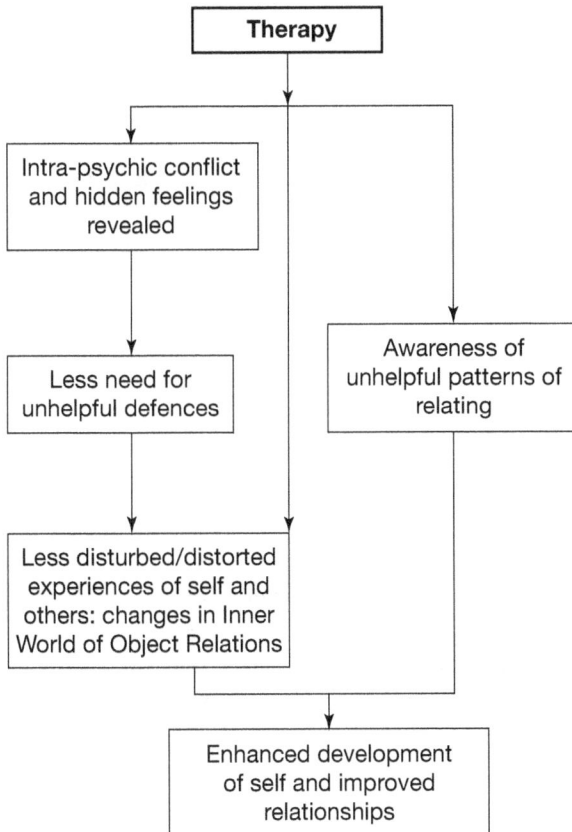

Figure 4 A Simplified Psychodynamic Rationale for Change: The Impact of Therapy

past developmental arrest, towards a secure and less damaged self through the experience of a new self-selfobject relationship.

The practice of psychodynamic therapy exists across a spectrum of brief, often time-limited therapy or counselling to long term and sometimes open ended psychodynamic or psychoanalytic psychotherapy or psychoanalysis. Across this spectrum, frequency of sessions will vary from usually not less than once a week for brief therapy, to a maximum of five times a week for full psychoanalysis. In some instances, the experience of therapy may involve a long term emotionally committed developmental relationship. This context may sometimes be needed when the nature of early trauma has resulted in particularly vulnerable aspects of self, strongly damaging inner worlds of object relations, powerful developmentally early defences and maybe significant aspects of dissociation.

In briefer and time-limited approaches to psychodynamic therapy, the existing security of self-development will be sufficient for developmental gains to be made within a shorter-term relationship and for the relatively more accessible aspects of conscious and unconscious experience to be explored and understood together.

Whatever path is taken within brief or longer-term therapy, the changes that evolve will reflect changes in the functioning of psychological defences, in the experience of feelings and emotions, in the perception of self and others, and changes in unhelpful patterns of relating. All of these changes will fundamentally involve changes within our unconscious inner world of object relations.

Summary

In Chapter 8 we have defined and discussed a wide range of psycho-dynamic concepts, mechanisms and processes associated with the functioning of conscious and unconscious mind, the core relevance of emotion, and the fundamental importance of human relating. We have also considered psychodynamic approaches to human development, the central importance of the therapeutic relationship, and the related value of re-enactments and repeated relational patterns. Finally, we looked at a simplified psychodynamic rationale for change. Content has reflected both psychodynamic and psychoanalytic theory and different schools of thought have not been particularly differentiated.

Cognitive and Behavioural Theory

9

Cognitive behaviour therapy, CBT, is the general umbrella term used to refer to those therapies that particularly address conscious cognitive processes and behaviour. Therapies involving a primary focus on conscious thoughts, attitudes and beliefs usually include direct attention to behaviour as well; and over the past forty years cognitive behaviour therapy has come to include an increasing number of interventions that have their primary origins in behaviourism. This chapter will look at the core principles of those cognitive behaviour therapies that are led by a primary focus on cognition and Chapter 10 will overview the core principles of those that have been developed primarily from a behavioural perspective.

A recognition of the limitations of earlier behavioural approaches in the treatment of depression, and a primary focus on cognition rather than on behaviour or unconscious processes, led what has been referred to as the cognitive revolution and in particular Aaron Beck's development of cognitive therapy for depression (Beck et al.,1979; Hawton et al., 1989; Joseph, 2010).

This chapter will consider the theory and practice of traditional cognitive therapy and CBT (Beck et al., 1979; J. Beck, 2011; Curwen et al., 2018; Greenberger & Padesky, 2015; Kennerley et al., 2016; Sanders & Wills, 2005). It will also look at the importance of damaging core beliefs and early maladaptive schemas (Young, 1990); the relevance of unconscious processes and cognitive-interpersonal cycles (Safran,1998); Constructivist Psychotherapy with its emphasis on developmental experiences and the importance of personal meaning (Guidano, 1991; Mahoney, 2003; Neimeyer, 2009); Mindfulness Based Cognitive Therapy influenced by the Buddhist practice of meditation (Segal et al., 2002); and Compassion Focused Therapy (Gilbert, 2010).

Traditional Cognitive Therapy and CBT

From a traditional cognitive therapy perspective, it is conscious cognition that is seen as the primary factor affecting human well-being versus distress. Our thoughts, beliefs and attitudes influence how we feel and how we behave, and in turn our feelings and the consequences of our behaviours influence our thoughts and beliefs, creating generative cycles that maintain or maybe escalate existing cognitive, behavioural and interpersonal patterns, or change them.

Thoughts are very powerful things and the essence of cognitive therapy was established when Aaron Beck focused on the relationship between the thoughts of depressed people and their depressed mood. Such thoughts involve negative content in relation to our views of ourselves, the future and the world around us; they are often just outside our immediate conscious awareness, and are known as negative automatic thoughts or NATs. The nature of these thoughts is influenced by the underlying beliefs that we hold about ourselves and others, and at the heart of the multitude of such beliefs about our everyday experience are deemed to lie relatively few fundamental or core beliefs, longstanding, deep and often rigid cognitive structures. Core beliefs automatically and powerfully shape the ways in which we interpret things that happen to us, and the meaning that we attach to our experiences. All will affect our thoughts, the ways we feel and what we do.

Cognitive therapy also draws on the cognitive science concept of schemas (Bartlett, 1932) to help conceptualize the ways in which people make sense of and interpret what happens in their lives, on a moment-to-moment, and day-to-day basis. Schemas are deemed to be unconscious memory structures, involving constellations of knowledge, beliefs and assumptions about the nature of specific phenomena such as our self, other people, and aspects of the world around us. They organize information about past experiences and guide the processing of new information (Safran,1998). Schemas and associated beliefs develop throughout our lives and are influenced by the nature of our experiences, being particularly affected by what happens to us in childhood. Together with resultant beliefs and automatic thoughts, schemas are seen as the cognitive conduit of the adverse psychological effects of damaging environments.

Theoretical distinctions are made between thoughts, conditional/intermediate beliefs (attitudes, assumptions and rules for living that often function on an 'if ... then' basis), and underlying unconditional core beliefs and schemas that function as basic truths (Curwen et al., 2018; Sanders & Wills, 2005). Beck (1999) sees core beliefs as fundamental beliefs about self and others that result from the existence of particular schemas, with negative core beliefs falling into the three categories of helplessness, unlovability and worthlessness.

A central aspect of cognitive therapy theory lies in the belief that unhelpful negative automatic thoughts are most likely to represent a distorted perception of reality. This is particularly argued by Beck in his early work on depression (Beck et al., 1979), where they are defined as thinking errors, and are seen as the dysfunctional consequence of the state of depression that also serve to maintain it. These automatic thoughts reflect negative beliefs about the self, the world we live in, and the future, which persist at least in part through our natural tendency to attend to aspects of our experience that are consistent with existing beliefs, and not to notice, or take into account, experience that contradicts them.

Life experiences, particularly any that are difficult or challenging, are responded to through the lens of these distortions or biases. Our conscious cognitive responses to bodily and physiological experiences can be influenced in the same way. We may overestimate the difficulty or sense of threat that an experience or situation poses for us, and/or underestimate our capacity to deal with it, as well as falling prey to a myriad of beliefs and negative thoughts about others and ourselves. The aim of CBT is to alter unhelpful distorted conscious thinking and enable people to adopt more realistic, adaptive and flexible perspectives. Categories of typical distortions or cognitive biases may be described, such as extreme thinking, selective attention, relying on intuition, and self-reproach (J. Beck, 2011; Kennerley et al., 2016). Work within therapy seeks to address individual patterns of unhelpful thoughts and to pay attention to the life experiences that may have influenced them. It is commonly recognized that thoughts and feelings exist in mutual two-way interaction with each other, with feelings influencing thoughts just as much as thoughts influence feelings.

Therapy aims to involve a collaborative relationship between therapist and client, that is characterized by therapist warmth, genuineness and empathy (Beck et al., 1979; Kennerley et al., 2016). It is described as generally brief, structured, psychoeducational, empirical and parsimonious with an emphasis on minimal intervention, starting at the level of symptoms and automatic thoughts, and moving on to work with underlying beliefs and their origins if this is needed. It is also recognized that thoughts themselves often directly express underlying conditional/intermediate beliefs and sometimes core beliefs, in which case the latter are automatically being dealt with at the same time (Sanders & Wills, 2005).

A core characteristic of cognitive therapy and CBT is the use of explicit case conceptualizations or formulations that are shared with clients and function as a central component of therapy. Cognitive behavioural formulations often involve a diagrammatic picture of the relationship between the client's thoughts, feelings and behaviours that clarifies the ways in which unhelpful symptoms are generated and maintained. They may also include bodily experiences and physiological reactions, and if deemed useful will address the core beliefs that underlie the client's automatic thoughts, and the early experiences connected with those beliefs (J. Beck, 2011; Blackburn & Twaddle, 2011; Kennerley et al., 2016; Persons, 1989; Sanders & Wills, 2005). They may be based on a standard diagrammatic structure, or reflect a structure that evolves in relation to the client's particular circumstances and history. Formulations are often generated by therapists and are then shared, confirmed and/or modified in collaborative discussion with clients. They make sense of the person's difficulties in cognitive behavioural terms, and provide hypotheses that may be tested out during the process of therapy. Simple symptom related cognitive conceptualizations may be used at the start of intervention, followed later by formulations that address the nature and origins of core beliefs (Sanders & Wills, 2005). At the end of an initial assessment period formulations contribute to the decision to undertake therapy or not, and support the development of an initial plan for intervention, which may include a problem list and related individualized goals for therapy, if this is deemed to be helpful.

A clear characteristic of CBT is its open and explicit nature. The basic theory behind the model and what may be expected to happen during therapy is described to the client in straight-forward terms, and discussion of client feedback about their experience of the therapist and the therapy is recommended on a regular basis. Assessment involves a structured discussion of current difficulties that includes the nature and severity of symptoms; key cognitive, behavioural, physiological, emotional and environmental aspects of the problem; its history including how it started, what keeps it going and the potential roles of life events and stresses; the family, work and relational context of clients' lives; and clients' developmental history and general health issues (Kennerley et al., 2016; Sanders & Wills, 2005).

Attention is also given to assessing the client's suitability for cognitive therapy, looking at factors such as the appropriateness of the cognitive model to their situation and the sense that it makes to them, their ability to access and differentiate their thoughts and feelings, their ability to take responsibility for change, their optimism/pessimism about therapy, and the strength of factors that may interfere with progress such as their degree of avoidance or unhelpful intellectualization (Curwen et al., 2018: Sanders & Wills, 2005). Standardized symptom measures such as the Beck Depression Inventory, BDI (Beck et al., 1961) and the Brief Symptom Inventory, BSI (Derogatis & Melisaratos, 1983) are often used pre and post therapy, and sometimes on a session by session basis. Simple personalized measures based on specific aspects of client problems or overall perceptions of well-being may also be used to help monitor change processes.

Therapy generally adopts a time-limited and brief approach and sessions usually proceed on the basis of an overt agenda agreed between therapist and client at the start of each session. The extent to which therapy adopts a clear, focused and predefined structure may vary depending on the degree to which the therapist is following a manualized protocol-led version of CBT, or implementing a rather more flexible application of cognitive behavioural theory. Homework in the form of therapeutic tasks is usually a part of therapy, with the activity being discussed and agreed between therapist and client based on the content of the current session and focus of therapeutic work, so that active work on the process of change takes place within the everyday world.

The identification of feelings and thoughts is fundamental within CBT, and diaries are often powerful tools in this respect. Emotions may be the initial focus of record keeping, enabling clients to become more aware of them and find words to describe and label them, followed by the identification of the thoughts that they are automatically associated with (Greenberger & Padesky, 2015; Kennerley et al., 2016). Diaries record the strength of the conscious beliefs that these thoughts reflect and the strength of the feelings associated with them, also noting the situations that prompt them and what happens subsequently.

Once clients are able to record their feelings and thoughts, the therapist's task is to enable an empathic and non-judgmental approach towards exploring the client's way of thinking. It is in these respects that cognitive behavioural therapy involves a process of collaborative empiricism, drawing on the value of rational and logical thinking to appraise, challenge and hopefully change unhelpful cognitions that have been observed and recorded in the everyday world (Beck et al., 1979; J. Beck, 2011; Curwen et al., 2018; Greenberger & Padesky, 2015; Kennerley et al., 2016; Sanders & Wills, 2005). It is hot cognitions, associated with strong difficult or uncomfortable feelings and emotions, that are seen as particularly likely to be associated with understandable but unhelpful cognitive distortions or biases. Appraisal and cognitive challenge may be facilitated by looking at the origins of these biases, their pros and cons, and the evidence for and against them, leading to the generation of new perspectives, new conclusions and more balanced views. This process may be supported by the use of imagery and role play, and generally adopts a Socratic approach to enquiry in which the use of Socratic questions prompts clients to think in particular directions and make helpful realizations for themselves (Kennerley et al., 2016). Diary records and discussions of thoughts, beliefs and evidence are often supplemented by behavioural experiments that seek to actively test out the basis of a client's conditional beliefs and assumptions.

Sanders and Wills (2005) describe an approach towards cognitive distortions or biases in which distortion is emphasized as a possibility not an assumption. Exploration, Socratic enquiry and guided discovery are used on an overtly neutral basis to open up the realities of clients' lives and deepen the ways in which they are known and understood. Pictures of who they are and the nature of the other people in their lives may then emerge that are available for comparison with their automatic thoughts and beliefs about themselves and others. The evidence from this broader view may be consistent with their negative perspectives or run counter to them. Sanders and Wills recommend that evidence in support of negative thoughts be investigated first to reduce the likelihood of clients resisting a perceived overt pressure to think differently.

Whilst thought diaries and the modification of cognitive distortions will be helpful in many instances this will not always be the case, especially in contexts where the negativity and threat of life circumstances are consistent with clients' thoughts and beliefs. In these instances, a cognitive approach needs to accept the reality of those life circumstances and take a more functional and pragmatic approach to the role of helpful and unhelpful thinking in terms of coping with real-world situations. Certain changes in cognition may help to support the ways in which people can cope with adverse realities, and clients may be helped to change their thinking on that basis.

The cognitive and behavioural therapies also draw on behavioural methods when they are seen as appropriate in relation to client needs. Such methods can include activity scheduling to support clients in increasing their daily activities and their experiences of enjoyment and achievement; problem solving; fear reduction methods such as graded exposure/systematic desensitization and modelling; relaxation techniques to reduce tension and anxiety; and distraction as a strategy to reduce a focus on depressive thinking, or to reduce attention to anxiety related experiences. It is important to ensure that these methods do not inadvertently become used as safety behaviours which clients adopt in the belief that feared consequences will be prevented, thus strengthening the cognitive basis of their anxiety or depression and preventing the disconfirmation of associated unhelpful beliefs.

A Focus on Unhelpful Core Beliefs and Maladaptive Schemas

Cognitive behavioural therapy techniques have been developed to focus on conditional assumptions and rules for living, and to move beyond them to address the deeper levels of unconditional core beliefs associated with underlying schemas overall, and particularly the early maladaptive schemas that are assumed to be associated with problematic personality development and related problems. Core beliefs are intrinsic and familiar parts of the person we know ourselves to be, and a non-judgmental, guided discovery perspective is particularly important in this context.

Conditional assumptions and rules for living may be explored by using the questioning style of the downward arrow technique (Burns, 1980; Kennerley et al., 2016; Greenberger & Padesky, 2015) and by exploring the meaning of client imagery associated with difficult aspects of life experience. In the downward arrow process the client is repeatedly asked what they fear happening, and what that would that mean to them until the base-line negative assumption or belief underlying the initial conditional assumption or rule for living is identified.

Base-line assumptions and beliefs can then be addressed in similar ways to negative thoughts, by looking at evidence for and against their value and validity, by Socratic enquiry and through behavioural experiments. The generation of new and more helpful rules may then be supported (Curwen et al., 2018; Kennerley et al., 2016; Padesky, 1994; Mooney & Padesky, 2000). Sometimes realizing the existence of a rule and its related assumption for the first time may be enough for it to lose its power, and the same may be the case for underlying core beliefs. This may particularly be the situation when clients have previously experienced reasonably good psychological functioning, and when connections have been made between assumptions and beliefs and the impact of past adverse experience (Sanders & Wills, 2005).

Core beliefs will often emerge as clients naturally talk about their life and childhood experiences and express the beliefs they hold about themselves and their lives. It is a specific decision whether such beliefs are actively addressed within CBT, and some authors such as Blackburn and Davidson (1995) see this work as relatively infrequent on a routine basis, with most CBT taking place at the level of automatic thoughts and rules for living.

Similarly, Sanders and Wills (2005) consider that direct and active work on core beliefs need not be involved in CBT unless they predispose the client to relapse, or are associated with marked personality disturbance. In keeping with the collaborative transparency of cognitive behavioural approaches, they recommend explicit discussion between therapist and client regarding decisions to directly address core beliefs and/or early unhelpful schemas in these ways. Core beliefs are a central part of who we know ourselves to be; they may sometimes be held with particular rigidity and be very resistant to change, and particularly damaging ones may also be strongly related to trauma and emotional deprivation in childhood.

Core beliefs and schemas identified within therapy can be incorporated in the overall formulation of client difficulties. If they are addressed, therapeutic work towards reducing their impact and modifying them involves a range of techniques including positive diaries to support the recognition of aspects of experience that run counter to them; continua work where a belief is defined on the basis of a continuum from one extreme to the other, so that the concept or personal characteristic involved may be explored in more refined and realistic ways; and the use of schema flashcards in schema therapy, which provide the client with on the spot reminders of alternative more positive and realistic schema related beliefs. The exploration of their early origins, and the use of active interventions such as role play, may also support these processes of change (J. Beck, 2011; Curwen et al., 2018; Kennerley et al., 2016).

Schema Therapy (Rafaeli et al., 2011; Young, 1990; Young & Klosko, 1993; Young et al., 2003) addresses the early maladaptive schemas and problematic behaviours associated with personality related problems, such as Borderline

Personality Disorder, BPD, resulting from psychologically damaging and traumatic developmental environments, and unmet core emotional needs. Young et al. (2003) identify different modes of behaving and coping that have potentially unconscious, and maybe dissociated origins within the self. Each mode of behaving is associated with dominant emotional states, underlying schemas and coping reactions. Three of these represent the ongoing internal psychological existence of a damaged child: the Vulnerable Child (the wounded core of the self), the Angry Child, and the Impulsive Child. Three adult maladaptive coping modes are defined: the Detached Protector, the Compliant Surrenderer, and the Overcompensator, plus two internalized parent modes, the Punitive Parent and the Demanding or Critical Parent. In reflection of healthy functioning, two further modes are provided: the Contented Child, and the Healthy Adult.

Eighteen typical early maladaptive schemas are defined in five general domains relating to disconnection and rejection; impaired autonomy and performance; impaired limits; other directedness; and over-vigilance and inhibition. Interview, self-report inventories, guided imagery, self-monitoring of events, thoughts, feelings and behaviours, and the observation of schema driven relational patterns in the therapeutic relationship may all be used to assess dysfunctional life patterns and predominant modes of being, their associated maladaptive schemas and the origins of those schemas. Assessment culminates in a written schema-based case conceptualization, developed collaboratively with the client in a way that carries both emotional meaning and intellectual understanding. This conceptualization includes the developmental origins of problems; unmet core needs; predominant modes and schemas and their triggers; core cognitions and distortions; and the goals and focus for change (Rafaeli et al., 2011).

The process of working towards these goals draws on a range of cognitive and behavioural strategies. Cognitive strategies include reframing and reattribution; schema flashcards providing summaries of healthy cognitive responses to schema triggers; the use of diaries; and schema dialogues in which the evidence in support of or against the validity of a schema is enacted as a dialogue between the schema-based mode of the client and the healthy adult mode. Behavioural strategies include schema flashcards providing instructions for alternative behaviours, and rehearsal of those behaviours; behavioural homework; client self-reward for healthy behaviours; and the withdrawal of sessions in the face of consistent and problematic lack of behaviour change.

The theoretical basis and practical application of Schema Therapy also explicitly includes concepts and processes from a range of therapeutic approaches beyond the cognitive and behavioural, including attachment and object relations theories and the experiential therapies.

Attention to Unconscious Processes and Cognitive-Interpersonal Cycles

In all of the above descriptions of cognitive behaviour therapy, client and therapist work together as observers of the client's conscious cognitive and emotional processes, and use a range of structured techniques and methods to actively engender helpful changes in conscious cognition and behaviour, and potential change in underlying schemas. Safran (1998) challenged this emphasis on conscious cognition and sought to expand the realm of cognitive therapy to include a recognition of the importance of pre-conscious, unconscious and associative processes. He also sought to apply that recognition to a consideration of the interpersonal context of cognitive functioning, the role of emotion in the motivation of human behaviour, and the ways in which the unfolding nature of the therapeutic relationship may be utilized from a cognitive therapy perspective.

Safran takes as his starting point the approach to interpersonal psychoanalysis proposed by Harry Stack Sullivan, largely because the nature of Sullivan's thinking and writing appear consistent with concepts within cognitive therapy theory (Sullivan, 1953). Safran (1998) believes that the capacity for cognitive therapy to influence beneficial change would be increased if it took Sullivan's concepts into account.

The key point of overlap between Sullivan's work and cognitive therapy is deemed to lie in his concept of personification. A personification is an unconscious mental representation of the self, consistent with the cognitive concept of a self-schema, which has the capacity to unhelpfully distort perceptions of self and others. Sullivan proposes three broad categories of personification in relation to the nature of the self and to self-esteem, *good-me*, *bad-me*, and *not-me*. He also describes the way in which he sees these personifications as being protected from any events that may challenge them, with the anxiety associated with such events prompting the functioning of security operations. These processes distort how such events are experienced, or exclude them from conscious awareness. In particular, internal emotions may not be fully processed. Events that remain outside of awareness and emotions that are not fully processed adversely affect the personal and interpersonal functioning of the individual. Various self-protective processes may result from the functioning of security operations including the avoidance of interpersonal situations, processes of dissociation, the transformation of anxiety into other emotions, and blaming others or putting them down in order to enhance self-esteem.

When such security operations are prompted by adverse early experiences with parents and/or other caregivers at the very early stages of schema/ personification development this can result in considerable disruption of developmental processes, particularly in relation to the synthesis of emotional experience. When it has not been possible for appropriate and needed synthesis to take place, this can lead to a later tendency to experience primitive, explosive, age inappropriate emotion and behaviour in adulthood (Safran, 1998; Sullivan, 1953). Sullivan sees healthy development and good adjustment as being associated with flexible personifications of self and others and poor adjustment with more rigid personifications, and very tight distinctions between *me* and *not-me*.

At the interpersonal level Sullivan sees interactions between individuals as being influenced by the personifications and associated security operations of each person involved, with the power of these personifications potentially leading to the evolution of damaging and self-perpetuating characteristic patterns or dynamisms between self and others. Safran draws on this position in proposing that enduring interpersonal cognitive-affective schemas involving cognitions linked to powerful emotions, and influenced by security operations, similarly lead to repeated dysfunctional cognitive-interpersonal cycles, and problematic relational patterns. These cyclical patterns involve generalized representations of self-other relationships which developed during childhood and functioned adaptively at that time to maintain relatedness to parents and/or caregivers under potentially dire emotional circumstances (Safran, 1998; Scarvalone et al., 2005).

From the basis of Sullivan's theoretical position, Safran argues for a widening of cognitive therapy theory and practice to include recognition of the central role played by emotion in the development and maintenance of psychological problems; the unconscious processing of emotion and cognition; and attention to the cognitive-interpersonal cycles that unfold within everyday lives and the therapeutic relationship.

As potentially unhelpful/dysfunctional patterns of interpersonal behaviour emerge between therapist and client, therapists are encouraged to be aware of their reactions and behaviours and actively endeavour not to repeat the complementary responses a client might have experienced in the past (Marcotte & Safran, 2002). In a context of sensitivity and acceptance, the nature of the interpersonal cycle is discussed with the client, looking at their feelings and cognitions during the experience. The cyclical aspects of the patterns are clarified, their connection with similar patterns in the client's everyday life, and the ways in which the processes feed back into maintaining the underlying cognitive-affective schema. Cognitions associated with damaging self-schemas are actively challenged and direct efforts made to support behaviour change within sessions and by setting related homework tasks. The opportunity to experience schema inconsistent responses from another person is seen as central to the process of developing new cognitive-interpersonal schemas, and new models of self-other interaction.

In addition, previously avoided primary adaptive emotions may now be felt and lived with and their associated memories explored and understood. These experiences, plus the active development of alternative cognitive structures and behaviours, all contribute to the evolution of new cognitive-interpersonal schemas which support healthier and more constructive relationships with self and others.

Constructivist Psychotherapy

Constructivist psychotherapy is a further member of the broad-based family of cognitive behavioural therapies which have their theoretical base articulated primarily within cognitive theory (Guidano, 1991; Mahoney, 2003; Neimeyer, 2009; Neimeyer & Mahoney, 1995). In contrast to the structured and focused attention paid to specific thoughts, attitudes and beliefs within cognitive therapy and traditional CBT, constructivist psychotherapy is a more process oriented, collaborative and developmental approach in which personal meaning holds centre stage. Influenced by Personal Construct Theory (Kelly, 1963), it sees our beliefs about ourselves, other people and the world we inhabit as reflecting our own individual ways of making sense of and interpreting our observations and experiences from childhood onwards. We make our own human constructions of reality, and feel, think and behave accordingly. Early developmental experiences in childhood may have led to constructions of reality/life narratives and processes of meaning-making that were useful in guiding life within problematic childhood social worlds, but may later lose their utility and prove unhelpful in adult life.

Constructivist psychotherapy argues that symptoms fulfil a function in the life of the individual, and are related to unconscious underlying emotional truths, which make it necessary for them to be maintained in spite of the suffering they may cause. This is termed the pro-symptom position, which is seen as involving unconscious self-protective processes and identifications, as well as issues related to self-esteem.

Therapy seeks to build an empathic encounter and connection between therapist and client supporting their collaborative exploration of the ways in which clients perceive and construe themselves, their own identities and their relationships in the context of their unique social worlds. Laddering can be used to help identify constructs associated with core concerns, drawing on methodology from personal construct theory. Clients are asked to identify a significant bi-polar construct, followed by repeated questioning about the pole that they prefer to be associated with, why it is important to them and what advantages it has. The nature of emotionally significant past and present life experience is explored, so that important and recurring relational themes may be identified. Therapy is recognized as a developmentally important and reparative experience with the potential for secondary emotions to give way to underlying primary ones and their often-powerful meanings and sense of emotional truth.

Overall, this is a facilitative therapeutic approach seen as enabling clients' innate potential for growth and development, rather than being reliant on therapist prescriptions for change.

Mindfulness-Based Cognitive Therapy

Mindfulness-Based Cognitive Therapy (Crane, 2009; Segal et al., 2002) draws on the Buddhist principles of acceptance, compassion towards ourselves and our capacity to experience a deep connection with the present moment whatever it involves. Clients are enabled to step back from their automatic and potentially unhelpful reactions to the context of their lives. Calmly living and feeling in the moment is seen as removing a source of suffering. From a Buddhist perspective, suffering is associated with the wish for reality to be other than it is, and in this way adds to existing difficulty and pain. Accepting current reality removes that pressure and sense of constant dissatisfaction, and the compassionate acceptance of ourselves as we are takes away the punishment and criticism we can so often dole out to ourselves. This does not mean that we might not also decide to do things that we know may help our situation improve, if it is feasible to do so, but it does mean that action is undertaken from a very different starting point. It also involves the potential capacity to accept and live the best we can with things that cannot be changed.

Defensive strategies may gradually and naturally become less needed and dissolve, with painful hidden experience becoming known and felt, held within our own acceptance, compassion and understanding (Crane, 2009). Acceptance may then become the cognitive and emotional base from which change naturally evolves, as the unhelpful impact of stress, resistance and tension are eased.

Compassion Focused Therapy

The final therapeutic approach to be discussed as part of this review of cognitive and behavioural theory, is Compassion Focused Therapy (Gilbert, 2010; Gilbert & Irons, 2005; Irons & Beaumont, 2017). Although reflecting a broad, integrative underlying theoretical base, Compassion Focused Therapy is generally defined as coming under the CBT umbrella. It is described theoretically in terms of its foundation in evolutionary theory, neurophysiology and brain systems research, Buddhist approaches towards compassion in relation to human suffering, and attachment related caring and soothing. In practical terms, it draws on the value of the therapeutic relationship, recognizes the primary importance of emotion above cognition, and utilizes CBT techniques particularly mindfulness and skills training approaches.

Gilbert (2010) differentiates between aspects/systems of brain function that were established at an early stage of our evolutionary development and systems argued to have evolved far more recently: old brain and new brain. Our old brain is described as carrying within it the capacities we rely on for basic survival and reproduction, incorporating primitive threat-protection systems, and the complex processing of threat and trauma related experience such as emotional memories. It is seen as resulting in unhelpful, intrusive and disruptive ongoing threat related experiences involving self-criticism, rumination and worry that cause us distress and disrupt our day-to-day functioning. Our new brain is described as carrying our capacities to feel calm, safe, content and soothed, as well as our abilities to mentalize; to think about, understand, stand back from and reflect on our own mental processes and those of others. All of these capacities are seen to be related to care and compassion, and their existence within each of our minds has depended on our parents' abilities to love and care for us within good attachment relationships whilst we were growing up. In evolutionary terms, compared with other mammals, Gilbert sees our need to be cared for in this way as a fundamental and primary human need.

Compassion is defined as the ability to validate, empathize and be in tune with our own distress and the distress of others; to accept, care about and soothe ourselves; to tolerate and not avoid difficult emotions, feelings and memories; and to be open to the hidden feelings that may underlie self-criticism and shame in a spirit of non-condemning acceptance. It also involves taking the responsibility to move towards constructive change in a non-punishing way that does not involve self-criticism, but maintains an attitude of warmth, self-acceptance and care.

For those of us who experience high levels of shame and self-criticism, this internal state of soothed comfort, warmth and compassion is very hard to access. Shame as part of the threat-related system, intrinsically results in powerful self-focused attack, which may be our only way of dealing with the attacks we have received from others, and help protect us from unbearable emotion. However, shame may also prevent us from recognizing our own negative behaviours at times, including the hurtful things we may do to others, actions which may later prompt painful and intense experiences of guilt. In these respects, shame and guilt bear complex relationship to each other: a capacity for healthy and compassionate guilt can enable us to recognize and tolerate what we have done, and to change in ways that may remedy those hurts and stop us from repeating them.

In addition to the above aspects of old and new brain systems, Compassion Focused Therapy theory differentiates a further constellation of brain functions described as a resource seeking system led by internal drives and relating to consequent experiences of pleasure and excitement, including all those resources that fuel human survival, and enable us to grow and thrive. Our common human experience of mixed reactions to events in our lives, where feelings and thoughts may contradict each other, and logic and emotion may be in conflict, is deemed to result from the existence of these different brain systems, with each leading to potentially different states of mind. The ability to mentalize and become aware of these potentially divergent motivations, emotions, thoughts and behaviours is seen as enabling us to achieve a greater sense of coherence within our self-experience.

Psychological distress is understood to be associated with our fear and threat related brain systems, and related processes of defence and self-protection. The aim of therapy is to moderate and reduce the activity of this threat response system, by increasing the activity of our new brain in terms of its soothing, calming, emotion regulation and metalizing functions. Distorted, unhelpful cognitions that contribute to distress are understood to be the result of defence related, self-protective cognitive processes rather than being judged as irrational thoughts or errors in thinking. They have resulted from understandable psychological processes, as part of efforts to make sense of often dire circumstances, and to avoid and survive aversive, painful experience. In this context our personal histories assume crucial importance, as do our emotional memories, our compensatory strategies and our schemas of self and others.

Compassion Focused Therapy theory takes the view that unconscious processing has a major impact on our emotions, cognitions and behaviours, and supports the position that our minds are not influenced by conscious cognitive processes until a relatively late stage of the overall information processing sequence. Therapy aims to help us understand the natural origins of our problems, in a way that does not blame us for what has evolved in our lives, but does not deny our own responsibility for who we are, how we behave, and how we may move forward in more constructive directions.

When we are treated with the care and compassion that we need so much, our experience of the warmth and emotional validation provided by others enables us to feel soothed, and to experience a calm sense of safety, connectedness and belonging, in which unhelpful self-protective processes, negative emotions and behaviours are moderated and reduced. We also become more able to redirect our attention to exploring and taking action in the world around us. In this context validation makes a central contribution to our abilities to understand and reflect on our own emotions, and not be overwhelmed by them. At a physiological level these relational experiences are assumed to achieve their benefits through the release of endorphins and oxytocin. These neurobiological processes are also particularly addressed by polyvagal theory (Dana, 2018; Porges, 2011).

The therapeutic relationship in Compassion Focused Therapy is advised by these factors and is seen as playing a key role in relation to engagement, communication and listening, so that feelings of safeness and connectedness may develop within clients as they are heard, understood and validated from a position of empathic compassion; a position that may then become an internalized part of themselves. At the same time the importance of limits and boundaries is clearly recognized as important. Transference and counter-transference within the relationship are recognized as important, particularly in the context of shame and the ways in which it may powerfully influence clients' perceptions of themselves and their therapists and the processes that unfold between them. Therapists' own attachment styles and underlying schema organization are similarly seen as having significant influence.

From this caring and compassionate base, therapists will develop and share an individualized formulation and understanding of client difficulties in the context of their life and relational histories and the theoretical base of the therapy. A range of structured approaches based on the principles of skills training and behavioural practice, are advocated to actively facilitate and support the development and generalization of the client's compassionate self. More active therapeutic work will involve attention to thought monitoring, evidence-based challenge of unhelpful cognitions, and the use of behavioural experiments, graded exposure, problem solving, and other aspects of cognitive behavioural practice.

Summary

The cognitive and behavioural therapies overviewed in Chapter 9 are all led by a primary focus on cognition, and all seek to support constructive changes within conscious mind. Across the range of therapies involved, it is within the detailed descriptions of practice that we come to appreciate the subtleties and nuances of the theoretical bases that underlie them. Beyond the more traditional approaches to CBT, which primarily rely on cognitive theory and a focus on conscious cognition backed up by attention to behavioural methods, we find a wide range of theoretical positions reflected within therapy practice, as discussed in relation to Schema Therapy, cognitive-interpersonal cycles, Constructivist Psychotherapy, Mindfulness Based Cognitive Therapy and Compassion Focused Therapy.

Behavioural and Cognitive Theory

10

This chapter will consider those therapies within the CBT umbrella that are led by behavioural theory. It will discuss core aspects of behaviourism, overview its contributions to psychotherapy practice, and look at several therapies in which behavioural theory takes the lead: stage one of Dialectical Behavior Therapy, DBT (Linehan, 1993; Swales & Heard, 2009), Acceptance and Commitment Therapy, ACT (Flaxman et al., 2011; Hayes et al., 1999), Behavioral Activation, BA (Martell et al., 2010) and Functional Analytic Psychotherapy, FAP (Kohlenberg & Tsai, 1991).

Core Aspects of Behaviourism

Overall behaviourism follows the principles of empiricism and logical positivism whereby it is only phenomena that can be observed, measured and thus investigated by scientific experimental methods that can contribute to theories of human psychological functioning. It focuses our attention on the role played by the environment and learning processes in the generation of human behaviour, and generally sees overtly observable behaviour as the legitimate focus of psychological investigation (Hawton et al., 1989; Joseph, 2010; Watson, 1924). However, different approaches to behaviourism make varying judgements about the nature of its legitimate subject matter (Moore, 2001). Externally and publicly observable behaviour may be seen as the only subject matter that should relate to theoretical understanding. Mental/cognitive human experiences that can only be subjectively observed, such as images, thoughts and feelings, may be totally excluded from theoretical consideration but may also sometimes be included. If they are included the way in which they are theoretically conceptualized may vary. They may be treated as behaviours in themselves, together with language/verbal behaviour, or they may be deemed to be the collateral by-products of the environmental and genetic influences that generate behaviour (Skinner, 1974).

The major distinction to be made within behavioural theory is between the associationist, stimulus response psychology of classical conditioning (Pavlov, 1927; Watson & Raynor, 1920) and the reinforcement-based learning processes of operant conditioning (Miller & Konorski, 1937; Skinner, 1938, 1974; Thorndike, 1927). Classical conditioning, also sometimes referred to as respondent conditioning (Kanter et al., 2009), describes the process whereby a conditioned stimulus becomes paired by association with an unconditioned stimulus. The former then elicits from the subject the reaction that would naturally be produced by the unconditioned stimulus. The persistent presence of a stimulus that would usually prompt an unconditioned response results in habituation and the response is no longer elicited. This process is particularly associated with the theoretical understanding of fear and anxiety experiences and the nature of the enduring consequences of physical and emotional trauma. Associations are forged between past fearful events and their stimulus context, and can exist at an unconscious level (Swales & Heard, 2009).

The basic aspects of the principles of operant conditioning, also at times referred to as instrumental conditioning, were first developed in parallel during the early years of the twentieth century by psychologists in Russia, Eastern Europe and the USA (Iversen, 1992). The key protagonists were Ivanov-Smolensky (1927), Miller and Konorski (1937) and Skinner (1938), with their work following on from the earlier work of Thorndike in recognizing that positive, beneficial consequences increase the frequency of the behaviour that elicited them, an observation that was defined as the Law of Effect (Thorndike, 1927). In all instances the principles were developed in relation to experimental behaviour in animals, and later generalized to humans. The core concepts of operant conditioning are positive reinforcement, negative reinforcement, extinction, punishment, and schedules of reinforcement.

The frequency of any behaviour is influenced by the nature of the consequences of that behaviour. If the consequences are experienced as positive and rewarding, the frequency of the behaviour will increase: positive reinforcement. If an unpleasant experience is ended by the behaviour this will also increase the frequency of that behaviour: negative reinforcement. If these previously experienced reinforcing consequences are removed, the frequency of the behaviour will decrease: extinction. If the consequences of a behaviour are experienced as negative and unpleasant, the frequency of the behaviour will decrease: punishment. The frequency and regularity of reinforcement: schedules of reinforcement, influence the durability of related changes in behaviour. Schedules are commonly either ratio or interval schedules, with an intermittent schedule of reinforcement resulting in the most durable changes in behaviour. New and complex behaviour may be developed by a process of shaping, involving the positive reinforcement of successive approximations to that behaviour. From the perspective of radical behaviourism, the totality of the nature, pattern and regularity of reinforcing or punishing experiences from early childhood onwards constitutes the learning history and contingencies that gradually shape our complex human behaviours; the person or the self that we are, is seen as being the sum total of the repertoire of those behaviours. Our behaviour is not influenced by our goals for the future, but solely reflects our experiences of past conditioning (Iversen, 1992; Skinner, 1974).

A further core characteristic of radical behaviourism is the place that is given to the mental, emotional and cognitive elements of human experience. Methodological behaviourism excludes mental events from its analysis and understanding of human behaviour, whereas radical behaviourism as developed by Skinner accepts that mental events exist, that they matter and that they need to be taken into consideration rather than be ignored. However, whilst accepting that self-observation of thoughts, perceptions, feelings, memories, and mental events is both possible and potentially useful, they are all considered to be produced by our bodies as the collateral products of our human genetic and environmental learning histories, and as such are not seen as playing any causal role in relation to our behaviour (Skinner, 1974). We have ways of experiencing, thinking and talking about ourselves and how we function as human beings, but our behaviour in all these respects is influenced by our histories, and the words we use in saying things to ourselves and others will be shaped by our personal histories and the histories of our verbal communities. Our verbal behaviour is powerfully reinforced by the effects it has on other people and on ourselves, and the meaning attributed to the words we use is seen to lie in their antecedent histories, with no meanings being exactly the same in the speaker or the listener. Skinner refers to mental events as 'the world within the skin' and sees them as having the capacity to reflect useful information and clues regarding past and current behaviour and the environmental conditions affecting it, and about conditions that may relate to future behaviour.

Hayes et al. (2001) extend Skinner's perspective on the operant development and maintenance of complex verbal behaviour in their description of Relational Frame Theory. The capacity to describe different types of logical relationships between physical and conceptual entities, such as equivalence or comparison, is seen as being established through the reinforcement of multiple exemplars of particular relational positions, resulting in the generalized ability to apply the consequences of these relational rules to other problems whose solutions share common features. Relational frames are described as higher-order classes of operant behaviour and are the product of a history of reinforcement. Novel verbal responses and new words, which have not themselves been directly reinforced, may then be generated by the interaction of such relational frames (Flaxman et al., 2011; Hayes, 2004; Ingvarssonn & Morris, 2004). Logical reasoning and associated verbal behaviour, together with the generation of novel ideas and new words, are seen as coming under indirect operant control through the automatic application of generalized rules that were acquired though operant conditioning.

Behavioural Contributions to Psychotherapy

Within psychotherapy practice, behaviour therapy particularly draws on the theory of classical conditioning, and behaviour modification and applied behaviour analysis particularly draw on the principles of operant conditioning (Joseph, 2010). In addition, Mowrer's two-factor theory of fear and avoidance (Mowrer, 1951) and Bandura's social learning theory (Bandura, 1977) and self-efficacy theory (Bandura, 1997) all play key roles in the nature of behaviour therapy interventions, as does Wolpe's principle of reciprocal inhibition (Wolpe, 1958).

Mowrer recognizes that fear can be acquired by classical conditioning with avoidance then developing and being maintained by operant conditioning. Bandura proposes that individuals often learn behaviour through observing others by a process of modelling, and that their capacities to learn and to perform are influenced by their expectations of their own abilities, their self-efficacy. Wolpe puts forward the view that a response can be weakened by being paired with a different, incompatible response, a process of reciprocal inhibition. Behaviour therapy makes a particularly significant contribution to psychotherapy in the treatment of problems relating to fear and anxiety in which a fear/anxiety response has become associated with a currently non-threatening stimulus. Reflecting Mowrer's two-factor approach and his own principle of reciprocal inhibition Wolpe (1958) describes the procedure of systematic desensitization, which uses physical relaxation to inhibit the fear/anxiety response whilst following an exposure-based approach towards altering the association between fear and the conditioned stimulus. Facing and experiencing feared and anxiety provoking situations and objects, enables the fear response to habituate and the avoidance response is no longer maintained by negative reinforcement. Exposure therapy usually involves a graded hierarchical approach, in vivo or in imagination, from the least to the most feared situation, with or without the use of relaxation, which may be supported by modelling. Flooding, immediate and sustained exposure to the most feared situation is an alternative that tends to be seldom used.

Within cognitive behavioural approaches to anxiety management, the importance of avoidance, the basic principles of exposure therapy and the potential value of relaxation are augmented by attention to negative automatic thoughts and intermediate beliefs. The physiological component of the anxiety/fear response and the evolutionary origins of our flight or fight reactions are also given an integrated place within the model of anxiety that is shared with clients. The general principles of exposure therapy may be relevant in relation to a wide range of practical and interpersonal experiences and situations that cause people distress and tend to be avoided.

Broadly based behavioural approaches to psychotherapy such as those reviewed by Kanfer and Goldstein (1986) draw on the core psychological mechanisms of both classical and operant conditioning theories, as well as accepting the meaningful validity of our inner worlds of thoughts, emotions, hopes and fears, goals and wishes. Written in the relatively early days of the cognitive revolution, Kanfer and Goldstein's work provides a comprehensive overview of behaviour therapy approaches including modelling, operant fear-reduction, self-management and biofeedback methods, as well as emerging cognitive and cognitive-behavioural approaches.

Behaviour modification and applied behaviour analysis reflect the application of radical behaviourism to human behaviour to achieve changes that are deemed beneficial to society (Baer et al., 1968). Behaviour change protocols are developed following the observation of specific behaviours and their environmental contingencies. They are currently particularly valued in addressing problem behaviours within learning disability populations and amongst people diagnosed with autistic spectrum disorders, as well as within general education (Axelrod et al., 2012). The terms applied behaviour analysis and functional analysis are also sometimes used interchangeably, and both involve the observation and recording of the antecedents of a behaviour, what is happening for the person and within their environment at the time the behaviour takes place; the behaviour itself, and the consequences that follow on from that behaviour, what happens for them and in their environment after they have behaved in that way. This is commonly referred to as the ABC sequence. Antecedents may also be referred to as discriminative stimuli which evoke behaviour because the learning history of the individual has led them to represent the likelihood of particular reinforcing or punishing consequences. This analysis can reveal the unique and personal ways in which the behaviour of an individual is being reinforced, reflecting the function that it is fulfilling for them, and enabling changes in the environment to be made that are most likely to result in desired changes in that behaviour.

Functional analysis in the psychotherapy context also puts emphasis on the aetiology of psychological problems, those early and past experiences that are likely to have contributed to their development, plus more recent trigger experiences and events. It also crucially addresses the ways in which current antecedents and consequences may result in the maintenance loops, or vicious circles that may maintain them (Owens & Ashcroft, 1982).

Amongst those therapies within the CBT family that are led by behavioural theories, stage one of Dialectical Behavior Therapy and Behavioral Activation both draw on applied behaviour analysis and functional analysis and apply radical behaviourism to private mental events, taking the position that cognition and thinking, affect and feelings, expressions of emotion, wants and needs are all behaviours influenced by the same principles as overt observable behaviour. Functional Analytic Therapy works towards changes in unhelpful relational patterns entirely from the theoretical base of classical and operant conditioning. Acceptance and Commitment Therapy advocates the acceptance of previously avoided distress, applies Relational Frame Theory to cognition, meaning and verbal behaviour, and utilizes skills training, shaping, graded exposure and other behavioural methods to help clients follow through their commitments to change.

Dialectical Behavior Therapy

Marsha Linehan developed Dialectical Behavior Therapy to address the challenging situation of suicide risk amongst some people diagnosed with Borderline Personality Disorder (Linehan, 1993; Swales &Heard, 2009). It is stage one of the overall four-stage approach that particularly draws on classical conditioning and applied behaviour analysis to help address this high-risk context, and achieve behavioural stability. Subsequent stages draw on a wider range of psychotherapeutic approaches to address other aspects of Borderline Personality Disorder once behavioural stability has been established and risk reduced. Behavioural analysis and interventions address the roles played by behaviour, cognition and emotion in the experience of problematic events. These therapeutic processes are accompanied by the secular application of the principles of acceptance that originate within Buddhism.

Invalidating developmental environments are seen as playing a significant aetiological role resulting in continuing self-invalidation, the prevalence of intense emotion with high sensitivity and reactivity and marked difficulties in regulation, intolerance of stress, personal and interpersonal skills deficits, unhelpful and sometimes self-destructive attempts to avoid or escape unbearable suffering, and the prevalence of unrelenting crises and inhibited grieving. Diagnosis of Borderline Personality Disorder is seen as reflecting the existence of a set of problematic behaviours rather than defining the person, and all behaviours, no matter how dysfunctional, are assumed to reflect a valid and understandable response to difficult experience from the perspective of the client. Therapy involves an ongoing dialectical balance between empathic acceptance and validation on the one hand and an active behaviourally led push towards change on the other.

Behaviour is considered to be anything a person overtly does, thinks, feels or imagines. Applied behaviour analysis, or chain analysis, of repeated examples of target behaviours reveals their patterns of reinforcement or punishment and the functions they fulfil, with the personal impact of environmental events being mediated by the individual's learning history. Factors are identified that maintain problematic behaviours and/or limit client capacities to use more skilful approaches to deal with situations they find challenging. A problem-solving approach is then taken towards finding new behavioural solutions to problem events. Within the therapeutic relationship it is considered important for therapists to manage their responses to client behaviours on an operant basis in ways that reflect contingencies that might occur in everyday life. This might involve relaxing aspects of limits within therapy such as time or frequency in response to positive changes, and tightening those boundaries, or imposing some aspects of punishment, such as a break from therapy, if self-damaging behaviour is unresponsive to intervention.

Stage one focuses largely on the overt high-risk behaviours associated with suicidality or aggression and behaviours that interfere with the process of therapy. Chain analysis and the management of contingencies are also used to address problematic emotions and thoughts related to risk, in addition to cognitive approaches involving the verbal challenge of unhelpful thoughts and beliefs.

Classical conditioning is also addressed in relation to the intense fear that may be triggered by the places, sounds or smells associated consciously or unconsciously with past traumatic events. Emotions are deemed to be warranted or unwarranted in terms of the actual threats present in the current environment. Exposure-based approaches are used to establish new learned associations, reducing trauma driven fears and anxieties, and other aspects of intense emotion. Skills training also plays a core role in stage one, and draws on traditional behavioural approaches to social skills and assertiveness training, the practices of mindfulness, self-acceptance, relational problem solving and the regulation of intense emotion. Training takes place on a group basis and one-to-one telephone coaching.

Acceptance and Commitment Therapy

Acceptance and Commitment Therapy (Flaxman et al., 2011; Hayes, 2004; Hayes et al., 2001) is referred to as a modern-day behaviour therapy, in which behavioural theory is seen to apply to cognition and affect as well as behaviour, and seeks to explain a wide range of private experiences including thinking, feeling, wishing, remembering and the experience of self. It adopts a behavioural skills training approach towards the mindful acceptance of and gradual exposure to distressing emotional experiences such as anxiety, fear and depression, draws on Relational Frame Theory to reduce the unhelpful impact of evaluative aspects of self-directed verbal behaviour, and focuses on a commitment to developing behaviours that are consistent with how people would value themselves as being. Therapy explicitly does not seek to change the form or frequency of unwanted thoughts and emotions. It aims to increase psychological flexibility, enable psychological contact with the present moment and increase people's capacities to live more rewarding lives even in the presence of undesirable, distressing thoughts, feelings and sensations.

Distress is seen as a normal part of human existence. It is the experiential avoidance of distress and the associated persistent efforts to control and remove it, that are seen to contribute to the problems that people experience. Therapy investigates the effectiveness of clients' current control related strategies, gradually challenging them and identifying the ways in which they are making problems worse. Clients are then offered the alternative of becoming more willing to accept and experience distressing and unwanted emotional states and physical sensations, increasing their capacities to live with them in the present moment, and decreasing their experiential avoidance. This process is supported by a structured approach towards making undefended contact with previously avoided emotions, and giving people some sense of distance between themselves and the emotion they are relating to, referred to as diffusion.

One way of doing this is to adopt a position in which clients imagine themselves as the observer of their own thoughts, emotions and physical states, a position that therapy refers to as experiencing the self as self-in-context as opposed to self-as-content. This position as an observer of our own inner experiences overlaps with aspects of mindfulness and associated meditative experiences. Diffusion might also be achieved by imagining an emotion such as anger as being a physical object outside of ourselves. From this perspective clients can think about and describe the emotion, which they are later asked to welcome back again into themselves.

Clients may also be supported in staying in touch with difficult painful feelings and other private events as they naturally emerge during therapy sessions, talking about what they notice within their bodies and sitting with those previously avoided thoughts, sensations and emotions.

As well as involving our own inner states, present moment awareness also involves becoming more aware of and tracking the environmental antecedents and consequences that relate to aspects of our behaviour. The more clients are aware of the environments they are functioning within, and the contingencies relating to what they do and say, the more likely they are to make effective changes to that behaviour.

Principles derived from Relational Frame Theory are applied to the verbal content of negative, self-critical thoughts. The human capacity to reflect on experience and apply logic to perceptions of the self in comparison based and negative ways, through the functioning of relational frames, is seen as a particularly important source of human psychological pain and suffering. Theory proposes that verbal constructs are generated that do not reflect reality, but are experienced as real by a process of cognitive fusion: the meanings that become attached to words is seen as arbitrary with no basis in truth. From this perspective, suffering can be reduced if words associated with self-criticism are rendered meaningless by the process of defusion, for example by saying a significant word over and over again, breaking the usual rules of language until the word becomes just a set of sounds rather than a meaningful entity. Dealing with self-critical thoughts is particularly important because they can be barriers that reduce the capacity for people to behave in ways that are consistent with their values.

Values are verbal statements about any states of affairs that an individual would wish to experience repeatedly throughout their lives. Such states of affairs would be associated with ongoing experiences of positive reinforcement, hopefully on a long-term basis. Therapy process seeks to enable clients to identify and clarify what is important to them in these respects, and to describe their values in terms of their own potential ways of behaving. Commitment involves the systematic planning of specific goals and actions that are consistent with the individual's values and putting these into effect, usually through a graduated process of behavioral activation. Identifying what is really important to people, how they would like to see themselves, and be seen and remembered by others, helps to increase motivation to act in a committed way to gradually change behaviour, whilst at the same time experiencing aspects of psychological distress that are not defended against, but remain in present moment awareness and are lived with. This process may also be supported by a range of approaches to skills training such as social and communication skills, problem solving and skills of daily living, if any such skills deficits are not primarily due to experiential avoidance or other psychological contexts that act as barriers to effective functioning.

Behavioral Activation

Behavioral Activation has its origins within two early behavioural approaches to depression (Ferster, 1973; Lewinsohn, 1974), which argue that depression is caused and maintained by the loss of stable sources of positive reinforcement and by the accompanying negative reinforcement associated with the avoidance of aversive experiences (Kanter et al., 2009; Martell et al., 2010). It aims to activate the operant behaviour of clients in ways that will enable them to change their current environments, establish diverse stable sources of positive reinforcement and, over time, create new learning histories that will then evoke and maintain more functional behaviour in the longer term.

In relation to thoughts and beliefs, Behavioral Activation holds thinking to be a behaviour under operant control and seeks to identify the historical and present events that lead to particular thoughts acquiring functional control over behaviour. From a behavioural perspective, unhelpful thoughts can have the capacity to affect the reinforcing nature of an experience and in this way make their own contribution to loss of positive reinforcement.

As well as recognizing the importance of the loss of positive reinforcement, therapy also acknowledges the important role of punishment and associated learned helplessness (Seligman, 1975) in the aetiology of depression. It is the prolonged and inescapable punishment often found in the childhood histories of people suffering depression that is of significance in this respect. Learned helplessness leads to the generalized stimulus of the punisher becoming aversive and evoking fear and avoidance, with widespread negative consequences particularly in terms of finding and maintaining intimate relationships.

In taking a behavioural approach to cognition and affect, classical/respondent conditioning theory and stimulus response psychology is applied to expressions of emotion such as sadness, anger, excitement, and crying. They are seen as respondent, unconditioned responses that are automatically triggered by negative environmental events and ones which may be maintained by operant conditioning. In addition, all behaviours associated with depression may be maintained by currently reinforcing consequences, as well as reflecting processes of secondary gain.

Behavioural explanations of depression carry with them the explicit message that this personal state of affairs is caused by normal human psychological processes, which makes sense in the context of people's lives; it is understandable, not abnormal. Behavioural theory is described as non-blaming in this respect and Kanter et al. (2009) see this position as an important factor in supporting therapists' capacities for empathy towards their clients and their struggles. It is also seen as supporting an empowering focus on the possibility of action and change within clients, even in the face of seemingly overwhelming histories.

The activation of operant behaviour associated with subsequent positive reinforcement is based on a functional analysis of client behaviours using the principles of applied behaviour analysis. Discussion of clients' histories, the contextual environments of their current behaviours, and information from people who are close to them, support the identification of current and historical variables leading people to behave in the ways that they do, and provide a picture of the effects their behaviours have on the environments that surround them. It is assumed that the important variables may not be those that clients themselves identify since they may be unaware of the processes of reinforcement that function within them. More accurate pictures are deemed to be gained from the perspective of external therapeutic observation and analysis. Clients' stories are an important source of information in this respect, but are also seen as being influenced by the operant contingencies of the current environment and the vagaries of memory. Empathic understanding and acceptance of those stories, however, is seen as important to the secure development of the therapeutic relationship.

As discussed earlier, functional analysis typically assesses antecedents, what is happening at the time; behaviour, what the person does; and consequences, what happens immediately afterwards. It enables hypotheses to be made about the nature of reinforcement maintaining problem behaviours. Changes are then targeted towards all three components of this analysis. Attention is paid to the stimulus control function of the current environment, behaviour is changed by activation assignments and skills training, and consequences are addressed by contingency management.

As with Acceptance and Commitment Therapy the nature of activation assignments is influenced by the identification of client values, which increases the likelihood that the consequences of carrying out the behaviour will involve elements of positive reinforcement. Values in terms of what people want from their lives, what will give it meaning and purpose, are seen to have evolved as complex products of their histories, and therapy aims to alter clients' environments in ways that will generate and maintain behaviours that are consistent with those values.

Again, in similarity with Acceptance and Commitment Therapy, there is an emphasis on the acceptance of current distressing emotions and feelings, with clients making changes in their behaviour whilst continuing to experience that respondent distress. The role played by experiential avoidance is recognized, and attention paid to the private inner consequences of behaviour. Problem behaviour may be maintained by the avoidance of aversive private events such as painful thoughts and emotions, which clients may not necessarily be aware of. In both these respects mindfulness is used to help clients become more able to live with their difficult thoughts, feelings and emotions, be prepared to make changes before such distress has decreased, and be more able to behave in ways that would previously have been avoided in order to protect themselves from difficult thoughts and feelings.

The problem behaviours targeted may be directly experienced within the therapeutic relationship. At such times it is seen to be of value to acknowledge and discuss them and make the connection between these lived experiences and similar situations in the everyday life of the client. The context is seen as a live opportunity for therapists to prompt and reinforce the activation of alternative behaviours, and in this respect bears some similarity to Functional Analytic Psychotherapy (Kohlenberg & Tsai, 1991; Tsai et al., 2014). In general, the therapeutic relationship is seen as an important context for providing instruction, guidance and coaching. The validation, empathy, and care that are provided are also seen as important and non-specific factors that generally facilitate therapy and reinforce/support the clients' continued attendance, but are not considered to play a part in the mechanisms responsible for the effectiveness of Behavioral Activation.

Functional Analytic Psychotherapy

The final therapeutic approach to be included in this chapter is Functional Analytic Psychotherapy, developed in America by Kohlenberg & Tsai (1991) and described by Tsai et al. (2012) as a behavioural approach that is founded securely within the principles of operant, contingent reinforcement. These principles are seen as accounting for the central place of the therapeutic relationship within client change processes. Theory and practice is designed to enhance the power of that relationship, increasing therapists' capacities for genuineness, intensity, compassion and effectiveness, all of which are seen as functioning as the springboard for client change, an approach that is described as having the ability to supercharge other CBT approaches to therapy.

Behaviourism is described here as a philosophy of contextualism that provides a powerful way of understanding the unique experience and behaviours of each individual, replacing the term radical behaviourism with contextual behaviourism. Private events, including cognitions, emotions and other internal and unconscious experiences are all accepted as part of human existence, and are seen as behaviours influenced by the typically unconscious processes of classical and operant conditioning across the life span. It is external experience that shapes all of our internal responses and our overt behaviours through the cumulative effects of our reinforcement history, and reinforcement is a ubiquitous constant throughout our human lives. Therapy accepts that cognition can have causal effects in relation to our behaviours, and acknowledges the stimulus properties of private events. Thinking and other cognitive experiences may sometimes have an impact on behaviour, and at other times may not be involved at all. All human behaviour is seen as explicable in these ways, and as existing as the result of natural human psychological processes. Similarly to Behavioral Activation, this acceptance of all behaviour as being explicable in the context of our lives is seen as an important factor in relation to human distress and disturbance, and as having the capacity to support a deep non-judgmental empathy between therapist and client.

In common with other behavioural approaches, our human self is seen as the sum total of all our ways of behaving and is considered to be under both internal and external /environmental control, with the capacity for beneficial internal private control being supported by confident expressions of self as opposed to confused, inaccurate and dependent ways of being. Therapy aims to shape private control and reinforce self-expression. Within our expressions of self, the meaning and function of overt behaviours and particularly verbal statements are seen as crucially important. Meaning is defined as the function of a behaviour in terms of what it accomplishes in relation to the individual, and such understanding may be supported by a behavioural functional analysis of antecedents and consequences. It is recognized that such functions and meaning may be hidden outside of our conscious awareness, and that their expression through overt behaviour and verbal statements may not be deliberate or necessarily related to any insight into the history that led to them.

Emotions and feelings are seen as types of sensory actions or behaviours and as physical bodily states, both of which are the result of unique operant and classically conditioned learning histories. The external environment is seen as the ultimate cause of these bodily states and it is assumed that we are not born with any intrinsic awareness of what emotions are, this being something we are taught by adults. Emotions and feelings have a crucial place within therapy, since they are seen as indicating that people are in touch with their experience of themselves within their worlds. It is therefore considered important that they can be felt and expressed freely and that the various ways in which their experience and expression may be restricted are taken into account, such as being cut off from aspects of emotional experience and the tendency to avoid situations that prompt particular negative or positive feelings.

Within the therapeutic relationship the therapist is seen as an interpersonal stimulus playing a crucial part in the functional behavioural context of the client's life within therapy sessions; eliciting, evoking and consequating client behaviours. The therapist's eliciting function refers to the prompting of classically conditioned responses within clients, of which emotional behaviour is considered to be a prime example. In that context, therapists' care and compassion and associated non-verbal behaviours are described as being designed to elicit/support respondent emotions, which may be connected with a wide range of triggers such as bereavement, abandonment, or anxieties about illness and death. Therapists evoke operant behaviour in their clients, and this is particularly significant when the evoked behaviour functions in therapy in a way that is similar to their everyday lives. Such behaviours by clients in relation to their therapists are referred to as clinically relevant behaviours or CRBs. Functional Analytic therapists actively seek to evoke CRBs, and pay particular attention to identifying any that emerge on a spontaneous basis.

Therapists consequate client operant behaviours when they respond to them and provide reinforcement or punishment. They pay attention to these naturally unfolding patterns, and apply reinforcement or punishment on a strategic basis to foster constructive change. These patterns of reinforcement are made explicit and are openly available for discussion and understanding within therapy. Whilst therapist responses may be made on strategic basis, it is seen as crucially important that natural reinforcement is experienced by clients rather than something that has been planned on some arbitrary basis by the therapist. Natural reinforcement is seen as reflecting consequences of behaviours that could occur in someone's everyday environment, and as being founded in therapists' genuine feelings of compassion and care.

Three different types of CRBs are defined: CRB 1 in which aspects of clients' presenting problems emerge between therapist and client during therapy sessions, which are seen as often involving emotional avoidance and difficulty in expressing honest feelings or personal needs; CRB 2 in which behaviour within sessions reflects improvements in CRB 1 behaviours; and CRB 3 in which clients express interpretations of their own behaviours, and their own functional understanding. CRB 1 behavioural patterns are made explicit between therapist and client, and understood in terms of their function and the relevance of that function in relation to past experience. This understanding is then used to support the possibility of change and the process of trying out different behaviours within the therapeutic relationship and in clients' current everyday lives. Therapist reinforcement of target behaviours as evidenced by a CRB 2 is seen as crucial in supporting early stages of change that may not receive such reinforcement in the outside world.

A context of intimacy, trust and attachment within the therapeutic relationship is essential to the capacity of clients to reveal deeply and often secretly held aspects of themselves and their lives, to become more able to express previously avoided emotions, and to explore hidden meanings; in this context a growing capacity for intimacy is often seen as constituting a CRB 2 for the client.

Summary

In Chapter 10 core principles of behaviourism have been reviewed and its contributions to psychotherapy practice, looking at the application of longstanding behaviour therapy methodologies and more recent developments. Relatively detailed discussion of stage one of Dialectical Behavior Therapy, Acceptance and Commitment Therapy, Behavioral Activation and Functional Analytic Psychotherapy has highlighted ways in which radical behaviourism, applied behaviour analysis and functional analysis directly address unhelpful behaviours, support the development of more constructive ways of being, and address aspects of conscious cognition, hidden feelings and relational interactions.

Contexts and Environments: **11**
The World Around Us

Whilst the theoretical approaches discussed so far have often made reference to aspects of the environments in which we live, especially our relational worlds, they have varied in the extent to which wider aspects of the world around us have been taken into consideration. In this chapter we will look in some greater depth at the psychological importance of environmental factors that have been the subject of psychosocial research within Western society, which will not particularly represent the contexts of minority ethnic groups and their cultures. This focus reflects the limits of feasibility within the current work, as well as the availability of related psychosocial research, and does not diminish the importance of the environmental and cultural contexts of other societies, or the importance of the multi-cultural nature of Western society. In this context, Shiraev and Levy (2016) provide a valuable overview of cross-cultural psychology. Chapter 12 will then consider the importance of our place in the lifespan in relation to our individual development, the environments we are part of across that lifespan, our interactions with them and the consequences for our psychological well-being, on a similar basis.

We each live in and interact with a unique and complex total environment. It may appear to have a lot of aspects in common with the environments of the other people around us, but the subjective experience of those common aspects will be different for each one of us. The nature of our current relational, social, demographic and cultural environments can also all play crucial roles in our capacities to experience constructive and beneficial psychological change when it is important for us to do so.

If our developmental past has been damaging for us, we may now be lucky enough as adults to inhabit a social milieu that is different in important respects compared with the problematic, emotionally deprived and/or abusive environments we grew up in. The on-going psychological consequences of those early experiences, however, may distort and spoil our capacities to live well within this current place. They may impede our potential to thrive in a world that could otherwise support us in doing so. But under propitious circumstances, particularly if we are relating to other people who are naturally able to understand us and modify their own behaviours, beneficial change may still naturally emerge simply because we are living in a different and better place; or it may need the involvement of a therapist to help it start to happen.

Alternatively, we may be living in a current psychosocial environment that truly repeats the damage of our earlier lives. Psychotherapy may be able to help effective change take place, but it may be much harder to achieve, and significant changes in our environment may be required to enable individual change to take place and be sustained. In addition to their direct impact, damaging adult relationships may also deny us access to other resources that are needed or may be essential to support our psychological development and growth. Finally, a damaging adult relationship, rather than repeating past experiences of hurt, may be psychologically damaging to us for the first time.

Overall, a wide range of relational, demographic and cultural factors, and life events influence our developmental processes, the person we come to be, and the nature of the lives we lead. All may play their part in the nature and generation of psychological distress, and may be important factors to take into account within psychotherapy. All may support associated processes of change, or limit the extent to which change is possible. We will start with an overview of the broad-based psychosocial literature, followed by a specific look at the importance of gender and the significance of sexual orientation and gender identity. The overall consequences of discrimination and the context of cultural difference will also be acknowledged.

Contributions from Broad-Based Psychosocial Research and Literature

In our current adult lives our psychological well-being is likely to be influenced, directly or indirectly, by the other people in our lives and our relationships with them, by the nature of the places in which we live and work, our financial situation, our own personalities and characteristics, our age, gender, sexual orientation and gender identity, ethnicity, disability status, marital and parental status, and by the cultures we are immersed in. Extensive psychosocial research from the 1970s onwards, particularly in the context of depression, validates some of the crucial and often complex roles that our environments and our interactions with them play in our psychological lives within Western society. Key reading is provided by Brown and Harris (1978/2011); Goldberg and Huxley (1992); Goodman and Lusby (2014); Gotlib and Hammen (1992a, 1992b); Hammen and Shih (2014); Harris (2001); Rutter (1991) and Scott et al. (2014).

Although its empirical base in logical positivism means that much of this research is unable to reflect the unique nature, meanings and nuances of individual situations, it is able to provide evidence in support of categories of life contexts which are statistically associated with vulnerability to psychological distress, and types of events that may trigger its onset. Contexts may also be associated with the absence or reduction of distress by supporting resilience or enabling restitution. Each aspect of research contributes to our collective appreciation of the factors that may influence the unique lives of individuals. From within this wide range of research, empirical evidence has emerged in support of three sources of adult vulnerability to psychological distress, particularly the experience of depression: firstly our distal, childhood environment within our families, secondly our current psychological selves, and thirdly our proximal, adult environment.

In significant ways clear overlaps and triangulation exist between this research and the theories that guide and influence our practice of psychotherapy, with the psychosocial literature often supporting premises to be found within our different theoretical approaches. Research has supported the damaging consequences of poor and inadequate parenting including emotional and physical neglect; unresponsive care; lack of warmth; punitive rejection; care that is intrusive, harsh or coercive; overly stringent reward criteria; neglect/deprivation following the loss of a parent; physical and sexual abuse; trauma; and parental marital discord especially if this has involved aggression, taken place repeatedly, has been unresolved, or has involved the child. These factors have generally been conceptualized as resulting in adverse effects on the child's developing cognitive representation of self and the world, leading to a range of cognitive vulnerabilities. In relation to the self these have been framed as reduced self-esteem, self-worth, self-confidence and efficacy, a general devaluing of the self, sensitivity to rejection, emotional dependency, hopelessness and helplessness, an external locus of control, and unrealistically high standards for self-reinforcement. In relation to the other people in our lives, cognitive vulnerability includes our perception of others and our relationships with them, resulting in interpersonal vulnerability and associated patterns of dysfunctional relationships. The total individual sum of these factors is seen as constituting a diathesis for adult distress/depression, in interaction with adverse provoking life events and in the context of the third source of vulnerability, our current social and demographic environment.

In relation to our adult environments, psychosocial research has collectively validated the potentially unhelpful consequences of poor housing, economic stress/poverty, unemployment, chronic stressors, on-going minor stressors/daily hassles, and a lack of opportunity to find sources of personal and meaningful value for ourselves. We may also be made more vulnerable to distress if we are limited in our capacity to have power and influence over the nature of our lives. Research into relational contexts has repeatedly identified the crucial importance of having a stable, intimate, confiding relationship that can and does provide sustained support at times of crisis. The nature, quality and size of our social networks, their perceived helpfulness and our satisfaction with them are also relevant to a supportive environment that reduces our vulnerability. These contexts have been particularly supported by the seminal research of Brown and Harris in the mid-1970s on depression in women, which has been republished in recent years (Brown & Harris, 1978/2011). Harris (2001) provides an update on this work, considers the integrative place of genetic and hormonal factors, and provides her own perspective on key points for clinical practice.

Research into the nature of adverse life events that may provoke distress/depression in the context of the above vulnerability factors has given a particularly central place to the experience of loss. Loss may take many forms, it may be the loss of someone who matters to us through conflict, separation or death and bereavement; it may be loss through the disruption of our social networks and the loss of friendships and family; it may be the loss involved in losing our job, or losing physical capacity; it may be what has been termed loss of a source of value, some change in our lives which means that we are no longer able to be part of something that we had a high level of investment in and that gave us a personal sense of value in ourselves. Such losses may be experienced as irreparable, with no means of replacement, and Harris (2001) identifies associated experiences of humiliation or entrapment, as significantly adding to the risks of subsequent depression. In addition, and unsurprisingly, experiences of threat and danger have clearly been identified in association with problems related to anxiety.

Research has recognized that the nature of our psychological selves and our interpersonal functioning may well mean that we make our own contributions at times to the unfolding of events and experiences that can prove so stressful to us. Such events are termed dependent events, and those that are assumed to have occurred with no contribution on our part are referred to as fateful or independent events. Psychosocial research has often made empirical distinction between the two, and in general the sources of vulnerability identified above have been associated with increased rates of both dependent and fateful adverse life events (Harris, 2001). The impact of painful life experiences will be no less because we have played a part in them evolving; indeed in some respects we might imagine further adverse psychological consequences, such as increased self-blame and hopelessness, if we are aware of personal contributions to our own suffering and loss that we have been unable to circumvent.

Our psychological functioning as influenced by our childhood will affect the life choices and decisions we make, the path we follow into adulthood and the nature of our subsequent adult social and demographic environments. Sometimes these pathways will result in exactly those practical and relational contexts that further increase individual vulnerability to distress in the context of adverse life events, and an increased likelihood of such events taking place. The daughters of mothers with depression show an increased likelihood of developing problematic but committed relationships by age 20 with men who have their own issues and problems, illustrating one such pathway (Katz et al., 2013). In this type of situation a stable, intimate and confiding relationship with their partners may be less likely, problems with home environments, employment, lower incomes and supportive networks may all be more likely, and together with the individual psychological vulnerability of the young women themselves could mean that risk may be increased on all fronts. In addition, teenage childbirth is more frequent in young women with depression (Hammen et al., 2011). In similar ways many of us may play our own, unwitting and unconscious parts in contributing to the evolution of unique, complex and highly variable constellations of vulnerability and risk. And whilst we may make direct contributions at the time to the stressful events that then happen to us, in general we will also be more likely to have bad things happen over which we have no control at all.

When bad things happen research has also shown that the impact of the event, and its capacity to destabilize, is greater if it matches, and bears similarity to past and/or present origins of personal vulnerability in individually meaningful ways (Goldberg & Huxley, 1992): painful relational experiences may bear similarity to the ways in which we were treated in our childhoods; a current experience may repeat a similar damaging event in our recent past, or be a more severe version of an ongoing stressful context (Brown et al., 1987). In similar vein, current events that frustrate and diminish our capacities to be involved in areas of our lives that we are particularly committed to will also show an increased capacity to destabilize us, particularly when they involve the loss of a source of value. These findings validate the current personal meaning and significance of adverse and stressful events, as well as the enduring psychological consequences of the past.

The psychosocial research outcomes available to us support a complex process of individual diatheses interacting with provoking life events, and is probably best encompassed by a transactional perspective which recognizes that interpersonal processes and the environmental contexts in which we live can both contribute to the occurrence of those life events. The nature of our psychological vulnerability resulting from our developmental experiences, will interact with the provoking agents that unfold within our lives, and the environmental and relational contexts of those lives will influence whether or not we are significantly destabilized by them.

Our resilience to the impact of adverse events will depend on the quality of our past developmental experiences and our current relationships (Goldberg & Huxley, 1992; Goodman & Lusby, 2014; Rutter, 1991), and we will derive protection in the present from the more severe impact of events if we are involved in a secure, intimate, personally satisfying, confiding relationship that effectively supports and cares for us in times of need and crisis (Brown et al., 1987; Goldberg & Huxley, 1992). In addition, Goldberg and Huxley (1992) pay attention to restitution and recovery from psychological destabilization, reviewing the research that identifies personal and environmental factors associated with it. These include less vulnerable personalities, which may be associated with memories of better maternal care in the past and fewer rows with others in the present; a decreased rate of undesirable events; no decrease in social support; close confiding relationships that provide crisis support; social advantages such as good housing and better incomes; and fresh-start events, defined as important life changes that engender new hope and new possibilities.

The Particular Relevance of Gender and Sexual Orientation

Our gender is a universal and central aspect of our human selves, and one that plays a significant part in the nature of our individual identities. Our biological sex leads to genetically based physical and physiological differences between female and male, and to potentially complex interactions between genetics, biology and our cultural and relational environments that mediate the effects of gender on the nature of our psychological selves. The nature of our sexual orientation as heterosexual, bisexual, lesbian, gay or an orientation within the wider range beyond these categories, will also be inherently important in these respects, as will our gender identity which may be consistent with our biological sex, cisgender, or different from it, non-cisgender. All of these factors will affect our beliefs, expectations and attitudes in relation to ourselves and other people, and how other people behave towards us.

From the overall perspective of Western culture, research endeavours have looked at the gender related context of mental health problems and the experience of psychological distress in ways that overlap with the psychosocial research discussed above. Unfortunately, psychosocial research in the 20th century tended to treat men and women as homogeneous groups reflecting heterosexual and cisgender categories, as far as sexual orientation and gender identity were concerned, leaving those people within the LGBT+ (lesbian, gay, bisexual, trans and other orientations) spectrum as invisible, hidden sub-groups, and sexual orientation and gender identity as variables not deemed worthy of interest and study.

This brief overview will reflect gender related research that has valuably contributed to our understanding of the relevance of gender, but has not taken sexual orientation or gender identity into account. It will also refer to more recent approaches to considering the psychosocial situations of LGBT+ people, and will consider the potentially complex inter-relationships between our sexual orientation, sex roles, gender identities and psychosocial environments.

Overall in Western European and North American societies, women experience more psychological distress and difficulties associated with anxiety and depression compared with men, and greater co-morbidity (Craske, 2003; Gove & Tudor, 1973; Kuehner, 2003). Globally, meta-analysis confirms this sex difference in relation to depression across 29 countries, with greater differences being associated with low gender equity (Hopcroft & Bradley, 2007). Nolen-Hoeksema (2006) provides a comprehensive consideration of a range of interactive factors that may be associated with this greater distress.

In looking at the impact of environmental and demographic factors, heterosexual marriage and employment have been shown to relate to depression in different ways depending on gender. Marriage may be more beneficial for men than women. Employment is more straightforwardly associated with reduced depression in men, whilst for women its benefits are influenced by the domestic context of their lives. Employment may exist in conflict with the demands and needs of domestic and family life, particularly bringing up children, and be associated with higher levels of depression (Cleary & Mechanic, 1983).

Sex role stereotypes have their role to play here. The societies and families that we grow up in convey attitudes and perspectives towards us as male or female, and we are influenced in the development of our own automatic perspectives on ourselves as male or female human beings: what we expect of ourselves, how we believe it is acceptable to behave, what we think and feel about who we are, what we value in ourselves, the roles that are important to us and our attitudes towards other people. For example, in relation to emotion, parents have been shown to discuss emotion related themes with girls more than boys (Fivush et al., 2000). Research in the 1970s looked at the implications of masculine, feminine and androgynous (a mixture of masculine and feminine) sex-role stereotypes. The culturally recognized characteristics of masculinity are associated with the capacity for agency, and those of femininity with the capacity for interpersonal connection and communion (Bakan, 1966; Bem, 1974; Carlson, 1971). Either gender may endorse a traditional masculine or feminine stereotype, or reflect psychological androgyny with a balanced mixture of both. Overall, for both genders a feminine stereotype has been most strongly associated with depression, and androgyny with low levels of psychological distress (Bem, 1974, 1975; Hingley, 1981, 1983).

Our gender influences the nature of our biological and our psychological selves, with both being in interaction with each other. Culturally driven gender related expectations and attitudes influence how we think and feel about ourselves, our goals and wishes in life and our reactions to life experiences. They will also influence our behaviour towards other men and women, girls and boys, and the ways in which we are all treated by individuals, groups and organizations.

Within this constellation of influences it would appear that to be more traditionally feminine, with strong capacities for connection, emotional sensitivity and communion but without having similarly strong capacities for assertiveness, action and agency may carry an increased risk of depression and anxiety in the context of problematic environments and adverse life experiences, for both men and women. In some respects, it may be that men with a traditional feminine stereotype could be more vulnerable than women, since they may also feel inadequate and more critical of themselves as men for lacking traditionally valued masculine attributes. It seems most likely that part of the overall equation relating to the impact of our gender on our lives lies in the greater valuing of capacities for agency rather than communion within industrialized Western society.

From psychodynamic perspectives the importance of gender within psychotherapy has received some particular attention. Eichenbaum and Orbach (1983) discuss the benefits of female clients having a woman as their therapist, in relation to the overall transference relationship between mother and daughter, and the value of experiencing autonomy and separation from a woman. They also discuss gender related projection and projective identification within heterosexual couples, looking at the tendency for women to carry the feelings of insecurity and dependency for both partners. It may also be useful at times to consider the potential fear of women's power, and the possibility for characteristics that are experienced as unacceptable for one person to emerge particularly strongly within their partner by a process of projective identification. For example, a woman's hidden anger and forcefulness may emerge within and contribute towards her partner's aggression; whilst his hidden emotional hurts may fuel the intensity of her experiences of painful feelings. From these perspectives a hope for therapy may be that greater integration of these unacceptable aspects of self may emerge for both parties, so that the divides of agency and communion may to some extent be softened, with growth and development being facilitated on both sides. From a behavioural perspective, the potential lack of agency within women may be particularly addressed by assertiveness training that hopes to empower women, increasing their self-esteem, reducing self-blame, and increasing self-respect and self-determination.

In terms of the overall vulnerability to psychological distress across gender, the tendency for men to have greater problems in relation to substance misuse compared with women and to be twice as likely as women to successfully take their own lives, points towards a context in which men's psychological vulnerability may far too often remain hidden (Williams et al., 2014). Part of the difficulty seems to lie in the gender related barriers that can make it much harder for men to recognize and acknowledge emotional/ psychological issues, experiences and problems (Englar-Carlson & Stevens, 2006; Kingerlee et al., 2014; Meth & Pasick, 1990), and for them to get support if they do: "women seek help - men die" (Möller-Leimkühler, 2002, p. 3). Men may experience a decreased sensitivity to their own and others' feelings, or become intolerant or confused in the face of emotion. The rational may become too highly valued compared with the emotional aspects of human living, with feelings being defended against in ways that disguise them from self and others. In this context intimacy may become a challenge and be automatically avoided, and alcohol or other addictive substances may be used to avoid problematic emotions, maybe even before they are consciously felt. The outcome may also be a greater prevalence of stress-related physical disorders, as well as a prevalence of anger-related problems, since anger may be the more acceptable emotion in a valued masculine world, and a natural outcome of thwarted or ineffective agency (Meth & Pasick, 1990).

None of the above research included sexual orientation or gender identity as research variables. As an overall group, research has indicated that LGBT+ people in the UK and the US experience disproportionately high rates of psychological and mental health problems such as depression, anxiety and suicidality, potentially associated with aspects of discrimination and the experience of violence (Bidell, 2016). Research by Blair and Holmberg (2008) has supported the positive association between social support, romantic relationships and mental well-being for sexual minority populations, echoing the research outcomes from psychosocial research in general.

In terms of the relationships between gender, biological sex, sexual orientation, sex role stereotype and gender identity, various combinations may emerge for individuals, which will be part of their unique personal selves, and be influenced by the nature of the social and physical world around them. We will each be affected by the overall social contexts of our lives, as we grow up and as we live our adult lives, and our sexual orientation and gender identity will be in there somewhere, maybe hidden within our own normalized assumptions, or existing as a central, maybe stark and ever-present influence on us, our psychological well-being and our relationship with the world around us.

In all of the above respects gender becomes an issue to be held in mind and considered in relation to every client that we see, as well as the potential significance of sexual orientation and gender identity. Sometimes the ubiquity and familiarity of gender difference within our lives, and assumptions about sexual orientation and gender identity, may mean that we take some of these contexts for granted, rather than using our understanding to help us think more deeply as therapists about the person before us, and the woman or man that they are in their own eyes, ours and the eyes of others.

The Context of Difference and Discrimination

Psychosocial contexts of difference and discrimination can lead to psychological distress and potentially serious mental health problems in a very wide range of circumstances. Any context in which we are negatively discriminated against can adversely affect us, with such discrimination often reflecting the misuse and abuse of power. This may particularly happen in relation to our age, gender, gender identity, sexual orientation, race, religion, disability or mental health problem. In all contexts we face the potential for bias, misconception, overt prejudice, dislike and even hatred. These may result in inappropriate, invalidating and often unfair treatment and in extremes, abuse and even physical attack, with unhelpful and maybe powerful and damaging consequences in terms of our psychological well-being.

Summary

This chapter has highlighted the importance of the world around us, particularly recognizing the significance of our relational worlds in the past and the present, the impact of adverse life events, the importance of our current close relationships and the attitudes towards us of friends, colleagues and wider society. All of these factors interact with our current psychological selves. Our gender, gender identity, and sexual orientation; our disability status; our ethnicity; our religion and our age all play important parts in these respects. We are also significantly influenced in our psychological wellbeing by the overall financial context of our lives, the quality of our homes, the nature of our employment, and our access to resources that can enhance our sense of who we are, bring us together with other people and provide satisfaction and pleasure. This chapter has overviewed a sample of the often-complex literature in relation to these contexts.

Contexts and Environments: Our Place in the Lifespan

12

As well as living in our own unique social and demographic environments and being potentially affected by the range of contexts discussed in Chapter 11, each of us exists at any one time at a particular juncture of the time-limited span of our human lives. The place we occupy in this respect will be associated with particular age-related psychosocial and practical environments, types of events and transitional experiences, and over our lifespan we will change in our capacities to interact with those environments.

We are born, we grow, we age, we develop, and at any point we may die. Finally, death comes to us all. We are continually adapting to both subtle and major changes in the context of our lives, the capacities of our minds and the physical nature of our bodies, as we grow up and grow older; the process of psychological development, the challenges and opportunities presented by transition, transformation and adaptation, and the benefits of consolidation are always with us. We have the potential for growth and development until the very end of our lives, at whatever age that takes place for each of us. These core principles can advise and support us as psychotherapists in relation to our clients at every point in their lifespan.

Models of Lifespan Development

Various approaches, models and metaphors have been described to support us in thinking about the nature of these psychological contexts, and the changing nature of our lives at different points in the lifespan. Multiple environmental factors interacting with each other and with our individual psychological and physical selves will influence our developmental processes, our functioning, the life events we are faced with and the quality of our lives. Sugarman (2001) and Hendry and Kloep (2012) provide discerning overviews of a wide range of both traditional and rather more progressive approaches. It is not feasible to provide a similarly intensive coverage here, and this Chapter will largely be restricted to a discussion of themes and issues that seem particularly important or useful in the context of therapeutic practice.

With the aim of conveying the complex ecology of the environments that influence our early development as children, and later lives as adults, Bronfenbrenner (1979) considers us all to be affected by a set of interacting immediate and increasingly distant, organizational and cultural influences, each nested within the others, with us at the centre; much as a Russian doll exists inside a number of other increasingly larger dolls. Most immediately around us we have our family, then our adult peer group or our school classroom as children, our work place if we are employed as adults, and any other organizational structures that may be available to us if we are not employed or have retired. These contexts, and other social and leisure contexts, constitute a network of personal settings, and what happens in each of them may affect the nature of what happens in the others, our experience of them, our processes of development and our experience of ourselves. Our differing immediate environments influence each other, and are influenced by those of the larger institutions of our societies and the cultures that they reflect, including economic, educational, political, governmental, mass media and religious institutions. The culture that influences all levels of this nested ecological system is portrayed as the outermost layer of our psychosocial Russian doll.

This is a model that can be applied to societies and cultures the world over, and is an ecological system in which the nature of the personal settings around us, our relationships with them, and the influence on us of wider institutions and culture will change as we move through the span of our human life; all will play their part in the nature of our developmental processes and the nature and quality of our everyday lives. In his final work, Brofenbrenner emphasizes that individuals, on their own and collectively, influence the people and institutions of their ecology as much as they are influenced by them (Brofenbrenner, 2005). It is within this complex transactional bioecological context that our therapeutic interventions in whatever form they are applied, will always be taking place.

Other models and frameworks provide a sense of structure to the unfolding patterns of the individual, family, social and occupational contexts of our lives from birth, though infancy and childhood, adolescence and into adulthood, older age and our ultimate age-related dying. Within these models our lifespan tends to be divided into the specific stages of childhood, adolescence, early, middle, young-old and old-old adulthood. Between and often within these stages we are faced with transitions from one relatively steady, familiar state to new and probably unfamiliar ones. Detailed attention may be paid to the nature of individual psychological development across these stages, with our development at each stage being understood as involving the achievement or not of particular developmental tasks, and our involvement in the range of roles that we might fulfil, such as worker, service user, parent, friend, son or daughter, spouse or lover. Typically, the processes and outcomes of each stage are influenced by the outcomes of the stages that have preceded them.

In many instances stage related models of development and change across the lifespan have been advised by aspects of empirical research. Whilst this valuably provides a basis in the reality of human lives, it will reflect only the lives of those people selected to be participants in such projects, and the results of group-based data analyses. Within this data, individual differences and uniqueness may be lost and many aspects of socio-demographic context may fail to be represented. Whilst potentially guiding our thoughts towards some of the possibilities for development and growth within our clients' lives, their content may not relate to the unique context and unpredictable unfolding of those lives, and assumptions and expectations in those respects may be actively unhelpful at times. They also have the potential to be overtly damaging when seen by people as pointing towards their failure to achieve the expectations of so-called normal development.

They may also be at risk of reflecting rather negative cultural positions at different points in the lifespan, particularly in relation to older age and the processes of change towards the end of life at that time. Sugarman (2001) provides a very salient example of this when she tells us of the views of Cumming and Henry in the 1960s who saw social role disengagement, and shrinkage of the life space from 65 years onwards as the normal healthy approach to ageing. They classified people between 70 and 75 with a large number of roles and/or a high daily interaction with others as unsuccessful disengagers (Cumming & Henry, 1961). We have certainly moved on from that dramatically biased and negative position, which did prompt serious criticism at the time. However, it does illustrate the extent to which theoretical positions can be distorted by culturally based belief systems. We could still argue that in general, positive and enabling attitudes towards adults in the 65-90 plus age range are sadly lacking, particularly in Western society.

Developmental theory continues to focus most intensively on the capacities gained during the earlier phases of the lifespan, limiting the extent to which the developmental tasks of young-old and old-old adulthood may be addressed from a constructive perspective, failing to recognize the vitality and capacities of older adults, their contribution to society, and the huge challenges many face and deal with, in terms of disability, loss and isolation: challenges that many people may have found overwhelming at earlier, younger stages of their lives, as might the younger people who currently live alongside them.

Maybe to develop such models would challenge lifespan theorists to include contexts of loss, lack of opportunity, and personal incapacity or disability within the earlier stages of the lifespan as well, rather than by default tending to present those stages as only involving positive opportunities for growth and development, sometimes in rather idealized ways. It would also mean that our societal and global difficulty in accepting mortality and death would need to be faced. Whilst fearful of death and disability, we are often fearful of old age, and potentially avoidant and maybe critical of older people, a situation that has been seen to reflect the principles of terror management theory (Martens et al., 2005), and which draws on Ernest Becker's ideas in his classic text *The Denial of Death* (Becker, 1973). This is a situation that can involve older adults themselves just as much as younger people; currently in older adulthood we are the only age-related group that tends not to identify positively with their own age-group. Our negative stereotypes can end up being applied to our peers, and sometimes to ourselves, both with unhelpful and damaging consequences.

The rest of this chapter will be devoted to an overview of Erikson's approach to stages of human psychosocial development and ego identity (Erikson, 1980; Erikson & Erikson, 1998), and attention to aspects of current life span models that may valuably support the capacities of psychotherapy to promote constructive change and development. The chapter will end with a look at some of the more recent developments in relation to older adulthood.

Erikson's Approach to Psychosocial Development

Erikson's work was advised by psychoanalytic theory during the 1950s to1970s and devoting this space to his work reflects my belief that it still holds a unique place in its exploration of core internal psychological changes that play potentially fundamental parts in the development of our human self across the lifespan. He sat somewhat at a crossroads in terms of Freudian psychoanalytic theory, supporting the importance of a psychosocial rather than psychosexual basis to psychological development, whilst at the same time still seeing aspects of Freudian oedipal theory, and the traditional requirements of masculinity and femininity as factors influencing the nature of developmental process and the psychological conflicts and crises that may be experienced along the way.

In certain respects, his work connects with aspects of attachment, object relations and humanistic theories as well as broader based psychodynamic approaches. It also puts clear emphasis on the importance of individual experiences of achievement and ability, capacities to cooperate with other people, and the central importance of being genuinely valued by significant others. In these respects, it is in effect an integrative approach to life span development and has much to commend it in support of our current approaches to psychotherapy. Erikson's work encompasses the following stages of development:

Basic trust versus basic mistrust: Basic trust is seen as being acquired during the first year of life and depends on the ways in which we are cared for by those most important to us. If we receive what we need in terms of sensitive love, care and physical attention, regulated by mutuality and reciprocity, we will come to experience what Erickson refers to as a reasonable trustfulness in others, and a simple sense of ourselves as trustworthy; we will have a fundamental and implicit sense of trust in the capacity of the world around us to fulfil our needs, and in our own body's capacity to fulfil its physical functions, defined by Sugarman (2001) as a sense of inner certainty as well as outer predictability. Without basic trust the way is open for fundamental and deep anxiety to interfere with all of our subsequent human psychological development; it constitutes the basis of our existential security and is the bed-rock for our secure development of self.

This position is fundamentally consistent with the importance of the secure, attuned attachment relationship, and Winnicott's position in relation to the crucial place of mirroring in infancy, and the reliability of the total maturational environment (Winnicott, 1965/1990). The consequences of an absence of basic trust echo Balint's concept of the basic fault (Balint, 1968).

Autonomy versus shame and doubt: With growth and physical development comes an increasing capacity for infants, children and young people to assert their own autonomy, and Erikson sees the ways in which parents deal with this as being of crucial importance. Both tolerance and firmness are essential within the context of sensitive, caring mutual regulation. The balance between love and hate, between cooperation and wilfulness, and between freedom and self-expression and its suppression, are all involved in the parental balancing act of support for the child's autonomy alongside necessary limit setting, firmness and protection. Erikson's ultimate hope for the child is for self-control without loss of self-esteem, from which he believes he or she will gain a lasting sense of autonomy and pride, rather than the lasting doubt, inadequacy and shame associated with parental over-control, however that may be motivated. Parallels may be seen here with Kohut's concept of optimal frustration (Kohut, 1977, 1984).

Erikson believes that the gaining of basic trust and the safe experience of autonomy free of guilt and shame, are the essential ingredients that enable the child to develop the sense of being a person.

Initiative versus guilt: The child that is a person, with a capacity for being an autonomous self now develops his or her capacity for initiative in discovering the sort of person they may become, in all sorts of respects. This process is assumed to start at about 3 years of age, and includes identification with parents and other adults, and imitative play and exploration as social relationships are made with other children. It is closely associated with the continuing evolution of autonomy.

Initiative may be impeded by guilt, and sometimes valuably so when parents and an evolving conscience rein in certain behaviours, but it may be thwarted to a damaging extent if overwhelmed by parental and moral concerns. It is seen as the basis for curiosity about the world surrounding the child and for his or her enduring sense of ambition and capacity for independence. The capacity for a sense of conscience and morality also needs to develop alongside this evolution of initiative, and is supported by constructive capacities to experience guilt and shame in relation to the needs of others.

In parallel with Winnicott's concept of the defensive, self-protective false self (Winnicott, 1986) and Rogers' ideas about conditions of worth versus organismic valuing (Rogers, 1951/2003), Erikson recognizes the risk that parentally induced excessive guilt and shame, and too much conflict with parents around the issue of initiative, may result in self-restriction that stops individuals from developing to their full potential.

Industry versus inferiority: Here Erikson focuses on the evolving capacity for the child to learn, create and make, in essence to be busy with an activity, watching how others do things and trying it out for themselves, in ways that often involve co-operation with other children, and at a time that often naturally coincides with starting school. He sees the child's sense of identity as evolving from being based on what he or she receives from others at the stage of basic trust, what they choose to do at the stage of autonomy versus shame, what they can imagine they will be at the stage of initiative versus guilt, to being what they learn and come to know and produce at the stage of industry versus inferiority.

Rather than the basis of identity changing between stages, this can best be envisaged as an additive model, with each stage adding a further basis on which our sense of ego-identity is founded. We now start to have a sense of who we are that is fed by the knowledge and skills we learn, that become assimilate into our sense of self. Children will be markedly influenced in these respects by the nature of their learning and educational environments and relationships, and the cultures that underpin them.

The ways in which such environments balance the natural play related tendency for children to guide their own discovery and learning, with the prescriptions of what any one culture defines as needing to be learnt, is seen as crucial. Too much prescribed learning may destroy an individual's natural desire to learn and to work, but too little leaves them under-stimulated and deprived of essential and exciting knowledge and abilities. Both are needed for children (and adults) to gain a sense of capacity, ability and creativity that they can be proud of, a positive sense of self related to achievement and industry, which reduces the risk of inadequacy and inferiority and fosters natural creativity. In addition, Erikson sees the impact of unequal opportunities across gender, race, and wealth versus poverty as resulting in lasting harm to the child's (and adult's) sense of identity.

Identity versus identity diffusion/role confusion: This stage of development relates to the ending of childhood and the journey through youth and adolescence; the challenges of body growth, genital maturity, and new social and relational opportunities and experiences in the context of increased consciousness of self. Up to this time a growing sense of ego-identity has been evolving on the basis of the accrued processes of each developmental stage. Erikson defines this as the experience of a vitalizing sense of reality, and a sense of the self as having an equal place alongside others in terms of individual capacities to function effectively, which is appreciated and valued by other people. In a belief that is reflective of Carl Rogers' emphasis on the importance of genuineness, he emphasizes that this valuing has to be wholehearted and consistent, and relate to real accomplishment; it has to be genuine.

The nascent sense of identity achieved by the end of childhood faces the risk of identity diffusion or confusion if adolescent youth struggles to find a clear sense of direction within the sometimes-bewildering array of work related and professional options that may be available, or alternatively is faced with a social context in which few such options exist at all. Erikson sees the primary source of disturbance in young people as the inability to settle on an occupational identity: a painful context which itself may be defended against by alternative identity options based on intolerance of difference in others, or on over-identification with particular well-known individuals or powerful social/political groups.

Intimacy versus isolation and self-absorption: Late adolescence and young adulthood crucially include new experiences in terms of mutual psychologically intimate and often sexually intimate relationships. It is Erikson who points out that our capacity for healthy intimacy with another will be greatest when our own ego-identity is established on a secure foundation. The deep connection of intimacy challenges the nature of our boundary of self, and may only be possible if we have sufficient confidence that our own self will remain intact. If we avoid intimacy, we condemn ourselves to degrees of isolation, and may often live with a precarious balance between the two. Alternatively, we may bolster an insecure sense of identity by an intense attachment to another, which may result in contexts of inequality, dominance and subordination.

Generativity versus stagnation: Erikson primarily sees generativity within adulthood as the most important achievement at this stage of life. He defines it primarily in terms of support for, and creative investment in, the next generation, particularly in the context of parenting and education. It draws upon broad based capacities for creativity and altruism, and is reflected in active approaches towards influencing the positive nature of current and future human societies. The experience of being needed, of giving and taking care, and of producing and maybe leaving behind something that is good, are seen as crucial aspects of healthy adult human experience. In later life the generativity of adulthood helps us to live with the losses often associated with older age, and the final ending of our own lives. Creativity, and the production of something that may be of benefit to others, for as long as we are able, confers a sense of meaningfulness and value that we are deprived of, if it is absent from our lives. Without such generativity we may experience psychological stagnation, leading to personal impoverishment and ultimately to despair.

Integrity versus Despair and Disgust: Erikson describes a state of ego-integrity or ego-integration and fulfilment in this final stage of the life-cycle that can be the ultimate outcome of constructive development within each of the preceding seven stages. This is seen as existing in contrast to the experience of despair, and of a disgust and bitterness towards the world around us that may mask an internal despair, when development has been marred within earlier stages, and when generativity has not been able to evolve during adulthood. Integrity is seen as enabling us to accept our own lives for what they have been without unhelpful regret, and ultimately to be able to say goodbye to those lives when we die. Crucially in this respect, Erikson is one of the main theorists to appreciate our potential for positive processes of psychological growth and development up until the last days and possibly even the last moments of our life.

Lifespan Approaches in the Context of Psychotherapy Practice

Models of life span development usefully contribute to our thinking about the ways that people are currently living their lives, and what might be feasible and helpful for them to change. Are they being held back by some aspect of psychosocial development that could have taken place but has not yet unfolded for them? And if it hasn't why might that be the case? Has some life transition proved particularly challenging, or come upon someone at a totally unexpected juncture? Are there roles within their lives that they are struggling to fulfil, or that they have not contemplated or have actively avoided; how might these situations be understood and maybe helped to change? And conversely, are there roles and activities that particularly sustain their sense of self and identity and bring pleasure and joy into their lives? What are their thoughts and feelings about the point they are at within the life span, and does their perspective on the future play a part in the context of the present? This last theme will be one that can be important at any stage of the lifespan, but may also become particularly salient as we move towards older age.

Many approaches to psychotherapy, through their exploration of the ways in which people are currently experiencing themselves and the context of their lives, will automatically touch on a lot of the issues that lifespan development gives specific attention to. Its models in many ways will back up and endorse the importance of lifespan related content and process that we might pursue anyway, but they may also point us in directions that we might otherwise miss completely, and encourage us to think about all of them from a constructive developmental perspective at all positions across the lifespan, particularly ones that are very different from our own.

Our personal direct experience of living through different stages of the lifespan, the unfolding lives of our family members, friends and others, and the lives that our clients have described to us, may all feed into our capacities to empathize with and appreciate the lifespan related contexts that matter for the people who come to see us. The extent to which we are able to reflect on our own thoughts and feelings about the stages that we have not yet experienced will matter too. We may struggle to really appreciate the contexts of other people's lives at ages and life stages we have not yet reached, as well as those that take place in social contexts very different to our own. In any of these respects our capacities to truly listen and hear those clients will matter a lot.

Carl Jung's emphasis on the importance of living in tune with our current stage of life (Jung, 1960/2014), rather than trying, or being expected, to be at a different one, is salient here. Maybe we cannot expect people who are younger to truly appreciate what it might be to be older, because to do so might spoil their capacity to fully live their young life. Similarly, our experiences across the lifespan and our processes of learning, adaptation and change may make it a challenge for adults and older adults to identify with young people at times. These factors may sometimes influence the nature of relating that is possible in psychotherapy when therapists at one life stage are working with clients who are in a very different lifespan position, however caring, empathic and sensitively aware therapists may be.

Since the recognition of developmental processes is virtually always intrinsic to psychotherapy in the context of working with children and adolescents, it is with our clients in young, middle and later adulthood that our life span approaches are likely to be of particular benefit in prompting us to take aspects of current lifespan development and context into account. In doing so we may find existing traditional models useful but also lacking in important ways. As Sugarman (2001) discusses, many of our traditional models see development in terms of value-based ideas about improvement, relating to an 'onwards and upwards' process over time which is likely to be unrealistic and risk engendering negative judgements of self for many people. At times they may convey idealistic perspectives on human beings, such as Maslow's self-actualized person, that most of us would fail to live up to (Maslow, 1943).

Enabling people to realize their own potential as human beings is a very different thing compared with the perfect person being advocated as a norm. In addition, the potentially perfect person of our adult years may be felt to be at even greater distance from the person we experience in old-old adulthood, when physical abilities have been lost and dependence on others may be essential for current existence. The risk of idealization versus denigration across the life span is enhanced. However, these approaches do valuably point us towards the importance of recognizing positive constructive potential in all of us, which may enable us to flourish at any point in the lifespan in some way that has not been possible so far.

Our awareness of aspects of transition, challenge and change that may be experienced as we move through the lifespan can help us to explore possibilities with individual clients. We may think more about relevant lifespan related transitions, the potential for transformation, and periods of consolidation, life events, social roles, and associated practical and relational tasks than we might otherwise have done, and about potentially salient internal processes of psychological development that people may be struggling with at conscious and unconscious levels. The lifespan approaches of Baltes & Baltes (1990); Erikson (1980); Havinghurst (1972); Levinson (1978, 1986, 1996/2011); and Super (1980) would all be relevant in these respects, and Hendry and Kloep (2012) provide a particularly sensitive analysis of adolescent developmental contexts.

Within therapy it is important to recognize the overall value of the opportunity to reflect on the nature of our lifespan experiences to date. Talking and thinking about our lives so far may result in new understandings of how that life unfolded, that support a more positive, accepting and compassionate sense of who we are, whatever theoretical approach may be guiding the therapy we are involved in. Sugarman (2001, 2004) refers to the value of having an internal cohesive narrative of our lives; a story that defines us. The emotional tone of that story influences our sense of security and wellbeing, and that tone is seen as being laid down in infancy by the nature of our relationship with our care-givers, a context clearly echoing the importance of the secure attachment relationship. Whilst Sugarman recognizes the continuous revision of our life story that evolves over the lifespan, she sees older age as involving only revision rather than construction. A more positive approach to older adulthood would recognize the potential for construction up until the end.

Overall, from a therapeutic perspective we would recognize that valuable aspects of psychological development commonly associated with earlier stages of our life, may still be able to evolve later on in the lifespan, supporting our development at that time and leading to enhanced cumulative developmental experiences from that point onwards. For example, in terms of Erikson's approach, basic trust may have eluded us in infancy and childhood, but a genuine secure emotional attachment relationship within psychotherapy may still support its development, at least to some extent, at any age when we have grown up. Similar processes may be helped to unfold in relation to autonomy, initiative, and industry. All of this is consistent with Kohut's perspective on developmental arrest, and the paths so often followed within psychodynamic/attachment related therapies, as well as client-centred approaches; it is normal to be able to catch up on development at any time.

In relational contexts the more secure we become within our self the better able we may be to allow intimacy into our lives, and in the context of all these changes, creativity and generativity may be enabled to flourish. To the extent that we are able to grow in these respects, we will also be supported in approaching the later stages of our lives and its ultimate ending from a better place than before.

The Particular Context of Older Adulthood

It is within the context of older adulthood that we can find our available models of lifespan development to be particularly lacking. Some models pay both minimal and negative attention to the later stages of life. For example Hendry and Kloep (2012) refer to Levinson's view that from age 65 adults settle into a stable phase of old age and let go of commitments, and to Havinghurst's work as describing our developmental tasks from age 60 onwards purely as adjusting to ageing and coping with bereavement. Neither of these perspectives fire us with any particular positivity towards older age, or recognize our continued potential for growth and development, and may primarily reflect attitudes associated with the lifespan stage of the authors, and the culture of the time.

Jung believed that to try to live as if we were young when we are in the later stages of life would do damage to our soul (Jung, 1960/2014), and this may be true in some senses. It may certainly be unhelpful in some ways to deny the realities of older age and our ultimate dying; but to deny the person we are and might actually become, irrespective of our chronological age, and to be defined by the age we are rather than who we are, may be more damaging. We may psychologically kill ourselves off before our time.

Culture plays a strong role in fostering unhelpful attitudes and stereotypes in relation to older age as reflected in the range of papers included in Nelson's comprehensive volume addressing the issue of ageism (Nelson, 2017). Even when more positive and constructive theoretical positions recognize the vital importance and benefits to older adults of physical and social activities, and their capacities to become actively involved in these respects, the benefits of this awareness tend to be restricted. For many older adults, extra practical and financial resources may be needed to help overcome the aspects of disability, loss of abilities and maybe loss of confidence that limit their access to social engagement and involvement, especially when faced with the loss of old longstanding social networks, and the need to develop new ones.

Attitudes and expectations in relation to work are relevant in this respect. The workplace provides a large part of our social contact, involvement and experience of meaningful, constructive activity. Adults in their mid to late 60s are likely to choose to and/or be expected to retire, but some will wish to remain in active work, on an employed, independent or voluntary basis as long as they possibly can. Whilst many people find good alternatives and experience pleasurable, and meaningful lives after retirement and into older adulthood, not everyone wants to retire and many other people may never experience an alternative source of meaningful social involvement, constructive activity and sense of self.

Overall, we do not have a culture that particularly holds older adults in esteem, or places them and their lifetimes of experience and learning in positions that could be beneficial to society as a whole. We do not enable young and old to make contributions to society in ways that may be mutually supported and advised by each other; instead we typically categorize, separate and divorce one from the other, when integration might be so much more productive for both.

More enabling approaches to the later stages of the lifespan would also need to involve greater acceptance of sources of distress that cannot be changed, when loss of loved ones, one's own strength and abilities, and maybe one's independence can never be resolved or replaced. The processes of grief are very relevant here. Their resolution late in life may need to follow a different path compared with younger years, when alternatives and the possibility of re-engagement and re-attachment could always lie ahead of us. Grief in relation to more absolute loss is something different. Living through that grief may still result in the potential for a calmer psychological place to be reached; eventually we may not be able to look forward at this stage of life in the same way at all, but it may still be possible to engage in a rewarding way with the world around us, as we approach the final challenges of what we now refer to as old-old age or the fourth age (Baltes & Smith, 2003).

As with all challenging psychological processes the experience of a secure attachment relationship, the importance of love and care, are likely to play a crucial part in enabling this to happen. We could argue that the capacity to live through these processes constitutes a developmental task particularly relevant in late-late old age, and we can see them as being consistent with Erikson's thoughts about ego integrity versus despair. Furthermore, in the context of basic trust, we may be best supported in psychologically surviving the ending of our lives when we are nurtured by people who care for us at the end in ways that are similar to the attuned love and care we needed at the start. The nature and quality of our family lives, the close friendships we may be able to maintain, or still make, and the capacity of formal carers to truly care in older adulthood will be crucial for us all.

Hendry and Kloep (2012) particularly recognize the value of an ecological approach towards lifespan psychology recognizing complexity and context. This includes Brofenbrenner's model described earlier, and Baltes' emphasis on the potential for constructive development and growth across the entire lifespan, including powerful and positive impacts in the later years of life (Baltes & Baltes, 1990). This approach recognizes multi-directionality in which the same event can have different outcomes, depending on context, or different events may lead to similar outcomes. It also acknowledges that development very often involves loss as well as gains throughout the lifespan, and recognizes the importance of plasticity and the value of active training and skill development at all stages of life, especially in older adulthood.

In particular, Baltes and Baltes (1990) advocate a selection, optimization and compensation model which is relevant across the lifespan. Life goals need to be selected so that they may receive focused attention, and the effort and resources that may be needed to achieve these goals are then optimized to give the best chance of achievement. In some instances, this may involve compensation if there has been a loss of available personal resources for any reason, by the addition of other resources that may compensate for the loss. Adaptation is used in these respects to enable goals to be aimed for in response to developmental challenges at any point in the lifespan. Hendry and Kloep (2012) make the connection between the nature of our personal resource systems and our sense of security. If our resources are sufficient to deal with the challenges we face, our sense of security and contentment are enhanced, and in some respect we will have developed further as human beings, whatever our age.

Summary

In Chapter 12 we have acknowledged the continuing value of traditional stage related models of lifespan development as well as their limitations, revisited Erikson's classical approach to psychosocial development, and considered some more recent approaches, particularly in relation to older adulthood. The function of psychotherapy at any point in the lifespan is to enable and increase the individual's capacity to live their lives in constructive rather than unhelpful and damaging ways, if it is possible to achieve that within their socio-economic and relational environments. Our work in this respect may be advised and supported by theories relating to lifespan development, or it may run counter to some of those theories when they themselves have been unhelpfully influenced by counterproductive cultural attitudes and beliefs.

Part 3

Dialectically Integrated Psychotherapy

Introduction to Part 3: A Dialectical Approach to Theoretical Integration

13

Part 3 constitutes the theoretical heart of this work. It describes the analytical process that leads to the development of the Unifying Dialectical Model of human psychological functioning, the UDM, and the Dialectical Integration of Approaches to Psychotherapy, DIAP, meta-framework that constitute Dialectically Integrated Psychotherapy. The principles and aims defined at the start of the book are put into effect to establish a basis for theoretical integration across the five major approaches described in Chapters 6-10 which also takes into account the environmental and lifespan contexts discussed in Chapters 11 and 12. It is carried out on a dialectical basis and is supported throughout by Roy Bhaskar's critical realism as discussed in Chapter 4.

In Chapter 1 we recognised similarities and differences across our five major theoretical approaches to psychotherapy as we initially considered a brief interaction between myself and my client Joan. We then considered the metaphor of a theatre, in which similarities such as these become the overlapping areas of the spotlights projected by each of these perspectives onto the stage of human psychological functioning. The valuable, unique differences become the areas of the spotlights outside the overlaps. For the spotlights of validated and accepted theories to shine at the same time they need to be compatible with each other, and not in conflict; the light from one spotlight must not automatically cancel out the light from any other.

In thinking about the nature of the human mind, the reality that we only have one mind means that there is only one theatre of human psychological functioning and only one stage. In the terms of Bhaskar's critical realism, our one human mind is an intransitive object with an absolute reality. All our theories about this one human mind are individually moving towards the potential understanding of that same intransitive entity; they are transitive and fallible. If they all ultimately relate to the same intransitive object, and we judge them all to have validity, then they have to be able to work together within that single entity; they have to be compatible with each other. Their spotlights all need to be able to shine together at the same time, without any one of them being in conflict with another and cancelling it out.

The natural consequence of this position is a belief in the fundamentally unified functioning of our human mind, in which all psychological mechanisms and processes are working together in synchrony and unified harmony; in absolute reality incompatibility simply is not possible.

Sometimes aspects of different psychological theories can appear to be incompatible with each other, when on deeper inspection ways may be envisaged for them to co-exist and make mutual contributions to a common outcome. Sometimes incompatibility may exist simply in the eye of the beholder, and theories may come to be accepted as not actually in conflict at all. Sometimes aspects of one or more theories may be judged to have been ill-founded and be discarded, or may be adjusted in some other way that means incompatibility is no longer a problem. Sometimes it is simplified or polarized thinking that results in conflict and incompatibility; when complexity and the existence of continua are brought into consideration, compatibility and complementarity may become more feasible. Thinking about theory, incompatibility and compatibility in this way constitutes a dialectical process, as discussed in Chapter 4.

In Chapter 14 we focus on these issues of incompatibility and discuss the dialectic of compatibility, exploring examples of incompatible difference relating to the work of BF Skinner and Sigmund Freud. As practitioners and theoreticians, we are faced with the choice of whether to ignore or minimise the importance of incompatible differences within and between our theoretical perspectives, or accept their reality and attempt to resolve them in some way. This is of particular relevance when we wish to integrate the beneficial contributions of more than one approach to psychotherapy, and fundamentally important when we aim to bring that integration together on a theoretical basis. This chapter explores the cultural, social and individual psychological contexts that might have influenced these particular authors in relation to significant theoretical positions that have subsequently come to be challenged. In doing so we may be supported in accepting the potential fallibility of our own current transitive beliefs. The chapter also acknowledges and explores the clear issues of incompatibility and compatibility that exist across our major approaches in relation to the nature and pragmatics of therapy practice.

In Chapter 15 we turn all five of our theoretical spotlights on at the same time, and pay some detailed attention to the ways in which they overlap with each other. Theory is looked at purely on its own account, with no reference to the pragmatics of therapy practice, and from a position of epistemological pluralism; approaches that are again reflective of Bhaskar's critical realism. Our only interest at this point is the existence of overlap and difference between the psychological constructs, mechanisms and processes described by each of them, all of which are considered as stand-alone entities whatever their theory of origin. In this sense I am taking down the boundaries between the five approaches. Where substantial overlap exists, this is seen as representing theoretical triangulation, supporting the validity of the construct or process in question. I take the position that when descriptions of theoretical entities appear to be describing the same thing, they are doing so, whether or not that assumption is supported by their protagonists.

Eleven of the most substantial instances of overlap are discussed on this basis, and the cross-theoretical connections associated with each of them are identified. They include five psychological constructs that exist in common across our major approaches, which are referred to as core constructs, with theory neutral terms being adopted for two of them.

In Chapter 16 the different compatible characteristics of these five core psychological constructs, as described across our major theoretical approaches, are brought together to generate integrative descriptions of each of them. This work integrates theoretical positions that are normally kept quite separate from each other, on either side of their epistemological boundaries. In a reality advised by critical realism, there is no reason whatsoever why a characteristic described from one epistemological position should not co-exist with a different but compatible characteristic derived from another position, as part and parcel of the same entity. If they are in conflict with each other, our thinking about them first needs to resolve that conflict. Once any nature of conflict is resolved, our creative thinking is free to consider the richer, overall nature of each construct advised by the wider range of possibilities made available to us in a fundamentally dialectical process.

Chapter 17 describes a theoretically integrated model of human psychological functioning incorporating these core psychological constructs and other key aspects of overlap across our major approaches, the Unifying Dialectical Model. This model then sits at the centre of the Dialectical Integration of Approaches to Psychotherapy, DIAP meta-framework discussed in Chapter 18, which considers the ways in which each of our five major approaches to therapy influence the processes of the Unifying Dialectical Model to achieve constructive psychological change. The Unifying Dialectical Model and the DIAP meta-framework constitute Dialectically Integrated Psychotherapy. Chapter 19 then discusses some of the ways in which Dialectically Integrated Psychotherapy supports therapists in the provision of flexible theoretically integrated psychotherapy, adapted to the needs of individual clients.

Incompatible Differences and the Dialectic of Compatibility

14

This chapter will look in some depth at the nature of incompatible difference that may exist both between and within theoretical approaches. I will discuss two examples relating to the work of two of our most respected theorists, and use them to review some of the themes that may emerge when we are working with incompatible differences in order to resolve or transcend them in some way. Finally, some thought will be given to incompatible difference in the context of therapy practice.

The Issue of Theoretical Incompatibility

As discussed earlier, in the absolute context of our intransitive human mind, incompatible differences in the nature of mechanisms and processes do not and cannot exist, and all the ways in which our human mind works must be compatible, and not in conflict with each other. On the stage of human psychological functioning, only compatible aspects of our different theoretical spotlights can be on and shine at the same time. If we are not interested in turning these different spotlights on together, we may just adhere strictly to one theoretical perspective. If we do wish to integrate more than one approach within our theoretical understanding and therapy practice, the existence or perception of incompatible difference can limit the theoretical perspectives that we can include.

The challenge is greatest when we find certain aspects of a theoretical approach compelling in their validity and of clear value in practice, in conjunction with other theoretical approaches, while core principles of that approach may be incompatible. A pragmatic solution may be to just ignore the incompatible difference, which is probably what often happens. However, we know that no such incompatibility between mechanisms and processes can actually exist inside our human minds, and the theoretical cause of that incompatibility needs to be resolved rather than simply ignored. Such situations prompt us to question the premises of our current theoretical perspectives, with the possibility of discovering more valid theoretical positions that may bring us that bit closer to the intransitive psychological nature of our human minds. If two theoretical premises about the functioning of the human mind are incompatible, then something needs to change in relation to one or both of them, and either of them may simply be ill founded in some way.

In this current work I am treating the structures, mechanisms and processes described by different theoretical approaches as stand-alone entities that are supported by aspects of observed direct or indirect evidence, rather than seeing them as bound to any one particular theoretical perspective by their epistemological base. In doing so I am not ignoring the importance of the differences between our epistemologies, but see them as reflecting different ways of gaining knowledge of the same intransitive material, a position consistent with Bhaskar's support of epistemological pluralism. An approach to theoretical integration that is advised by critical realism should not ignore aspects of theory as if they did not exist, or run the risk of putting together descriptions of theory that are fraught with inconsistencies. It should face the current realities of incompatible differences between perspectives, and seek to resolve them on as sound a theoretical basis as possible, reducing the risk of the theoretical anarchy that can be associated with atheoretical pragmatism. The core task of dialectics is to find valid ways of moving initially incompatible differences between theoretical approaches to a position in which the differences are now compatible with each other.

Sometimes a theoretical position may only be experienced as incompatible with another perspective if it is applied in a polarized and dichotomous way. If a principle exists on a continuum, or is open to being variable in its application, then a potentially incompatible difference may become one that is more compatible with aspects of other theoretical positions, opening the way for dialectical integrative understanding.

On other occasions the resolution of incompatibility may involve coming to the conclusion that some particular premise is wrong. All approaches may need to accept their fallibility, and all may need to change to some degree. Both similarities between approaches and their compatible differences may then be drawn upon in support of theoretical integration.

When we are faced with making such decisions in relation to aspects of theory, their current validity and incompatibility, it is also helpful to consider what may have influenced their original development, taking political, cultural and personal contexts into account. We may need to accept and understand the fallibility of some of our most revered theorists, as well as ourselves. When we can understand and accept the possible background and motivations that may have influenced the development of theoretical principles that we have now come to question within approaches that we support, it may become easier to formally adapt or remove them.

Two Examples of Incompatibility and Fallibility in Relation to Theory

I will now share some of my thoughts and ideas about ways in which I think B F Skinner and Sigmund Freud might both have been influenced to develop theoretical positions that are incompatible with more recent developments and that in many respects we have moved on from. These examples involve incompatible differences both within and between individual theoretical approaches.

In relation to Skinner I will be looking at the theoretical status of private events and emotion within radical behaviourism, and in relation to Freud I will be looking at his theories regarding the structure of mind, and those relating to the Oedipus complex. Both have held pivotal positions in relation to the development of theory within their particular branches of human psychology, and have knowingly or otherwise contributed to powerful incompatible positions across our academic and applied communities.

B F Skinner: The position of human emotion and other private events within psychodynamic and cognitive theories on the one hand and radical behaviourism on the other constitutes a particularly powerful example of theoretical incompatibility. Within psychodynamic theory emotion is a primary influence within human experience and behaviour, and from a cognitive perspective thoughts and feelings are in constant causal interaction. From Skinner's radical behaviourist position, emotion, feelings and thoughts are all collateral by-products that have no causal function at all (Skinner, 1938, 1974). In the extreme this would remove the entire basis of our human capacity to understand and relate to each other with attunement and empathy. In terms of the roles of emotion and private events in human life the overall spotlight of radical behaviourism cannot shine at the same time as those of psychodynamic, humanistic, attachment and cognitive therapy theories.

Our theory related options are choosing between radical behaviourism and the other approaches, amending radical behaviourism to include the importance and causal power of private events, cognitions and emotion, or taking a pragmatic and instrumentalist approach that simply ignores the incompatible theoretical differences. Currently behaviourally led positions include private events by deeming them to be forms of behaviour.

If we step aside from these issues for a while, we may create some space to ask ourselves why Skinner as an individual person might have naturally adopted the behavioural position he did in relation to human emotion. Skinner seems to have been a sensitive and caring man who was deeply touched by human suffering. He developed the air crib in response to his wish to reduce the mutual distress of his wife and new baby daughter (Bjork, 1997), by creating a controlled physical environment that was seen by him as less challenging and upsetting than it would otherwise have been. It may, however, have reduced the opportunities for mother and infant to come together in the face of discomfort and for that discomfort to be experienced by the infant, recognized and contained by the parent, and resolved through the sensitive provision of comfort and physical care. From psychodynamic and attachment perspectives these would be seen as developmentally important experiences.

I started to wonder whether Skinner found it personally hard to experience human distress and suffering. His wish was to save humanity; he believed we could achieve a better society by paying sole attention to overt human behaviour, and to the control of the environment that influenced that behaviour; and at a theoretical level he removed emotion and all its individual complexities from the equation of causality. If we got the environment right emotion would take care of itself, but within theory it became hidden, almost as if it did not exist. Thinking about this I found myself feeling differently towards Skinner and much less frustrated by his theoretical position in this respect; I was more able to think constructively about the integrative contributions made by radical behaviourism and operant conditioning once I had reached this place in my mind.

In situations such as this we are in a position of choosing to accept some aspects of a theoretical perspective whilst rejecting others. It is this ability to discriminate between different components of a theoretical approach that is crucial to theoretical integration, and it is essential that we feel free to do so. It does seem important, however, that we are open and transparent about the theoretical decisions that we have made. In this context we may, in effect, choose to apply a filter to the spotlight of radical behaviourism, a filter that takes out the belief in the collateral, non-causal status of emotion and other private events, but allows those of operant conditioning and applied behaviour analysis to shine through.

Sigmund Freud: My next example of incompatible theoretical positions involves the continuing reference in psychotherapy literature and colloquial language to Freud's structural model of the mind (Freud, 1911-1940/1984) and to the Oedipus complex (Freud, 1905-1931/1977). Whilst the status of these aspects of theory has evolved and changed considerably over time, there continues to exist something of a theoretical disjuncture between Freudian understanding of the self and the human mind, and of oedipal relating, compared with other psychoanalytic positions, and more clearly between psychoanalysis and other perspectives. Whilst they may well overlap and echo the thoughts of others, I would like to share the thoughts that went through my own mind as I started to think more deeply about the ways in which Freud might have been influenced by social and psychological factors to develop these related aspects of theory.

The structural model of the human mind, involving the id, ego and superego, replaced Freud's earlier topographical position in which the only division was between conscious and unconscious mind. Within post-Freudian developments we have generally returned to his earlier model, with the terms id and superego largely having more metaphorical rather than structural meaning. Fragmentation now tends to be understood rather differently, often being associated with aspects of dissociation, and being reflective of unhelpful and damaging early experience. This position is particularly reflected in Fairbairn's approach to object relations theory and the aims of psychoanalysis (Fairbairn, 1940/1952, 1958). How did Freud come to believe so clearly in a compartmentalized and essentially fragmented ego?

When he retracted his affect-trauma theory of hysteria in the face of powerful negative reactions to his discovery of its connection with sexual abuse, Freud could still not deny the reality of what his patients had told him, the sex would not go away. He needed to find a way of explaining the memories of the sex that should not have happened. His answer was to propose that the repressed memories were the product of the child's wish to have sex with the adult (Brown, 1961). In effect Freud put the responsibility for an adult sexual act into the mind of a child, when a child just does not know, think or feel about the act of intercourse in the same way as an adult mind and body does. The capacity to wish for adult sex and to break the boundary forbidding it then became part of children's minds, and laid the ground for the concept of the id as an infantile part of the adult mind in which unfettered wishes for forbidden pleasures are deemed to originate; wishes and capacities that represent the adult wishes and behaviours that Freud's society found it impossible to bear.

In contrast to the id, Freud represented the internalized adults that children grew up with as constituting the super-ego, the authority figures that guide us in what is right and good to do and to be. The infantile id became the entity that holds what is bad and the adult super-ego the entity that holds what is good in a process of projection and splitting; in some instances this assumed internal representation of moral authority would actually represent a grown-up who has had inappropriate and damaging sex with their child.

These thoughts led me to wonder whether Freud developed a fragmented structural model of the mind as an unconscious consequence of his own psychological processes in the face of trauma, the trauma of uncovered abuse combined with the trauma of a rejection he could not live with.

Within the classical Oedipus complex, it was assumed that boys as young as 3 years old could want to have adult sex with their mothers and fear castration by their fathers in an act of jealousy and anger. In virtually all contexts people do not believe this today, but Freud did. As well as not having the knowledge or sexual maturity to want adult sex, it seems unlikely that a three-year old boy would naturally assume that his father would want to cut off his testicles for that reason. But an adult might wish to do this to another adult who has sexually abused a child. Maybe again the awfulness of sexual abuse, what it can arouse in the human mind and how this might be defended against, emerged as part of Freud's theories.

Through gaining the trust of his female patients and enabling some of them to remember the abuse they had suffered, Freud made an amazing discovery, but neither he nor the society he lived in were in a position to cope with it. The sex that Freud discovered, however, could not be overtly denied or 'put back in the box', and the conflict within him led to the unconscious distortion of psychological theory so that children became responsible although not blamed, the mind became fragmented, and the grown-ups of his time were restored to the position of respectable citizens.

Working with Theoretically Incompatible Difference

These two examples of incompatibility and fallibility in relation to theories that have been central to human psychology and psychotherapy reflect some of the varying contexts and outcomes that can relate to difference. As knowledge develops, earlier theoretical beliefs become replaced and the evolving positions may not be held on a coherent basis within any particular professional community. Choices may be made about aspects of theory that are questioned and maybe rejected, while others continue to be accepted and become more firmly grounded. Differences, particularly incompatible ones, may be ignored or minimized, so that the apparent coherence of a theoretical position may be enhanced. The requirements of logical positivism tend to push us in that direction.

Critical realism on the other hand encourages us to explore the nature of difference, and to look at ways in which we may generate hypotheses about understandable threads of connection, essentially through a dialectical process. Exploring the social and psychological origins of theoretical positions may help us to continue to appreciate and respect ideas and beliefs we later move on from, at the same time as letting them go.

We may also be able to reach less polarized positions in relation to apparently incompatible theories, and be more able to allow for mixtures of possibilities, rather than the answers to theoretical questions being provided in terms of one theoretical position or the other; we may become more able to think in terms of one position and another existing alongside each other. It may also be easier for us to recognize and accept that a theoretical position that is presented as uniquely different, may actually reflect aspects of understanding that are shared with other theories, past and present, although they may be framed within different terminology. We may also creatively reconsider and develop our theoretical positions in ways that resolve incompatibility and in doing so gain in validity. All of these options reflect aspects of a dialectical process.

As human beings seeking to develop understanding of ourselves, we may be particularly open to the influences of our own psychological functioning and needs within the theories we develop. This can apply to every one of us and no one is immune. We may also be influenced by a range of social, political, cultural and structural factors in our immediate and wider environments, and by our individual positions in the life span. We function within very complex open systems. In some respects, we could consider it surprising that we achieve as much consistency in the nature of our theories and our research outcomes as we do.

Issues of Difference Relating to Psychotherapy Practice

We will now turn our attention to issues of difference that relate to the nature and style of psychotherapy practice. The practice of psychotherapy varies considerably across our theoretical perspectives and can provide us with its own examples of incompatible difference.

The principles of therapy practice are developed so that therapists following a particular theoretical approach can influence a sub-set of psychological mechanisms and processes that are judged to be of causal relevance in relation to beneficial psychological change. The nature of the principles of practice will be influenced by the concepts of theory and the beliefs and attitudes of practitioners associated with each therapeutic approach. Different approaches may exhibit aspects of theoretical overlap and triangulation in relation to psychological structures, mechanisms and processes, but may show incompatible difference in the ways in which therapy is conducted.

Significant aspects of compatibility and incompatibility between the practice of different therapies may revolve around issues of structure, planning, control and the nature of interventions. Therapy sessions may be actively planned, structured and explained in advance, or allowed the opportunity to unfold along an unplanned and more unpredictable path. Interventions may directly and explicitly aim to access psychological material such as beliefs, thoughts, feelings, behaviours and patterns of interpersonal relating, or they may seek to facilitate clients in spontaneously revealing these aspects of themselves as they come to mind. Similarly, efforts to help people change may involve planned and overtly structured methods or rely on supporting and enabling the experience of internal psychological processes that then result in changes taking place. We come across the contrasting terms of non-directive versus directive, or exploratory versus prescriptive therapies in this respect. A directive, structured and planned approach to therapy tends to be characteristic of protocol led CBT whilst exploratory therapy that allows process to unfold is more characteristic of psychodynamic and humanistic therapies.

The mechanisms and processes to be addressed in CBT often involve conscious cognition, everyday life experiences and overt behaviours, and techniques are applied to focus attention specifically on them. Information and overt statements about the theoretical approach being taken, what clients might expect to happen, and psychological formulations of their difficulties all constitute aspects of the structure that CBT provides for clients. Overt education and teaching in relation to psychological mechanisms and processes, and their relation to symptomatology are key aspects of therapy. In psychodynamic and humanistic therapy, what the client naturally and spontaneously brings to the therapy conversation is the matter for discussion and attention. Therapeutic responses are designed to facilitate clients' increasing awareness of their own thoughts, feelings, and actions in relation to their life experiences, including those that may initially be hidden from conscious awareness.

From single-model perspectives, concern may exist that non-adherence to a pre-defined style associated with specific therapeutic approaches will reduce the capacity of a therapy to influence the mechanisms and processes that need to be addressed. From a psychodynamic position it may be assumed that the more therapists provide information and explanation, the more goals are decided at primarily conscious levels and set in advance, the more agendas are set and directive processes used to work with aspects of psychological experience, the less experiential space there will be for clients to discover their own naturally unfolding feelings, thoughts, beliefs, fantasies, expectations, wishes and goals. From the position of a protocol directed approach to CBT, the exploration and emergence of previously hidden emotional and relational experience could be seen as a distraction from the required focus on unhelpful conscious cognitions and the work needed to change them.

The more these differing styles of therapy are applied in strict and comprehensive ways, the more the resulting therapies become incompatible with each other in practical terms. If our options are presented as a forced choice between one of these positions or the other, we have to decide between them, and possibilities for practical integration within the same therapy are reduced.

Integrative therapists take a more flexible approach that enables them to use a mixture of styles involving such aspects as planning, structured attention to specifics, and the provision of information and explanation, in addition to allowing sufficient space, time and facilitative support for inner processes to unfold and be thought about. In this situation differences of therapy style are no longer seen as incompatible. This more flexible integrative stance may help us to consider the potential disadvantages of strict adherence to either style. These may include the negative effects of anxiety and uncertainty on client thinking processes in the absence of needed information and shared understanding, or the potential problems of therapist plans for action that clients may feel unsure about but unable to challenge. A broad based, integrative awareness of theory also supports our capacities to think about the style of therapy provision that may best serve the interests of individual clients, and to discuss the options with them.

Summary

In Chapter 14 we have looked at the challenge and importance of openly acknowledging the existence of incompatible differences between theoretical positions, and the benefits of their dialectical resolution. In relation to incompatible differences and the fallibility that may be associated with them, I have discussed my personal ideas in relation to key theoretical positions that were central to the theories of B F Skinner and Sigmund Freud. Finally, the chapter took a brief and introductory look at the relevance of incompatible differences in relation to psychotherapy practice.

In Chapter 15 we will move on to look at aspects of overlap and similarity in relation to psychological constructs, mechanisms and processes identified across the major theoretical approaches to psychotherapy considered in this work.

Overlaps and Theoretical Triangulation   **15**

This chapter focuses on overlaps and instances of theoretical triangulation identified across the five major theoretical approaches to psychotherapy presented in Part 2. Some such overlaps may be anticipated in advance because the developmental paths of two or more approaches may have been influenced by a common perspective. At other times overlaps can emerge between therapeutic approaches that do not have an influencing theory in common, and their overlapping theoretical beliefs may be expressed in quite divergent language. Connection and overlap between perspectives may be overtly acknowledged in some instances, but in others the practitioners and researchers involved may not recognize, or may actively reject, that possibility. As external observers, however, we may see things otherwise.

Those elements of theory that do not overlap, but are not incompatible with each other are all available to contribute to our understanding of human psychological functioning and to the processes of effective psychotherapy on a theoretically integrative basis.

An Analysis of Theoretical Content Across the Major Approaches

This work represents an enhanced version of the type of informal analysis that all of us might undertake as we read, think about and apply differing theoretical approaches to psychotherapy within our everyday practice. Based on the content of Chapters 6-10, I generated lists of key elements of theory associated with each major approach. Overall, I noted a total of 100 elements of theory: 19 for attachment theory; 14 for humanistic theory; 28 for psychodynamic theory; 19 for cognitive and behavioural theory; and 20 for behavioural and cognitive theory.

The lists generated are provided in Appendix 1, and as in all aspects of this work, in order to be manageable, it was not feasible for them to be fully exhaustive or reflect each theoretical approach in its totality.

Comparisons across these lists helped to support and advise my judgements regarding the overlap of theoretical elements across approaches. This work highlights the frequency of theoretical connections, and supports the identification of compatible and incompatible differences.

A few words are also relevant here regarding the theoretical status of unconscious mind. It is rare for cognitive behavioural theories to refer to unconscious mind, although aspects of experience outside our conscious awareness are clearly recognized, as well as the existence of psychological constructs and processes that do not function at the level of conscious awareness. If it is directly discussed, the nature of mind involved in this lack of awareness tends to be described as something that is very different from the unconscious mind of psychodynamic theory, and is generally deemed to be incompatible with it. In this work I take the position that the unconscious mind discussed by psychodynamic theory is not incompatible with the mind that is described as outside of conscious awareness within cognitive behavioural approaches.

Descriptions of Overlaps and Theoretical Triangulation

Overlaps and triangulation support the validity of theory. The compatible differences that are so often part of those overlaps, then provide us with fertile ground for enhanced and dialectically driven understanding. The above informal analysis of theoretical content supported me in identifying the following eleven instances of substantial overlap and theoretical triangulation across our five major approaches. In two instances the differing terminologies used by individual approaches have been replaced by new labels that are as theory-neutral as possible: unconscious internal models of self, others, relationships and the outside world and the constructive developmental relationship.

- conscious mind
- unconscious mind
- the innate capacity for growth
- the processing of emotion
- psychological defences
- the relevance of overt behaviour
- the importance of relational processes
- the importance of past experiences
- unconscious internal models of self, others, relationships and the outside world

- the experience of acceptance
- the constructive developmental relationship

The specific theoretical content justifying these judgements and decisions will now be discussed.

Conscious and Unconscious Mind: Our capacity for the conscious experience of thoughts, emotions, physiological and behavioural responses is a self-evident given for every one of us. All of our approaches to psychotherapy inevitably overlap in this respect, although the specific, focused attention that each theory gives to conscious mind differs considerably. That our minds can and do process experience at an unconscious level outside of our conscious awareness has to be based on the assumed outcomes of that processing. Brewin (1988/2014) and Williams et al. (1997) provide interesting research-based reviews of such evidence from the perspective of cognitive psychology.

The strongest position advocating for the existence and importance of our unconscious mind lies within psychodynamic theory, where powerful processes taking place outside conscious awareness are seen as fundamental to our human existence. Attachment theory overtly recognizes unconscious processing, and humanistic theory allows for aspects of self and experience to become hidden from conscious awareness. Within the CBT umbrella, cognitive therapy theory relies on the existence of latent schemas outside of conscious awareness. Mindfulness Based Cognitive Therapy, Acceptance and Commitment Therapy and Behavioral Activation all appreciate that feelings can become unhelpfully hidden from that awareness, all of which supports the existence of unconscious mind by implication. Functional Analytic Psychotherapy accepts the relevance of private events that exist at an unconscious level. Constructivist Psychotherapy, Compassion Focused Therapy and Safran's approach to cognitive therapy overtly acknowledge, allow for and work with unconscious processes, and Constructivist Psychotherapy explicitly refers to the existence of unconscious mind.

We also find largely implicit support for unconscious processes from within applied behaviour analysis and radical behaviourism, since the reinforcement and association processes of operant and classical conditioning, and the functions they fulfil are mostly not consciously apparent to us, taking place within our minds at an unconscious level. This reality is commented on within Behavioral Activation. The powerful and complex life-long learning histories that automatically feed into current psychological functioning also exist outside conscious awareness.

Whilst considerable inter-theoretical divergence exists regarding its nature and the types of structures, mechanisms and processes that may exist and unfold within it, all five of our major theoretical positions support the existence of unconscious as well as conscious mind.

The Innate Capacity for Growth: Three of our major approaches strongly overlap in advocating the position that all of us have within ourselves the innate capacity and potential to grow, develop and change. We may see this as being articulated most ardently within humanistic theory where it is defined as the actualizing tendency. Within attachment theory Bowlby clearly believes in the existence of this capacity, and from a psychodynamic perspective it ties in well with the classic concept of the life instinct and libido, which was re-defined by Rank as the autonomous striving of the life force, or the will, and is reflected in Winnicott's concept of the true self. It is also clearly supported within Constructivist Psychotherapy from a cognitive perspective. In total four of our major approaches make reference to our innate capacity for growth and development.

The Processing of Emotion: A strong consensus exists regarding the importance of emotion within human psychology and psychotherapy. It is central to so much of psychodynamic and analytic theory, and plays absolutely crucial roles within attachment and humanistic/experiential theories. Within the cognitive and behavioural therapies, access to emotional experience and the soothing of painful emotion is important within Compassion Focused Therapy, and has a core place within Constructivist Psychotherapy and Safran's work on cognitive-interpersonal cycles. It is mutually connected with cognition, cognitive distortions and schema activation and maintenance within more traditional cognitive therapy/CBT interventions, and there is a significant place for the experience of emotion within Acceptance and Commitment Therapy, Behavioral Activation and Functional Analytic Psychotherapy.

Overall within radical behaviourism, human emotions relating to pleasure, displeasure, anxiety and fear constitute the basis for the behavioural processes of operant and classical conditioning. To be either rewarding or aversive within the processes of operant conditioning, behaviour must result in experiences such as these, and although felt emotion as a private event is excluded from the traditional theoretical base of radical behaviourism, emotional reactions lie at the heart of behavioural theory. Similarly, the effects of classical conditioning result from the association between external or internal events and either positive or aversive emotions.

In a range of respects, all of our major theoretical perspectives endorse the central, and fundamentally important place of emotion within human psychological existence and processes of change. In this context Greenberg and Safran (1987) provide a comprehensive review of the ways in which emotion is embedded within psychodynamic, cognitive behavioural and experiential psychotherapy traditions.

Psychological Defences: Defence mechanisms are conscious or unconscious self-protective mental processes whereby feelings and thoughts that cause discomfort, inner conflict, anxiety and distress may be avoided and become hidden from our conscious awareness, or disguised by aspects of distortion so that we no longer experience them in the same way. The term used here is taken from psychodynamic theory where defences constitute fundamental and core understanding, since the same term is often used from within other theoretical positions and has common colloquial understanding.

Attachment theory considers defences primarily from the perspective of the evolving attachment relationship in childhood and the defensive exclusion of emotions and our own needs in the context of insecure attachment. Client-centred theory similarly pays primary attention to defences in the context of our early developmental relationships, and the exclusion of experience from awareness.

Amongst the cognitive behavioural therapies, Mindfulness Based Cognitive Therapy recognizes the existence of painful hidden experience; Constructivist Psychotherapy describes the importance of self-protective processes associated with hidden emotional truths; Safran (1998) acknowledges the functioning of schema related defences/security operations; Compassion Focused Therapy sees cognitive distortions as resulting from defence-related processes; and the powerful influence of avoidance and escape from unbearable suffering is recognized as an underlying motivation for problem behaviours within Dialectical Behavior Therapy.

From a position influenced by radical behaviourism, Behavioral Activation uses the term experiential avoidance to refer to the avoidance of aversive thoughts and emotions which people may not be consciously aware of, and Acceptance and Commitment Therapy discusses the similar experience of emotional avoidance.

All of the above positions are consistent with the basic nature of psychological defences, which are theoretically supported across all of our major approaches.

The Relevance of Overt Behaviour: Behaviour is automatically important across every approach to psychotherapy. We cannot enter the therapy room and talk about ourselves, our difficulties and the lives we lead without talking about our behaviours, even if the actual term is never used. We tend to see the cognitive behavioural therapies, particularly those led by behavioural theory, as the approaches that particularly take behaviour into account and seek to influence it directly. Therapies influenced by attachment, humanistic/client-centred and psychodynamic theories all pay their own intimate attention to behaviour in terms of the ways in which clients' live and experience their lives and their relationships, the ways in which they behave towards themselves and others, and the nature of the varying activities of their lives, but not in terms of the specific details that behavioural theory addresses. Behavioural approaches seek to effect change explicitly by focusing on behaviour directly, while other approaches influence it indirectly and more implicitly.

The Importance of Relational Processes: In different ways four of our five major theoretical approaches pay attention to the specifics of relational processes and the ways in which they evolve between people. For example, within psychodynamic theory we find the principles of transference and countertransference, repeated relational patterns and re-enactments which are echoed by attachment theory. Within the cognitive and behavioural therapies relational processes are specifically addressed by Safran's approach to cognitive-interpersonal cycles. Within behaviourism the operant conditioning and patterns of reinforcement that maintain our lives largely involve relational processes. Much of the theoretical attention to behaviour within behavioural and cognitive theory has an influence on relational processes, and Functional Analytic Psychotherapy specifically addresses operant relational responses to conditioned interpersonal behaviours within therapy sessions.

The Importance of Past Experiences: The principle that our past experiences influence the ways in which we behave in the present has a central place within all of our different theoretical approaches to the human mind and to the process of psychotherapy. All of our major theoretical approaches believe that the past matters, that memories are held within us, and that these memories and the learning associated with them influence us in the present time; whether this relates to the processes of classical and operant conditioning coalesced into a complex learning history, simpler processes of association, the schemas of cognitive therapy theory, the inner world of object relations of psychodynamic theory or the internal working model of attachment theory. Whichever way we look at it, our personal pasts matter enormously.

Unconscious Internal Models of Self, Others, Relationships and the Outside World: Psychodynamic, attachment and cognitive and behavioural theories, whilst using different terminologies, all support the existence of organized memory structures that develop from the start of our lives, are heavily influenced by our early developmental experiences, are maintained and modified during adulthood and influence our day-to-day experiences, behaviours and relationships, very largely without our conscious awareness.

The inner world of object relations is of core importance within psychodynamic approaches to therapy and the internal working model is central to attachment-based approaches. Schemas are crucial aspects of the cognitive and behavioural therapies, with self and interpersonal schemas having particular relevance within Schema Therapy and Safran's approach to unhelpful cognitive-interpersonal cycles. Constructivist Psychotherapy also refers to unhelpful unconscious constructions and meaning-making processes in a similar context, and the importance of schemas is clearly evident within Compassion Focused Therapy.

Functional Analytic Psychotherapy as a modern behavioural approach recognizes the existence of repeated patterns of inter-personal behaviour that originate in past relational experience and live on within our cumulative complex learning histories. These histories encompass patterns of contingencies and reinforcing or punishing experiences from early childhood onwards. They generally exist outside of our conscious awareness and influence our inferences, judgements and behaviours in relation to ourselves, others and the world around us.

Finally, humanistic/client-centred therapy refers to current relationships being coloured by the nature of past relationships. This rather general position is consistent with the concept of unconscious internal models, but is more limited than the examples above and is not seen as in itself justifying a position of overlap or triangulation. In addition, it is relevant to acknowledge the broader-based position of cognitive science in which schemas are seen as the unconscious memory structures that automatically enable us to identify and relate to the entities within our worlds.

In the context of this work on theoretical integration, the entities referred to above as the inner world of object relations, internal working models, schemas and complex learning histories are all judged to relate the same intransitive entity and are defined by the theory neutral term unconscious internal models of self, others, relationships and the outside world. Overall, I have judged this construct to be supported by four of our five core theoretical perspectives.

The Experience of Acceptance: Some attention will now be given to the concept of acceptance within psychotherapy theory and therapy practice, particularly as reflected in the work of Carl Rogers, and the therapeutic approaches advocated by Dialectical Behavior Therapy, Mindfulness Based Cognitive Therapy, Acceptance and Commitment Therapy and Compassion Focused Therapy.

Acceptance can be considered from two perspectives: firstly as referring to our acceptance of ourselves as who we are, and secondly our acceptance of the realities of life as it is currently experienced. In both contexts, acceptance is not being seen as the equivalent of resignation or defeat, or a denial of personal responsibility for our own actions and behaviours. It reflects an acceptance that a certain state of affairs in the nature of who we are and the lives we lead truly does exist; it is not being denied or wished away, or being dealt with by punishing and judgmental attitudes towards ourselves. Its existence is being accepted and experienced in all its reality.

It is in these respects that behavioural therapies such as Acceptance and Commitment Therapy tend to refer to radical acceptance. Seeing and accepting the realities of ourselves, accepting and not punishing ourselves for the problematic and painful aspects of who we are and the lives we lead, may be crucial to the process of change. This acceptance is associated with a reduction in unhelpful defences, and an increased capacity to experience the range of both painful and positive emotions that may be associated with those realities.

Our capacity to accept ourselves is supported by the empathic, attuned acceptance we receive from others. It will also be enhanced by new understanding that makes helpful sense of our problematic ways of being. It improves our self-esteem and self-concept and increases our freedom to become the person we have the natural potential to be. In these respects, it relates strongly to processes associated with psychodynamic, self-psychology and attachment-based theory and practice, although acceptance as a specific concept does not tend to be explicitly discussed within these perspectives.

There is a direct parallel between the way in which Crane (2009) talks about the compassionate understanding and acceptance that can result from Mindfulness Based Cognitive Therapy and the acceptance that is often movingly advocated by Carl Rogers from a humanistic client-centred perspective. Both Rogers and Crane understand that deep and true self-acceptance can facilitate a natural process of growth and change, and the reduction in negative thoughts and beliefs about the self which accompany such changes are usefully articulated by Crane from the cognitive perspective. The concept is similarly reflected within Compassion Focused Therapy (Gilbert, 2010). From Dialectical Behavior Therapy, Acceptance and Commitment Therapy and Behavioral Activation perspectives, acceptance of ourselves and acceptance of the current reality of our lives and our present suffering, are explicitly combined with overt, structured approaches supporting growth, development and change.

Overall, self-acceptance can reduce our internal barriers to positive change, enhance the likelihood that positive growth and development will occur, reduce some of the pain and distress in our lives and increase our capacity to value ourselves. Acceptance of the realities of the current context of our lives may reduce unhelpful negativity and enhance our capacity to make changes where possible, with a starting point that reflects the realities of ourselves and our world as they actually are. Whatever approaches help us to experience these aspects of acceptance, they hold an important place within the psychology of our human mind. Overall, its provision is supported by all five major approaches, with three of them making specific mention of acceptance as a concept and overtly addressing it as a priority.

The Constructive Developmental Relationship: Maybe the most powerful context of overlap and theoretical triangulation to emerge within the detail of the therapeutic approaches discussed in this work lies with the nature and importance of the human relationship that fosters and supports our psychological growth and development. In both overlapping and differing ways we find aspects of this relationship and their relevance to psychological development being recognized and described within all of our major theoretical approaches.

The empathic, genuine and accepting relationship between adults in therapy described by Rogers overlaps with and may be considered the absolute equivalent of the secure attachment relationship of childhood and adult life. The relationship principles of client-centred therapy and the maternal behaviour associated with secure infant attachment constitute a research supported example of triangulation within psychotherapy theory. They are added to by psychodynamic understanding, particularly in relation to Winnicott and Bion from an object relations perspective and Kohut from the perspective of self-psychology. Between them these three approaches assert similar but also unique and compatible understanding of developmentally secure relationships throughout the lifespan.

The very strong overlap between psychodynamic, attachment and humanistic theories regarding the central importance of developmental relationships is one that makes sense in terms of their historical connections. In establishing attachment theory, Bowlby was building on his psychoanalytic starting point, influenced by the object relations theorists, and in developing his client-centred approach to therapy, Rogers was influenced by the relationship therapy of Jessie Taft and the thinking of Otto Rank from post-Freudian psychoanalytic positions.

Whilst it is within attachment, psychodynamic and humanistic theories that we find the core base of explanatory theory regarding the developmental relationships essential to human beings, we also discover strong echoes of these themes playing key roles within therapy-based theories from other orientations. From within the CBT theoretical umbrella, we find very clear reflection of the value of empathic attuned acceptance, by others and of ourselves within Mindfulness Based Cognitive Therapy and particularly Compassion Focused Therapy. The importance of emotional needs being met in childhood, and the damaging consequences if they are not, is powerfully evident within Schema Therapy; the damaging developmental impact of invalidating environments as opposed to the validating context of empathic attunement is a core aspect of Dialectical Behavior Therapy theory; and empathy, validation and compassion are valued within Acceptance and Commitment Therapy, Behavioral Activation and Functional Analytic Psychotherapy. In addition, Constructivist Psychotherapy strongly asserts the importance of empathic encounter. Overall, we might say that the strongest and brightest overlap of our theatre spotlights, involving all of our major approaches, is generated by the relational context of our human psychological development.

Core Psychological Constructs

It is being assumed in this work that conceptual overlaps identified across the psychological constructs of our major theoretical perspectives represent instances of theoretical triangulation in relation to those constructs, and in instances of substantial overlap, the judgement is being made that they are addressing the same entity, whatever term they may be using to refer to it, with conscious mind automatically being recognized by all perspectives.

The unconscious mind of psychodynamic and analytic theory is assumed to be the same aspect of mind that contains the latent schemas of cognitive therapy, the complex learning histories and the processes of classical and operant conditioning of behaviourism, and the hidden painful experiences referred to by therapies within the CBT theoretical umbrella. The defence mechanisms of psychodynamic theory are assumed to be referring to the same phenomena as the experiential and emotional avoidance of more recent behavioural perspectives, the security operations incorporated into the functioning of cognitive-interpersonal cycles, and the unconscious self-protective processes of Constructivist Psychotherapy. The schemas of self and others of cognitive therapy theory are assumed to be referring to the same psychological construct as the internal world of object relations of psychodynamic theory, the internal working model of attachment theory, and the learning histories of behaviourism. Similarly, the relationship between therapist and client in humanistic client-centred therapy is assumed to be referring to the same relationship as the secure attachment relationship of attachment theory, the relational component of the good-enough maturational environment of Winnicott, the mirroring relationship of self-psychology, and the empathic/validating relationships of Mindfulness Based Cognitive Therapy, Compassion Focused Therapy and Dialectical Behavior Therapy.

On this basis, conscious mind, unconscious mind, psychological defences, unconscious internal models of self, others, relationships and the outside world, and the constructive developmental relationship are identified here as representing five core psychological constructs whose validity is supported by theoretical triangulation.

Summary

In this chapter, eleven aspects of theory demonstrating substantial overlap across our five major approaches to psychotherapy have been identified. Eight have been judged to overlap across all five approaches, and three across four of them. Five elements of theory have been proposed as core psychological constructs that are validated by this theoretical triangulation.

   In Chapter 16 we will explore the ways in which our understanding of these five core constructs may each be advised by an integrative synthesis of the associated compatible differences that each theoretical position has to offer.

The Integrative Description of Core Psychological Constructs

16

This chapter will bring together differing aspects of compatible theory across our major theoretical approaches to psychotherapy, on a dialectical basis, to define and describe the five core constructs identified in Chapter 15:

- conscious mind
- unconscious mind
- psychological defences
- unconscious internal models of self, others, relationships and the outside world
- the constructive developmental relationship.

I will be considering ways in which we may creatively bring together theoretical positions that are normally kept quite separate from each other, within the boundaried confines of their theories of origin. In the terms of Roy Bhaskar's critical realism, this work draws on aspects of different but compatible transitive knowledge gained from the perspective of different epistemologies in relation to what I am assuming to be ultimately the same intransitive phenomena.

So that narrative fluency may be maintained, I will not necessarily make specific connections between these discussions and descriptions and the theories that have advised them.

Conscious and Unconscious Mind

As discussed in Chapter 15, all of our core perspectives on psychotherapy are seen to directly or indirectly support the existence of unconscious as well as conscious mind. Our conscious mind is self-evident to us, but our unconscious mind is automatically harder for us to recognize and to define, it belongs to us but outside our conscious awareness. Its nature can only be surmised by inference, and differing characteristics are attributed to it across our range of major theoretical perspectives. It is a creature of our own imagination, but we do know that it exists.

Our core approaches seem to be in varying degrees of conflict in relation to these constructs. Some emphasize the importance of particular aspects of unconscious mind, while others give most attention to the functioning of conscious mind, and some completely minimize and almost deny the relevance of unconscious processes altogether. Sometimes the existence of unconscious functioning is implied rather that explicit, as in the use of the term latent in relation to the unconscious schema of cognitive therapy. The dialectic of this work seeks to transcend these differences, validate the existence of unconscious mind, and integrate the importance of both conscious and unconscious functioning as fully as possible, recognizing their completely inseparable and constant interplay with each other.

The functioning of our conscious mind includes those thoughts, emotions, beliefs, attitudes, attributions, perceptions, interpretations and memories in relation to internal experiences and events in the outside world that we are consciously aware of. It also involves all of our conscious reasoning, analytic processing and creative thinking. The moment-by-moment content of conscious mind results from a constant flow of content between conscious and unconscious, in fluid ever-evolving process. Our conscious thoughts influence the emotions that we feel, and vice-versa, with the connective processes between the two taking place outside our conscious awareness. At a conscious level our thoughts, feelings, decisions, and actions will appear to consciously connect directly to each other, but all the time they are being influenced by the immensely fast and smoothly harmonious mutual processes of both conscious and unconscious systems.

At times we consciously decide to exert control over what we are feeling and thinking. Sometimes we push away a feeling because it may seem frightening, uncomfortable or too painful to bear, or a thought that may raise anxiety, guilt, anger or shame that we would rather not experience, a conscious process of defence. We may at times consciously decide to think in certain ways because we believe it would be better or more justified to do so, or sometimes because we may be expected to by other people. We make both conscious, and not so conscious, decisions about what we do, what we say and how we behave, on our own and within our interpersonal relationships.

All sensory data about the world around us is processed at an unconscious level first to achieve object recognition, and to connect us with our accumulated knowledge of the entities we are relating to, both inanimate and animate, our relevant past experiences, and the nature of relating that may exist between us and them. These processes automatically guide our ways of relating to all contexts of our external world, they take place at extremely high speed, and blend seamlessly with our conscious awareness, thinking, feeling, decision-making and action. They involve the automatic processing carried out by the memory structures and associative networks of our unconscious internal models of self, others, relationships and the outside world. These internal models play a very large part in the functioning of unconscious mind and will be considered in detail in a separate sub-section. They function alongside and are influenced by a range of unconscious processes such as psychological defences, internalization, introjection, projection, projective identification, dissociation and the processes of association and reinforcement reflected in classical and operant conditioning.

Unconscious mind also draws on our internal models in creative ways that are not immediately influenced by the external world and conscious mind and unfold outside of the bounds of logic, time and other reality-based constraints: processes that may be reflected in our dreams, and are referred to as primary process thinking within the psychoanalytic literature.

It functions on a constant basis being influenced by our senses and interacting intensively with conscious mind while we are awake, and following paths of processing that are not influenced by those inputs and connections while we are asleep. Sleep provides a time solely devoted to the maintenance, generation and restoration of its internal structures and to their creative automatic processing free of the intrusion of the everyday outside world.

Psychological Defences

The existence of psychological processes that protect us from problematic emotion, distress and pain, has been recognized to varying degrees within all of our major theoretical approaches. Defences are essential and valuable aspects of human psychological existence, ultimately associated with psychological survival and fulfilling day-to-day, moment-to-moment self-protective functions in relation to events in our lives and the emotions they may prompt within us. Because of the ways in which they achieve their results, defences alter and distort our perceptions, feelings, memories and overall cognitive processes. At times these outcomes may result in unhelpful as well as beneficial consequences. They may function with our conscious awareness, as in the conscious and deliberate suppression and avoidance of a thought or feeling, or exist without us realizing that we are being influenced in this way, as in the case of unconscious and involuntary repression.

Defences will sometimes reflect the specific general mechanisms that are identified within psychodynamic theory, including denial, anger turned against the self, splitting, intellectualization, identification with the aggressor and many others. Each of these provides an example of the multiple, often unique ways in which defences may function, with the resultant constellations of cognitive, behavioural and emotional patterns fulfilling self-protective functions for us. At times, these defence related constellations may also involve complex unconscious phenomena such as projection, projective identification and dissociation.

How Defences Work: Defences and the avoidance of internal adverse experience that they achieve, essentially reflect a process of negative reinforcement within both conscious and unconscious mind in relation to an internal experience of anxiety, fear, pain or other emotional discomfort. They are associated with the conflict between an internal experience, such as a wish, a felt emotion, a thought, a belief, or an impulse to action and its anticipated negative consequences. The resultant intra-psychic conflict may be a simple one between an emotion and the distress caused to us if we experience it within our conscious mind. In other situations the internal conflict may exist because something we wish to do or to say might elicit an adverse reaction from another person. Whatever the basis of the conflict, the resultant internal signal anxiety triggers defence. All of these processes may be taking place outside our conscious awareness. If that is the case the wishes, needs, perceptions, thoughts, feelings and emotions associated with the intra-psychic conflict will not come into conscious mind, and our conscious thinking and behaving will be influenced in ways that maintain that position. Sometimes defences provide essential psychological protection, and at others they are unhelpful and destructive to ourselves and to our relationships. At times they form part of the automatic ways in which our unconscious mind enables us to survive the consequences of emotional deprivation, abuse and trauma during childhood, and the sequelae that live on in our adult lives, holding together a damaged and fragile self.

The Paradox of Unhelpful Defences: In some respects the existence of unhelpful defences involves the inherent paradox that a mechanism functioning to protect us may also be damaging for us at the same time. Thinking about the processes involved helps us make sense of this paradox. For example, a process of defence may lead us to avoid taking protective action to assertively stand up to someone who is treating us badly. The wish and need to be assertive in this way may be in conflict with the fear, maybe even terror, of being abandoned and rejected by someone who we are intimately involved with and dependent on. We may also fear the greater hurt of their retaliation. Signal anxiety may result in us holding back, we may accept their bad treatment of us and even come to believe that we deserve it, joining them in their negativity towards ourselves. Our need to stand up to them and the emotions associated with it, may be totally hidden from conscious awareness as if it did not exist. We may, however, feel sad, and experience aspects of depression, helplessness and despair; a price we are paying for protecting ourselves from the felt risks of loss, hurt and abandonment. We experience suffering, but that suffering may be part of a process that is protecting us from something else, and the something else is, at some level, experienced as something worse.

In the context of defence related processes such as these, our overt feelings may run counter to the unconscious emotions that are being defended against - for instance, our conscious feeling may be one of anxiety when the underlying hidden and unconscious emotion is anger, an anger we may be terrified of expressing. The reverse could also be the case: we may consciously feel and express anger, when our hidden feeling is an anxiety we cannot bear to feel. Sometimes we may refer to our overt emotions in these instances as being secondary, and our underlying hidden feelings as being our primary emotions.

This type of understanding helps us to appreciate the potential hidden nuances of psychological defences, and the very individual basis of the ways in which the processes of defence may relate to our emotions, thoughts, beliefs and behaviours. They may generate significant cognitive distortions and biases, contribute to the development of damaging core beliefs about self, others and relationships, and result in unhelpful patterns of behaviours in relation to ourselves and other people.

The Developmental Context of Defences: The ways in which our minds may protect us in the face of intra-psychic conflict and unbearable emotions vary according to our age and developmental experiences. Infant minds will respond to the emotionally challenging aspects of the world around them very differently compared with older children, who will in turn deal differently compared with adults, as the neurological and psychological substrates of our minds grow and develop.

The development of our minds in these respects is influenced by the nature and quality of our experiences, particularly those that unfold within our closest and most important developmental relationships. Defences develop from less mature and more distorting, to more mature and less distorting types of process, with individual mixtures of these immature and more mature defences existing during our adult life. The terms immature and mature as used here are not intended to imply any negativity or personal failure, they simply reflect the age and environmental contexts in which defences may have evolved. This development is primarily influenced by genetically guided brain maturation and the nature of childhood relational experience: the quality of parental care, the presence or absence of trauma, and the capacity of adults to contain our problematic infant, and childhood emotions. Sometimes parents actively and directly communicate to their children that certain realities either do not exist although they do, or must never be referred to. All of these environmental and experiential factors help us to recognize the connection between the focus and nature of current defences and our past experiences.

In infancy and childhood, defences can help to protect our developing self from emotion that it cannot cope with, from the loss or absence of the love and care we totally depend upon, and from the pain and anxiety of the fundamental existential insecurity of an unloved and inadequately established sense of self. In many ways they may be essential to our human living and psychological survival; in some contexts we would be lost without them. They continue to benefit us in related ways throughout our lives, but can at times become unhelpful and damaging, when their early or later benefits are actually no longer needed, and their remaining impacts cause us problems. At times we may be able to understand and accept ourselves only if we draw on these ways of thinking about defence related processes, and their appreciation may also prove essential to the empathy and acceptance we can experience towards ourselves and other human beings.

The Benefits of Changes in Unhelpful Defences: It is theoretically self-evident that benefits can result if unhelpful defences that are no longer needed, cease to exert their effects, or are replaced by other more helpful and constructive self-protective processes. This premise is supported to greater or lesser extents by all of the major theoretical approaches considered in this work. It is clearly central to psychodynamic theory, a strong part of humanistic, experiential and attachment theories, and evident as part of more recent developments within cognitive behavioural approaches. In all these respects, the belief is supported that human experience will be open to further and potentially helpful processing if the impacts of unhelpful defences are reduced.

Changes in our psychological defences result in the conscious awareness of hidden feelings of some nature, such as anxiety, fear, joy, excitement, sorrow and anger. Hidden memories, beliefs, thoughts, wishes, and needs can come to conscious mind, and all can then be experienced and thought about. As unhelpful defences cease to function, their unhelpful effects on what we think, feel and do may be eased, with the possibility of constructive emotional, relational, cognitive and behavioural change emerging as a natural outcome.

All theoretical approaches that recognize the importance of unhelpful defence related mechanisms and processes show a basic agreement about the context that can enable them to change: people need to feel emotionally and psychologically safe enough for the power of those defences to become reduced, and supported in living with and surviving the emotions that may emerge. This may happen spontaneously through developmental processes within ourselves, supported and enabled naturally by changes in the environmental contexts of our lives and relationships, as well as within the supportive context of the therapeutic relationship.

Unconscious Internal Models of Self, Others, Relationships and the Outside World

Our unconscious internal models will be described here by bringing together the different ways in which the four approaches that support their existence define their nature and consider their development from infancy onwards. Whilst developed independently, this work interestingly echoes and sits alongside Freeman and Martin's (2004) discussion of the cross theoretical understanding of schemas and their development, which I discovered after writing this chapter.

The Nature of our Unconscious Internal Models: As discussed in Chapter 15, I am using the overarching construct of unconscious internal models of self, others, relationships and the outside world as a theory-neutral term to encompass the self and interpersonal schemas of cognitive and behavioural theory, the inner world of object relations of psychodynamic theory, the internal working models of attachment theory and the behavioural construct of a complex learning history. It will also relate to the schemas of cognitive science and information processing psychology. I have taken the position that all of these are referencing current and incomplete transitive knowledge regarding differing aspects of the same intransitive phenomenon.

At a neurological level the processes associated with this construct will be taking place within highly complex associative, memory related networks. The term model has been chosen because it implies a sense of structure, of components being connected and functioning together in a meaningful and non-random way, that produces psychological outcomes. It does not imply any particular endorsement of attachment theory's internal working models above other theoretical approaches. The abbreviated terms internal models or unconscious models will be used for convenience in the following discussion.

Our internal models may be broadly defined as memory structures and networks, involving constellations of accumulated descriptive, functional, emotional and relational information and subjective states of being in relation to ourselves, others, our relationships and all aspects of the world around us. They interact with the sensory input available to us in relation to all the entities, inanimate and animate, that constitute our personal worlds, and our internal physical and psychological states. They support us in recognizing those entities, understanding how they may function, and being aware of the likely or possible outcomes of our interactions with them, influencing our associated thoughts, feelings, beliefs, reasoning processes and behaviours. Their outcomes at a conscious level will also be influenced by the creative and reasoning capacities of our conscious mind. Overall, they constitute a large, central and essential part of our psychological capacities to actively and interactively live in our worlds.

At an unconscious level, our internal models are generated, maintained and modified by a wide range of interactive and overlapping processes, all of which will unfold in the context of unconscious emotion. These will include memory creation; learning, conditioning and association; identification; internalization; projection; projective-identification; dissociation and our processes of psychological defence. They will also be influenced by our conscious processes of cognition as these evolve across the lifespan, involving our processes of thinking and reasoning, and our conscious experiences of emotion.

These internal models will function at differing levels of complexity, with the most basic level relating to object recognition, a primary function that works on a constant basis in response to every sensory input that we receive. As our knowledge of all aspects of our outside and inside world increases, that knowledge continually becomes associated with object recognition, increasing the complexity of existing models and generating new ones.

Our internal models will include memory related constellations of accumulated information and subjective states that represent general categories of objects and entities in our internal and outside worlds, as well as specific instances of those entities, and will at times connect to specific narrative memories relating to both of them. In simple terms, in relation to people we will have a generalized model of what a friend is, and specific models of the particular friends who are involved in our lives; a generalized model of a home and a specific model of our home. Each will influence the other.

At times our internal models will directly represent the reality of the world around us and ourselves, or they may provide us with distorted, less than accurate versions. Our psychological defences will influence both their development and their moment-to-moment functioning. In their flexibility and sensitivity, our models may be activated by current experience in symbolic as well as overtly direct ways. The subtlety and range of these processes are likely to be greatest in relation to the other humans in our world and our relationships with them. Their moment-to-moment activation enables and influences all our interactions with the world around us. They may lead us to perceive and interpret aspects of that world that reflect its accurate reality, or they may lead to inaccurate and distorted interpretations. Both may influence our functioning in helpful or unhelpful ways. Within the interpersonal realm, these processes of distortion are reflected within the concepts of transference and countertransference.

While we are awake our minds receive an intense level of sensory input, which ceases when we are asleep. Whilst awake our internal models will be activated in ways that are triggered by the nature of our current waking experiences. Different aspects of available models may be activated by particular experiences depending on exactly what is happening at the time, and our internal models will vary in their availability to be activated in this way. Most of the time we are consciously unaware of the ways in which they are working. At times, however, we may find that thoughts, feelings and memories associated with particular past experiences, and related to those underlying unconscious internal models, come to conscious mind and may help us make particular sense of ways in which we have responded to events in our lives.

When we are asleep all, or virtually all, of this massive conscious sensory input ceases and our unconscious models, free from the powerful influence of that input, and the processes of conscious mind, take us along totally self-generated paths, potentially involving primary process thinking, lacking the logic and reality of our conscious world, and at times revealed to us in part by the consciously remembered content of our dreams.

Models relating to the same object, and objects in relation to each other, may exist in multiple forms, including our internal models of self, with each of them comprising a different constellation of characteristics, relating to somewhat differing past experiences. These unconscious internal models representing differing aspects of the same entity may co-exist in more or less integrated ways. They may be affected by degrees of fragmentation that markedly reduce the associative connection between them, a situation consistent with the functioning of some defence related processes, and with the concept of dissociation. Some models or aspects of models may be completely dormant unless activated by very particular circumstances. In very extreme contexts, multiple forms may be responsible for the experience of Dissociative Identity Disorder, DID, in which entire networks of internal unconscious models relating to our self and our world may exist in isolation from each other, separated by impermeable boundaries and capable of functioning independently.

Overall, our unconscious internal models influence how effectively we live our lives and interact with the world around us in all respects. They fulfil essential functions for us, and depending on their pathways of development, they can be both helpful and constructive, and unhelpful and damaging.

The Development of our Unconscious Internal Models: The following discussion of developmental processes will relate primarily, but not exclusively, to our internal models of self, others and relationships.

Colwyn Trevarthen's work, as discussed in Chapter 6, tells us that infants are primed to selectively respond to the human face when they come into the world, and that within hours of birth babies demonstrate the innate capacity for dialogues of imitation and expression of emotion associated with human interaction. This implies that we carry within us the genetically based capacity to create the neurological associative structures that we are referring to as internal models, that these generative processes are active before birth and that for the human face we do not need to learn by seeing one - we know it already. It also tells us that these early structures include the processes of relationship from the very start.

From this earliest starting point, our experiences of self, others, our human relating and the rest of the environments we live in will contribute to those evolving structures in whatever way our bodies and minds can sense and perceive our inner and outer world experiences. Very early development will be based on sensory experience, physical, emotional, aural and visual, and will exist in non-linguistic forms of memory that are not related to language associated cognitive functioning. Young babies will hear the sounds of words and how they are vocalized, see the facial expressions that accompany them and experience the nature of the good or uncomfortable consequences of everything that happens in their physical and relational world. One way or another, emotion and sensation will hold full sway in the development of our very early inner world.

As our internal models start to develop, they will be influenced by aspects of our genetic endowment in contributing to the basis of our individual baby and infant patterns of likes and dislikes, what gives us pleasure, what upsets us, angers us or makes us sad, and these early evolving models will play their part in influencing the nature of the relationships that unfold with those who care for us. Internal models of self and of others will evolve in ways that are both separate from and intimately related to each other. The overall evolution of our unconscious internal models will be influenced by all the experiences of our early lives, relational and otherwise, with the processes of learning and reinforcement playing their crucial part.

As we grow, the nature of every developmental process in relation to our neurological and physical maturation, particularly our evolving cognitive and language-based abilities, and our capacities to move and to act on our environment, will impact on those evolving models. They will start to reflect our cognitive and linguistic capacities, including overt memories of specific events in relation to ourselves and others, and their emotional impact. Our models bear particular relationship to language and words as our cognitive capacities grow in these respects. Words and language are not essential for models to exist and function, but their elaboration and complexity will be much increased as language and cognitive capacity develop. As our neurological and cognitive capacities grow, it becomes increasingly possible for our models to involve much more extensive and complex representations of external and internal reality that are influenced by language and cognition as well as emotional and sensory experience.

We may refer to our very early unconscious internal models developing during infancy, before language development as non-linguistic and pre-cognitive immature models and those that have developed and evolved by the time we reach later childhood and early adulthood, under the influence of language and cognition, as more mature models. The nature of both immature and mature models will be influenced by their associated defences, which themselves will also evidence differing stages of developmental maturity, as discussed above in the section on psychological defences.

As language and thinking evolve for us in early childhood, we move from the non-linguistic unarticulated precursors of beliefs about ourselves and the world around us associated with these internal models, to a linguistically based capacity to express and to think about them. As soon as beliefs start to exist as part of our internal models, whatever their phenomenological nature, they will automatically influence what we attend to and what we remember, all of which will influence the continued evolution of those models. As core beliefs and our cognitive capacities become more established our tendency to attend to material that is in keeping with existing beliefs may result in more experiences feeding into our unconscious models that is consistent with them rather than inconsistent.

As our capacities for cognition develop, they will include our human capacities to think and to question, to seek to understand and make sense of our experiences. Whilst these thought processes themselves will be influenced by our internal models and defences, we are creative and constructive beings with aptitudes for analysis, reasoning and logic, all of which play their natural creative part in contributing to our emotional, cognitive and behavioural responses to the things that happen in our lives. We play a creative part in generating the nature of all of our interactions with, and experiences of, the world we live in. The nature of our conscious creative, analytical thinking and reasoning, and the outcomes of our behaviours and actions will all feedback into the evolving nature of our internal models.

To some extent our earliest immature models stemming from infancy and early childhood will persist alongside more maturely evolved models, and our adult internal models will always include some mixture of the two. Early immature internal models may be both helpful and unhelpful for us. Those that have evolved within secure attachment contexts without the damaging influences of emotional deprivation and/or trauma and abuse may well be the unconscious internal models that lie at the heart of our most secure bonds with others and our precious capacities for basic trust in relation to ourselves and the world around us.

Our internal models are powerfully influenced by the nature of our early relationships with those most important to us. The most helpful models of self, others and relationships, and associated psychological defences will be supported by constructive developmental relationships providing attuned and empathic relating, emotional containment, optimal frustration, genuine acceptance, unconditional love, and the absence of deprivation, trauma and abuse. These models will involve a valuing and accepting confidence in ourselves, reflecting our true, organismically-valued self rather than a self-protective, false and incongruent one.

Our models of self and others will carry within them a sense that it is possible for others to be trusted and for us to be cared for. The innate potential for growth and development within each of us will have been supported. These helpful and constructive internal models of self, others and relationships are not unrealistic or idealized, but rest on secure and realistic perceptions of the interpersonal worlds that have surrounded us. Clear, open and genuine interpersonal communication will enable any unhelpful and/or inaccurate internal models to be modified and changed in constructive directions, during early development and throughout the life span. It is within the environmental context of secure developmental relationships, and maturational environments in infancy and childhood, that our internal models have the best chance of developing from early immature models to more mature ones in constructive and helpful ways which support our capacities to thrive in our adult world.

Inadequate developmental relationships that fail in these respects, and may also involve contexts of early distress, deprivation, abuse and trauma, will most likely result in unhelpful damaging internal models of self, others and relationships. Our model of self will be influenced by self-protective processes, and the internalization of negativity; it will be false and incongruent in relation to our innate potential, and carry within it the enduring, and often intense need for those crucial aspects of relational developmental experience that were denied us. Within our models of others, negative attributes and expectations may be to the fore, and a sense of trust may not exist. In most contexts, internal models will reflect a mixture of constructive and damaging characteristics. The more problematic, depriving, traumatic and abusive our developmental relational environment, the more damaged and damaging our unconscious internal models are likely to become.

When inadequate developmental relationships have been present from birth onwards, they will impact on the nature of our early pre-cognitive and non-linguistic immature models from the very start of our lives, models that will naturally incorporate immature defences. Depending on the severity of deprivation, trauma and abuse, this can result in severely damaging, immature internal models, influenced by powerfully distorting immature defences. If the nature of the developmental relationship continues to be unable to provide the emotional environment necessary for their growth, and if deprivation and trauma continue to be part of a child's experiential world, these models will be maintained and strengthened, and their future more constructive development will be impeded. At times these models may be consistent with the bizarrely disturbing inner worlds of object relations that can be described within Kleinian theory, and have sometimes been assumed to have primarily innate rather than environmental origins.

Complex individual contexts of both immature and mature, constructive and damaging internal models will continue to unfold throughout our childhood and into adulthood. Immature models will evolve into more mature ones, but some of them will also endure. Mature and immature models will both exist as mixtures of damaging and constructive constellations, each incorporating mixtures of mature and immature processes of defence.

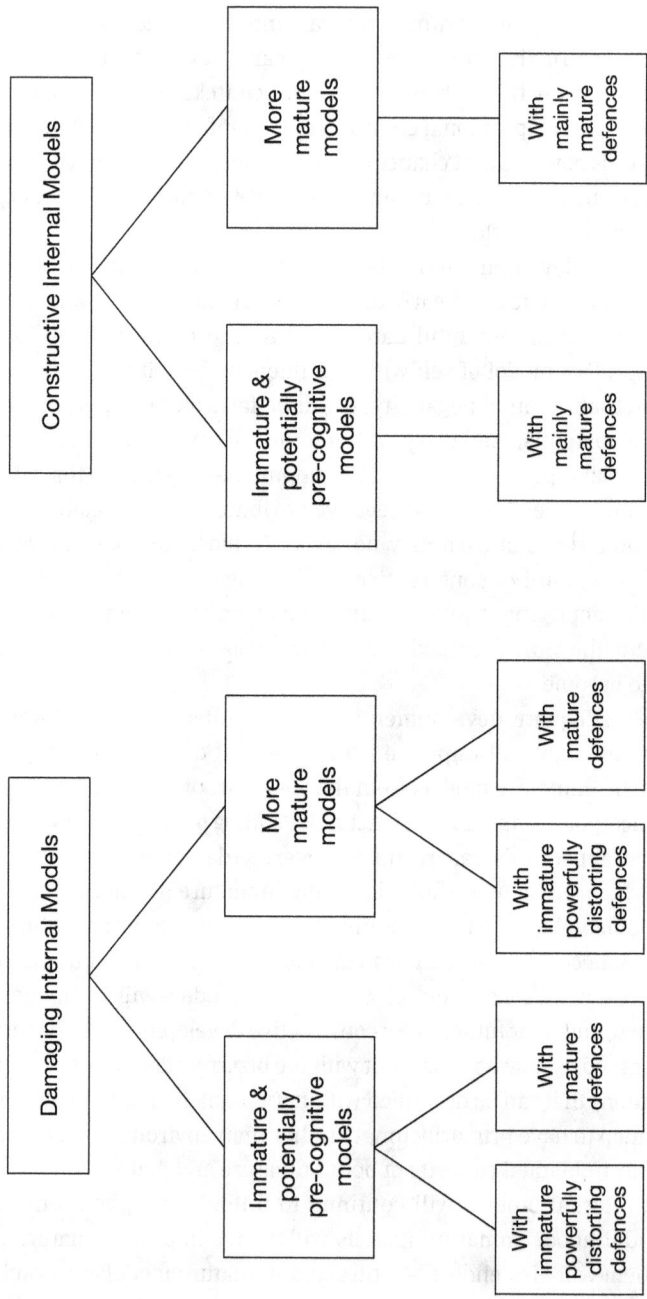

Figure 5 The Co-existence of a Range of Constructive and Damaging Internal Models Within Unconscious Mind

When our very early environments have failed us, the outcomes for our adult internal models will be influenced by the enduring nature of that environment, whether it continues to be as damaging, or provides something more attuned, caring and constructive as time goes on. Or it may become more depriving and abusive instead. Inevitably whatever the quality of those very important relationships, our internal unconscious models will still develop and change, becoming more complex, linguistic and cognitively-based mature models.

Their damaging nature may be maintained, reduced or enhanced. In adverse circumstances an increased proportion of early damaging immature models are likely to survive through to adulthood, having been deprived of what they needed to be able change, with powerful and distorting defences and continuing adversity contributing to their maintenance.

Figure 5 summarizes something of the range of models that might exist within us, indicating categories of potentially co-existing options, but not the gradations between them. Each will be accompanied by tendencies towards differing ranges and intensities of emotion, which in some damaging contexts may become overwhelming and very difficult to manage.

Alongside the context of our intimate developmental relationships, all of our experiences of the world around us will extensively enhance the detail and complexity of our internal models as we move through childhood, adolescence and into adulthood. Our models of self, others and relationships will be influenced by the myriad of relational experiences we have with other people, adults and children, intimate and otherwise, that unfold for us in all the environments, domestic, social, educational and work related, that are part of our lives across the life span. Across all contexts we will also learn about the ways in which it is deemed usual and acceptable to behave, and overall we will have extensive opportunities to learn more through literature, theatre, television and film.

Our development in all of these respects will also be influenced by our genetic endowments, by our life long experiences of learning about the physical, practical, cultural and political worlds in which we live, by our natural tendency to seek meaning and understanding, by all of our educational and training-based experiences, and by the unique experiences of what gives each of us pleasure, satisfaction and a sense of achievement, or causes us distress, pain and unhappiness. All of the skills, abilities and knowledge we gain throughout our lives, and the roles we fulfil within our families, our work and our other activities will become core aspects of who we know ourselves to be, and how we perceive and understand the nature of the world we live in.

In psychological terms the processes and outcomes of life span development as overviewed in Chapter 12 essentially involve development and change within our unconscious internal models of self, others, relationships and the outside world throughout our lives. Such processes will take us forward through extensive constructive development across the lifespan, but at times the transitions involved may present us with particular challenges. Pre-existing models may be at odds with the nature of changed life circumstances. Problematic or challenging life-events and contexts may reveal unhelpful aspects of our models of self, others and relationships that were not evident before. Sometimes previously adaptive and helpful models may no longer be of the same benefit to us. Losses of physical and cognitive capacities at any stage of the lifespan, through illness, accident and disability, and the ageing processes of later life, will also have their own unique place in these respects. The evolution of our internal models is central to our adaptation to such changes. At all stages our models will have the most straightforward potential to develop to the best of their constructive capacity if we have experienced the security of good developmental relationships from the start of our lives, and are fortunate enough for them to be there for us in the present. The enabling or disabling nature of our social and demographic environments will make all the difference too.

The Constructive Developmental Relationship

As discussed in Chapter 15 the term constructive developmental relationship has been adopted as an integrative, theory-neutral term that encompasses the theoretical contributions of attachment, humanistic and psychodynamic perspectives to the nature of relationship that enables human emotional connection and supports our psychological growth and development.

Rather than working to transcend differences between theoretical perspectives, or synthesizing their different but compatible contributions, in this situation we are largely looking at different ways of talking about the same thing, and using that convergence to strengthen the validity of our understanding. Drawing on all three perspectives, we enhance our appreciation of the constructive relationship that parents can provide for their children, that adults in close significant relationships can provide for each other, and we can provide for our clients.

Being loved and cared for unconditionally by someone who can experience genuine sensitive attunement and empathic connection with us, hearing, understanding and accepting who we are, lies at the heart of our human ability to grow and develop into the people we have the natural potential to be from birth onwards, supporting our innate capacity for growth. Our primary human motivation is to find relationship between ourselves and others, and we become who we are by developing and growing in the context of relationship. As recognized in Chapter 15, the actualizing tendency and organismic valuing of humanistic theory refer to the same potential and motivation to become a unique human self as do the libido, life instinct, life force and autonomous striving of the will of psychodynamic approaches, and the innate capacity for growth and recovery recognized within attachment theory.

All of these approaches believe in the existence of this potential within each of us. All believe that the developmental relationship between child and parent is central to the early and later unfolding of that potential. They overlap powerfully when they independently describe the nature of the effective relating that supports the sound development of this potential within each and every child, enabling each to follow his or her own unique path. Separately they have found themselves using similar terms when thinking about the need for children to adapt to whoever their parents are because they are totally dependent on them for love and care, and for psychological and physical survival. Repeatedly we come across terms and phrases such as defensive exclusion and distortion of self-development, which result in a false or incongruent self in which our opportunities to become our true, real or organismically-valued self, have been limited or even destroyed. Client-centred therapy describes the absence of empathic acceptance and valuing during childhood, and the imposition of conditions of worth as resulting in the defensive exclusion of experience from conscious awareness, echoing psychodynamic and attachment theories. These self-protective adaptations and distortions mean that our feelings, our wishes, our needs and maybe our passions and abilities become pushed aside and lost to ourselves, submerged within a false self, shaped by unconscious processes to be acceptable to those we need most. We become a self that is not congruent with the real or true self we would most naturally have become, and conditions set by others have defined what is seen as having worth within us. All of this will be reflected and held within our unconscious internal models of self, others, relationships and the outside world.

When our self-development has proceeded well, the crucial experience of being accepted for who we are by parents and others will have emerged as an automatic and natural part of their true and genuinely expressed empathy, attunement and acceptance in relation to us.

As therapists we learn about the nature and depth of empathic connection, and come to appreciate the particular importance of responses that are communicated and felt beyond and without words. We know the importance of emotional containment and the capacity to live with and survive the difficult emotions that come our way from the other person. We learn that it is important that natural disappointments, frustrations and limits are experienced, since it is through optimal frustration and impingement that others discover they are psychologically separate from us. We learn that it is crucial to be genuine, that we do not pretend, and whatever we do or say comes from a genuine basis within ourselves. We see that power matters, and that the misuse of power is inconsistent with and destructive of that relationship. We recognize the fundamental impact of the developmental relationship on the evolving nature of the other person's internal models of self, others and relationships, as discussed above. We know that it affects the need or not for unhelpful defences, provides crucial corrective emotional experiences, and supports the capacity of others to experience the separated existence of their own mind and the minds of others.

Psychodynamic theory, in particular, advises our understanding of the broad-based importance of corrective emotional experience within this relationship, and together with attachment theory addresses the importance of repeated relational patterns and behaviours. The latter are also sometimes recognized within cognitive and behavioural theory and are evident within behaviourally based Functional Analytic Psychotherapy theory. Their emotional connectedness, empathic attunement and attention to psychological needs makes constructive developmental relationships particularly fertile grounds for the re-enactment and re-living of relational patterns in both positive and potentially problematic respects.

At the end of therapy, and during breaks, we are supported in appreciating that experiences of separation and loss within the therapeutic relationship may carry particular meaning for people who have been painfully affected by loss and grief. Attachment theory may be particularly helpful to us in this respect, and issues of separation, loss and grief are also key elements of psychodynamic understanding. Relational experiences within therapy in these contexts may carry particularly significant capacities to influence our unconscious internal models of self, others and relationships.

As therapists we recognize the importance of our own current supportive attachment relationships, and the ways in which they help to make possible our own provision of that relationship to others, just as a mother/primary care giver is enabled in this way by the relationship with her or his spouse/partner. The relational system around us plays an important part in supporting and enabling our capacity to take on the challenge of engaging in healthy, constructive developmental relationships with others.

The nature and challenge of empathic connection and communication is made most real by the work of Carl Rogers, who brings us so personally face to face with the human reality of being touched by the felt experience of another person. Psychodynamic theory and humanistic theory echo each other in making us aware how important and helpful it can be to sense hidden meanings within therapy relationships through the nature and quality of our listening, putting into words experience and meanings which the other person may barely be aware of, which echoes core aspects of the advanced empathy of the listening skills literature. From Rogers we hear it emphasized that such communication needs to be done in a way that makes sure empathic attunement and connection are maintained, and offers understanding that can be rejected as well as accepted. Both psychodynamic theory and client-centred theory recognize that empathic connection that has been effective in these ways increases the rapport between the people involved, and sometimes markedly so.

Theoretical integration within the constructive developmental relationship will be echoed in practice within many approaches to psychotherapy. The approach to short-term dynamic interpersonal psychotherapy proposed by Haliburn (2017) provides a specific example. Although unfortunately in that work no acknowledgement is given to Carl Rogers or humanistic theory, the empathic connection, discovery of shared meaning and opportunity to grow described in Hobson's Conversational Model (Hobson, 1985) is explicitly integrated with attachment theory and interpersonal psychodynamic theory.

In a somewhat similar way Erich Fromm's classic text *The Art of Loving* reflects a coming together of psychoanalysis and humanistic philosophy in the context of essential developmentally important human love and care (Fromm,1956/2013).

The essence of a constructive developmental relationship, one that benefits another other person in our lives in these ways, be they client, child, friend, colleague, relative or lover, involves a meeting founded in genuine reality in which valuing, care, attuned understanding and emotional containment are experienced between us. This relationship can also involve a lot else, depending on the context of the situation; active support and learning, direct advice and guidance, or largely interpretive understanding may play their part, but the sound starting point and continuing basis for all of these is the empathic, attuned, containing relationship; the secure base, and we never stop needing it.

Summary

In Chapter 16 we have brought together aspects of the different but compatible theoretical positions of our major approaches, to define the core psychological constructs identified in Chapter 15, on a theoretically integrative basis. Conscious and unconscious mind, psychological defences, unconscious internal models and the constructive developmental relationship as defined and described here, will all play substantial parts in the Unifying Dialectical Model of human psychological functioning to be discussed in Chapter 17.

The Unifying Dialectical Model of Human Psychological Functioning   **17**

This chapter will describe the central component of Dialectically Integrated Psychotherapy, the Unifying Dialectical Model of human psychological functioning, the UDM. Following the principles of critical realism and a belief in the single, intransitive absolute reality of the human mind, valid theories about its functioning and associated processes of change need to be compatible with each other. Their processes and mechanisms should be able to work together. This model has been built on the basis of such compatibility, and draws on theoretical overlaps and compatible differences across our current five major perspectives.

In Chapter 16 we looked at theoretically integrative descriptions of the five core psychological constructs identified in Chapter 15: conscious and unconscious mind; psychological defences; unconscious internal models of self, others, relationships and the outside world; and the constructive developmental relationship. These constructs, as defined on this integrative basis, play significant roles within this dialectical model. It also incorporates the six further elements of theory identified as demonstrating substantial overlap across our major approaches: the relevance of behaviour; the importance of relational experience; the importance of past experiences; the processing of emotion; the experience of acceptance; and the innate capacity for growth and development.

In addition, the basic principles of vicious circles and maintenance loops found within applied behaviour analysis and functional analysis have advised its processes of feedback and maintenance. Our relational, social, demographic and lifespan contexts are also taken into account. In order to support theoretical neutrality and maintain narrative fluency, overt connections between specific components of the model and the theories that have advised them will generally not be made explicit in the following discussions. In most instances, the model is defined and discussed in terms that are as theoretically neutral as possible, and is offered as an example of a unifying approach on this basis.

This is a model of processes within our human self in interaction with the world around us. It is our self in its entirety that we bring to psychotherapy, and we will therefore start by briefly acknowledging the very complex nature of this human self.

The Self

From an objective position the self is an entity that is hard to define, although our use of the term is colloquially ubiquitous within much of human existence. It incorporates our conscious and unconscious minds, all their known and unknown processes, and the brain that generates them. It is inherently associated with the body that constitutes our living self, and all that our body contributes to our human experience of existence. We use psychological terms such as personality, self-concept, and self-esteem to try to label aspects of that entity we call our self, that unique set of perceptions, behaviours, emotions, beliefs, attitudes, thought patterns, abilities, vulnerabilities, creativity, physical attributes and all that encompasses the individual person that we are.

It is our self that experiences our life from day one until the end. To all our known intents and purposes, it is who we are, and it is unique. Its development is influenced by our environment and life experiences. Such influence is likely to start evolving during our intrauterine life and continues from birth until death, in interaction with our biological endowment, with genetics setting the upper and lower limits of our individual human potential. There may be variation in how coherent our sense of self appears to be, with our human functioning emerging in rather disconnected and fragmented ways at times.

We may also vary in how much our self is adversely affected by difficulty and challenge, in terms of its security and resilience or vulnerability. This is a self that is affected by and can exert its own influence on the world it lives in. However, whilst our own choices, actions and behaviour clearly influence the nature of our lives, we are also affected by much in our social and demographic worlds that we may not be in any position to influence. Those worlds in all their difference and complexity set the scene for our human existence.

The Unifying Dialectical Model of Human Psychological Functioning

The proposed Unifying Dialectical Model will first be discussed in relation to the broadly defined components illustrated in Figure 6, followed by a more detailed consideration of the processes influencing psychological change and development.

Within this unifying model, the self is represented as comprising our unconscious and conscious mind and our behaviours. All aspects of experience

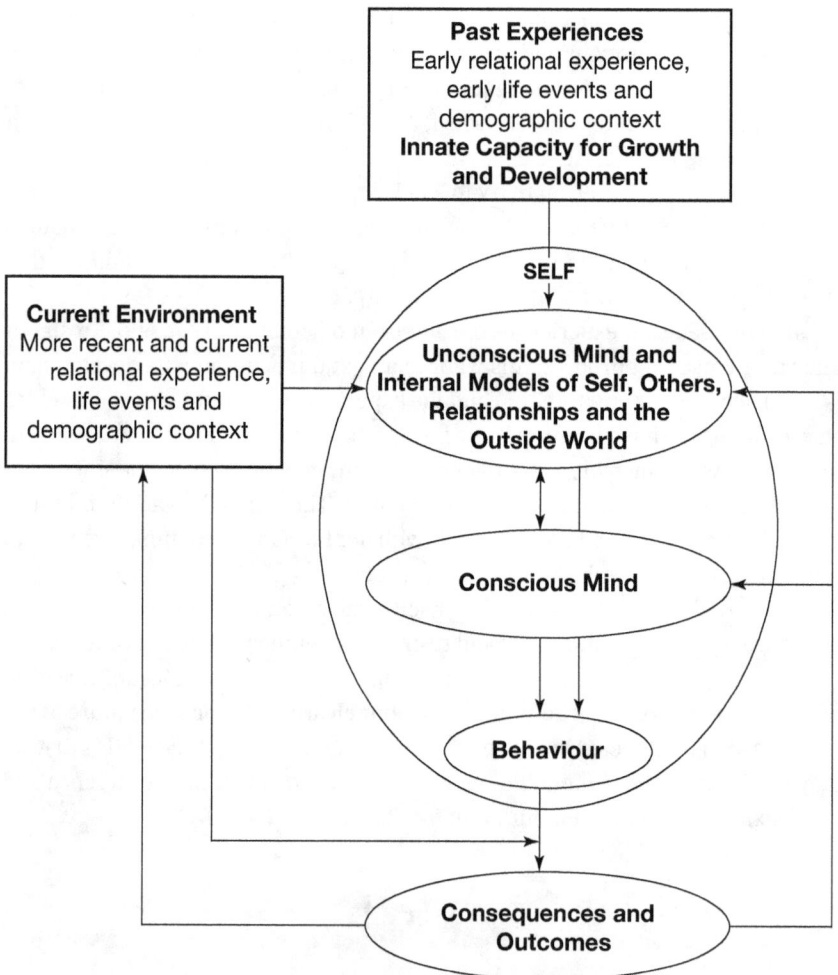

Figure 6 The Unifying Dialectical Model of Human Psychological Functioning

first impact on our unconscious mind, which is in constant and mutual interaction with conscious mind. Within unconscious mind our unconscious internal models of self, others, relationships and the outside world hold a central place at the heart of our human psychological functioning and associated processes of change.

Our internal models are broadly defined in Chapter 16 as memory related constellations of accumulated descriptive, functional, emotional and relational information and subjective states of being, relating to all the entities we interact with in our lives. They play a large, central and essential part in our psychological capacities to actively and interactively live in our physical and relational worlds. The nature of those models and their associated unconscious processes, particularly our psychological defences, have been influenced by our past experiences, especially our early developmental relationships, as well as our innate potential for growth and development. Our early lives may involve primarily constructive developmental relationships, or they may be influenced in varying degrees by unhelpful, damaging, and maybe abusive and traumatic relational worlds. The nature and quality of the early physical, practical, social, cultural and economic world around will us will also play its part, together with the impact of early life events. In addition, our adult internal models will be influenced by the more recent and current relational and demographic contexts of our lives, including the experience of recent or ongoing meaningful life events and relational experiences. In the context of our individual genetic endowment and innate capacity for growth, the interactive influence of all of these factors will result in our own individual mix of unique constructive or damaging, and immature or mature internal models, as discussed in Chapter 16.

The functioning of unconscious mind will also include unconscious cognitions, emotions, psychological defences, memories, wishes and needs, primary process thinking, identification, internalization, projection, projective identification, dissociation, the processes of association and the mechanisms of classical and operant conditioning. These phenomena will all be interacting synergistically and will contribute to the nature and functioning of our unconscious internal models. Together they will feed into our conscious emotions, beliefs, thought processes and actions. Everything we experience will initially be processed, extremely rapidly by our unconscious mind, with our internal models enabling, facilitating and influencing our overall capacities to process and respond to the events within our worlds.

Our conscious mind incorporates our conscious sensory perceptions, emotions, thoughts, beliefs, interpretations and memories. All of our conscious awareness of experience is available to our cognitive capacities of thinking, reasoning, creativity and decision making, the conscious processing of emotion, and the functioning of our conscious psychological defences. Conscious and unconscious mind interact with each other on a constant basis. The outcomes of our conscious cognitive processes automatically feed back into unconscious mind, maintaining and maybe changing the nature of our internal models. The mutual functioning of unconscious and conscious mind leads to our overt behaviours, which then have consequences and outcomes within our environments. These consequences and outcomes influence the ongoing nature of those environments, and feed back into both conscious and unconscious mind, maintaining or changing our internal models of self, others, relationships and the outside world.

As a core psychological construct, psychological defences are attributed significant roles within this unifying model as elements of both unconscious and conscious mind. In both contexts they influence the nature of our responses and behaviours in relation to moment-to-moment experience. Their integrative description provided in Chapter 16 supports our appreciation of the multiple ways in which they may have powerful effects, influencing the nature, functioning and maintenance of our unconscious internal models, the nature of unconscious and conscious experience and our overt behaviours.

Our behavioural responses and actions, what we do, what we express and what we say, will have consequences and outcomes involving ourselves, the physical and practical worlds around us, and our relational experiences with other people. The specifics of these consequences and outcomes will be influenced by the nature and quality of the current context of our lives, particularly the characteristics of the people we are most involved with. However they unfold, these outcomes will feedback to influence conscious and unconscious mind, maintaining our unconscious internal models, or contributing towards helpful or unhelpful changes.

The immediate consequences of our behavioural responses may also influence the overall nature of our current relationships and demographic environments. Changes within those environments may then have influence in the longer term, and make helpful or unhelpful contributions to the quality and impact of our life experiences in the future.

Positive psychotherapy outcomes depend on the constructive modification of our unconscious internal models and their functioning. The activation of unhelpful internal models may be reduced, and they may be enabled to change in helpful directions; existing more helpful models that are currently latent may become activated, and constructive new models may become established. It is the capacity to facilitate beneficial and lasting change within our unconscious internal models and their functioning that underlies the enduring effectiveness of any approach to psychotherapy.

Processes of Change within Our Unconscious Internal Models of Self, Others, Relationships and the Outside World

Change within our unconscious internal models requires changes in the feedback processes that maintain them within the Unifying Dialectical Model. These processes will involve the overall interactive influences of conscious and unconscious mind, the nature and consequences of our behaviours and actions, the nature of our environments and our place in the lifespan. Their discussion will also include the five further aspects of therapy theory validated by significant theoretical overlap and triangulation in Chapter 15: the processing of emotion, our psychological defences, conscious acceptance, relational experiences, and our innate capacity for growth and development.

Unconscious Mind: Our unconscious internal models can be influenced and changed by every-day events in ways that lie entirely outside our conscious awareness. Experiences in the world around us including the outcomes of our own behaviours will all be available to unconscious mind, creating new memories, affecting emotion and cognition, and influencing a range of processes such as identification, internalization, defences, associations and unconscious learning, all of which may modify the nature of our unconscious internal models. These influences may be transitory, or result in enduring change. Experience that is consistent with existing models will function to maintain them; experience that is different and inconsistent may have capacity to engender change, for better or for worse.

The Boundary Between Unconscious and Conscious Mind: Unconscious and conscious mind are in mutual constant interaction with each other, across the boundary between them. Material within unconscious mind will vary across a spectrum of accessibility to conscious mind, from one extreme to another. It may lie only just outside conscious awareness, and be able to drift in and out, or at the other extreme it may be completely concealed from our potential awareness by powerful and impermeable boundaries. Across this spectrum, our tendencies to become aware of unconscious material will be influenced by a range of factors, and will be particularly affected by the strength of our unconscious and conscious psychological defences. Increased access across this boundary, to material that normally lies outside our conscious awareness, is a very important part of our processes of change.

Conscious Mind: When experience becomes conscious rather than unconscious it is open to being processed in different ways. Through our conscious thinking, feeling, and making sense of the things that happen to us, our conscious mind has the potential to process and understand experience in ways that can feed back into unconscious mind and alter our internal models of self, others, relationships and the outside world.

In response to any event in our lives, big or small, we will probably experience an initial spontaneous conscious cognitive and emotional reaction, influenced by the unconscious models that are immediately activated. If we spend some time thinking about the situation, we may find that those reactions become modified; a different and maybe wider range of related unconscious internal models may influence our conscious thinking, and our processes of reasoning may lead to different conclusions about ourselves and others, we may start to feel differently and we may make different decisions about how to behave, for better or worse.

Sometimes we may make a deliberate effort to do this in a constructive way. We may actively choose to step back and reconsider our spontaneous, automatic cognitive responses in helpful ways, catching unconscious internal models in action. If we judge them to reflect unhelpful and inaccurate interpretations of current circumstances, we may change those interpretations, come to think and feel differently, and may make different decisions about what to do. Our capacity to do so will be supported by our abilities to moderate any associated strong emotions, and may also be enabled by the easing of any unhelpful self-protective mechanisms of defence.

In all of these respects, if such changes in conscious cognitive and emotional responses result in helpful and valuable experiences for us, we will have generated feedback loops into unconscious mind that support constructive processes of change within our unconscious internal models. If these altered ways of being turn out to have reliably beneficial outcomes, changes in our internal models will be maintained and may prove to be enduring. In this situation, our more helpful conscious cognitive and emotional responses to events in the world around us will then emerge automatically and spontaneously without the need for active and deliberate monitoring: sustainable change will have been achieved.

The Processing of Emotion: Emotion is an aspect of all our unconscious internal models, and plays a particularly important part in the processes of activation, maintenance and change within those models. Its accepted and contained experiencing at a conscious level, often through the easing of defence, helps feeling, thinking and meaning to evolve and change. This is likely to be particularly important in relation to strong and painful or uncomfortable hidden feelings. Emotions can then be processed and may become transformed, with meaning and the nature of our internal unconscious models changing along with them. Hidden positive emotions may become more accessible as well and all changes in experienced emotion will influence the range as well as the nature of unconscious internal models that become activated and available to the processes of conscious mind.

Emotion is a powerful and ever-present motivator for action or inaction at unconscious and conscious levels; our behavioural responses towards ourselves, others and the immediate world around us are all intimately bound up with emotion and meaning. Manifest changes in emotion and associated thought processes may lead to different and more constructive ways of being and behaving in relation to ourselves and others.

Psychological Defences: As discussed above and in Chapter 16, whenever unhelpful defences continue to have powerful effects within any of us, their functioning may play a major role in the maintenance of unhelpful unconscious internal models and associated ways of thinking, feeling and behaving. Experiences that might otherwise enable constructive psychological change to take place, may not be able to do so unless these defences are addressed. Sometimes changes will happen automatically once an unhelpful defence-related process is no longer taking place. Attention to the processes of psychological defence may prove crucial to changes in our unconscious internal models, both directly and indirectly.

Acceptance: Acceptance as discussed in Chapter 15 involves becoming more able to consciously accept the reality of ourselves as we currently are, and the realities of our current relational and demographic worlds. Both realities will probably have negative and positive aspects to them. Acceptance helps us to stop denying them, and stop railing against them or punishing ourselves for them. Instead we start to live in more valid connection with both their painful realities and the positivity they may involve. Psychological barriers to change may be reduced, unhelpful defences decreased, and negativity and self-criticism may be eased; our innate potential for growth may be supported and our behaviour towards self and others may change. All will influence our unconscious models of self, others and relationships.

Self-acceptance also involves an emotional sense of love and care towards ourselves, and has significant power to directly influence our internal models of self in this respect. In relation to our outside world, without actually accepting the realities of our current lives, it is probably impossible for us do anything about them, and when those realities are accepted, inevitably our internal models of that outside world start to change. Overall, acceptance supports processes of change that influence our unconscious internal models in a wide range of ways.

Overt Behaviour: New and changed behaviours will virtually always be involved in the development and maintenance of changes in our unconscious internal models. These altered behaviours emerge as the consequence of changes in cognition, emotion and defence, and other components of unconscious and conscious mind. They may become established by specific focused intent, through deliberate conscious decisions to behave differently, in social, relational and practical contexts. They may also involve the active learning of new abilities and capacities. As behaviours change, they make essential contributions to the development of the self and associated unconscious internal models. In so many ways we know ourselves by what we do and what we are capable of doing.

The nature of any behaviour reflects the nature of the internal models that have been involved in its production, and the process of that behaviour being put into effect may automatically play a part in maintaining them. In some ways this is illustrated by the behavioural concept of safety behaviours; if we do something to make ourselves safe that action in itself confirms that there was something to be scared of; supporting the validity of the underlying belief and the nature of the unconscious internal model that it is part of.

Choosing and deciding to behave differently in itself starts to make a difference. If we then experience valued outcomes, the natures of those outcomes have a powerful opportunity to influence the feedback processes relating to our unconscious internal models. We may experience a sense of success or achievement and come to see ourselves in different, more positive ways. We may elicit different, more positive and beneficial responses from others, and the nature of our relationships may improve. If we change our own behaviour towards others in constructive ways, they may change their behaviour towards us, altering the nature of relating and the experience of emotion and meaning between us, potentially influencing mutually functioning defence-related processes, and changing underlying unconscious mutual patterns of positive and negative reinforcement and punishment. Behavioural change that involves our exposure to previously avoided contexts unhelpfully associated with anxiety and fear, will have the potential to dissolve that association and open up a wider world of experience within our lives, at times radically changing the nature of our unconscious models. We may come to know ourselves and the world around us in a totally different way.

All of these processes will play their part in changing our unconscious internal models of self, others, relationships and the outside world for the better, and helping to maintain those changes; change in our behaviour is essential, and the impact of what we do and the outcomes of our actions should never be underestimated.

Relational Experience: The quality of the close relationships that we experience in our lives plays a major part in the development and maintenance of our unconscious internal models of self, others and relationships. If we are lucky enough to experience secure, empathic, accepting and emotionally containing constructive developmental relationships, these can support beneficial processes of change that enable our internal models to reflect more of our true rather than our defensively distorted false selves, supported by our innate potential for growth and development, as discussed in Chapter 16.

Repeated relational patterns play an important part in this context. Sometimes aspects of relational experience may trigger responses within us that create self-generated maintenance feedback loops, which may be problematic where unhelpful models are concerned.

For example, within a significant relationship we may experience an interaction that bears apparent similarity to a damaging context in our early experience, when it is actually happening on a different basis. Our internal models may lead us to respond in ways that are in keeping with the early situation, rather than the realities of the current one. Prompted by our reactions, the other person may then respond in ways that are similar to those we experienced in that early damaging past. From our internal perspective we are being treated in the same way again, our related models of self, others and relationships are maintained, and our current relationship is put under stress.

From differing theoretical positions we may see these mutually influencing processes as reflecting the concepts of transference and counter-transference, the impact of discriminative stimuli associated with the likelihood of particular reinforcing or punishing consequences, or as the result of self-fulfilling beliefs associated with early maladaptive schemas. All would be referring to the same underlying intransitive processes.

In other instances, the person we are relating to may truly be treating us in exactly the same damaging way as others did before; if so, the environment around us will be repeating that past and directly maintaining our related internal models. In many relational contexts the situation is likely to be some mixture of these two clear-cut extremes, with both parties making a contribution to the problematic perceptions and inter-personal behaviours involved.

Positive change can take place when a damaging relational context that bears similarity to the past starts to unfold but this time manages to move forward in a different and more constructive way. Something new happens, and at some level we become aware of this. If different and better outcomes are experienced then our internal models of our self and who we are, of other people and who they are, and our models of relationships can change. It is also helpful if we recognize and understand the nature of what has unfolded differently.

We may be in a stronger position to appreciate and think about these internal processes between ourselves and others, if we have sufficient capacity to mentalize and to recognize that other people have minds that are separate from our own. Clear and honest communication between us will help to update and transform our internal models in these ways, and genuineness, trust and empathic attunement will make all the difference. Unhelpful feedback loops can be changed. This overall beneficial, and transformative relational context will inherently need to involve the easing of unhelpful defences, enabling us to experience the nature of our interactions more fully and to connect with underlying emotions that may have previously been avoided, being more open to the impact of our thoughts and feelings. This is all most likely to be able to happen in the context of a constructive developmental relationship.

In these constructive circumstances, whatever way it happens, the other person involved in the relational interaction does not behave towards us in the problematic ways that our internal models will have led us to expect, and often to fear; we will have experienced a corrective emotional experience, as discussed in Chapter 8, and something about the foundation of our beliefs about our self and other people will be opened to change. If we live in a relational environment that is not currently directly replicating a problematic past, and involves others who are open to mutual processes of change, we will now have the opportunity for new, more rewarding and more intimate relational patterns to develop between ourselves and those who are important to us, and our internal models of self, others and relationships will be influenced in positive and constructive directions.

Corrective emotional experiences are commonly understood in this way, as involving the situation in which better emotional outcomes evolve compared with the past. However, it may also be the case that a relationship starts to repeat the actual reality of a situation of past emotional damage or abuse, but this time we may be able to deal with it differently, recognizing the nature of the other person's damaging behaviour towards us, and appropriately asserting and protecting ourselves. In a different, but equally important way this will also be a corrective emotional experience that will have the potential to constructively change our unconscious internal models of self and others, and how we relate to ourselves and to them.

The processes of corrective emotional experience and the capacity of another person to contain and understand the unhelpful emotional reactions that may be involved in our own self-generated feedback loops, may be of particular relevance when we are living with a background of emotional hurt and deprivation, abuse and trauma, where internal unconscious models may be functioning at pre-cognitive and pre-linguistic levels in significant ways. In these contexts, the emotional non-linguistic experience between people will be even more important. It may override things that are said, and it may make words redundant. It may be able to speak more loudly than words ever can. In this context trust, genuineness, and empathy will hold their most powerful place.

Environment and Place in the Lifespan: As overviewed in Chapters 11 and 12, our individual human potential unfolds in interaction with our developmental environments, and we live our lives in interaction with everything that constitutes our personal, inter-personal and demographic world. Every aspect of change in our unconscious internal models will take place in intimate interaction with our environment, which will play a significant part in supporting and enabling the processes of change. It will also influence the nature of change that is possible and how well that change can be maintained.

Sometimes people may actively be able to alter unhelpful aspects of their own environments, or those environments may change beneficially through some other process not under their control at all. At times, however, unhelpful aspects of the world around us may exist and it may not be possible for anyone to change them. Our processes of psychological change will always take place within the limits of our own individual potential, and the enabling or restricting influence of our relational, social and demographic worlds. Our potential to alter things that might be changed within our environments will vary across the lifespan, and will be influenced by our economic status and our physical and cognitive abilities. Early in the lifespan, before our independent capacities are sufficiently developed, and later if we lose them through illness and disability, or the changes of older adulthood, we will be dependent on others in this respect.

Across the lifespan we will experience changes within our developing selves and our environments that engender extensive growth and change within our unconscious internal models of self, others, relationships and the outside world. In general, many of these changes will be of enormous constructive value as we move from childhood into adulthood, becoming more able, capable and knowledgeable human beings involved in the social and practical worlds around us. Our environments may impede that development at times, with damaging consequences. In addition, internal models that have stood us in good stead may be challenged by our own developmental processes, or come into conflict with changes in the world around us, particularly during periods of transition and at times of loss. Our place in the lifespan will set an important context in relation to our overall processes of development and change.

The Innate Capacity for Growth and Development: All of the changes within our unconscious internal models discussed here will be influenced by our innate capacity for growth, which will be supported and enhanced by the developmentally constructive nature of our relationships.

Summary

The above material illustrates the use of current, transitive understanding of our intransitive human mind to generate a coherent Unifying Dialectical Model of human psychological functioning and processes of change, advised by the dialectical integration of five major approaches to psychotherapy: a model which has at its heart our unconscious internal models of self, others, relationships and the outside world.

In Chapters 18 and 19 we will look at a meta-framework supporting the Dialectical Integration of Approaches to Psychotherapy, the DIAP meta-framework, and discuss ways in which each of our major theoretical approaches to therapy practice may make their individual, or integrated contributions to processes of change within the Unifying Dialectical Model.

A Meta-Framework Supporting the Dialectical Integration of Approaches to Psychotherapy   **18**

Introduction

Following the discussion of the Unifying Dialectical Model, the UDM, in Chapter 17, this chapter will describe the second component of Dialectically Integrated Psychotherapy, a meta-framework supporting the dialectical integration of different approaches to psychotherapy on the basis of their individual capacities to facilitate changes in our unconscious internal models via the mechanisms and processes of the UDM.

In Chapter 15 a process of qualitative analysis was pursued in which the boundaries that conventionally divide our five major theoretical approaches to psychotherapy were lowered. This allowed us to examine the constructs, mechanisms and processes associated with each of them as theoretically neutral stand-alone elements, looking at the theoretical triangulation reflected in overlaps, and identifying aspects of compatible difference. Five core psychological constructs emerged from this work: conscious and unconscious mind; psychological defences; unconscious internal models of self, others, relationships and the outside world; and the constructive developmental relationship. They were defined on a theoretically integrative basis in Chapter 16 and play crucial roles within the UDM with our unconscious internal models sitting at the heart of our human psychological functioning. Changes within these internal models are assumed to underlie the enduring effectiveness of every successful psychotherapy, whatever its theoretical and epistemological base. The role of six other areas of theoretical overlap were also considered in relation to these change-related processes.

In this chapter the boundaries between our major approaches are reinstated as we consider their practical application within psychotherapy; they are put back into their metaphorical therapy boxes. As therapists we will each feel most comfortable when we are sitting within one of these boxes, or within a clearly integrative box that has expanded its walls to include aspects of other therapy theories that we also feel at home with. We need our metaphorical boxes, or therapy homes, so that we feel secure enough about what we are doing; therapy needs to be contained within a meaningful and manageable space.

We will now consider the contributions that each of our five major approaches to psychotherapy may make in influencing the feedback processes within the UDM and facilitating changes in our unconscious internal models.

The Dialectical Integration of Approaches to Psychotherapy, DIAP Meta-Framework

A simplified version of the self, focusing on the internal processes described by the Unifying Dialectical Model, sits at the centre of the DIAP meta-framework, illustrated in Figure 6. The client's self is flanked on one side by the total environmental context of their life and on the other by the therapeutic constructive developmental relationship, and is in two-way mutual relationship with them both. In all its complexity, the self plays a part in influencing the client's practical, demographic, social and relational environments. It similarly contributes to the nature of the constructive developmental relationship that will hopefully evolve during therapy. In this respect, the contributions that each individual client and the world they live in make to the unfolding experience of psychotherapy is clearly acknowledged.

Psychodynamic and attachment theories are linked together in this framework within the same overall metaphorical therapy box, reflecting their overlap in routine therapy practice. They feed into unconscious and conscious mind, and indirectly into behaviour, and together with humanistic theory they both feed into and support the constructive developmental relationship. Cognitive and behavioural theories relate particularly to conscious mind and behaviour, and behavioural approaches will sometimes directly seek to influence the environments we live in.

Each of our five major theoretical approaches is in a position to influence the nature of our unconscious internal models of self, others, relationships and the outside world, by influencing the processes of change within the Unifying Dialectical Model discussed in Chapter 17. The following discussion of the integrative and overlapping ways in which our major models may make such mutually supportive contributions will start with a consideration of the constructive developmental

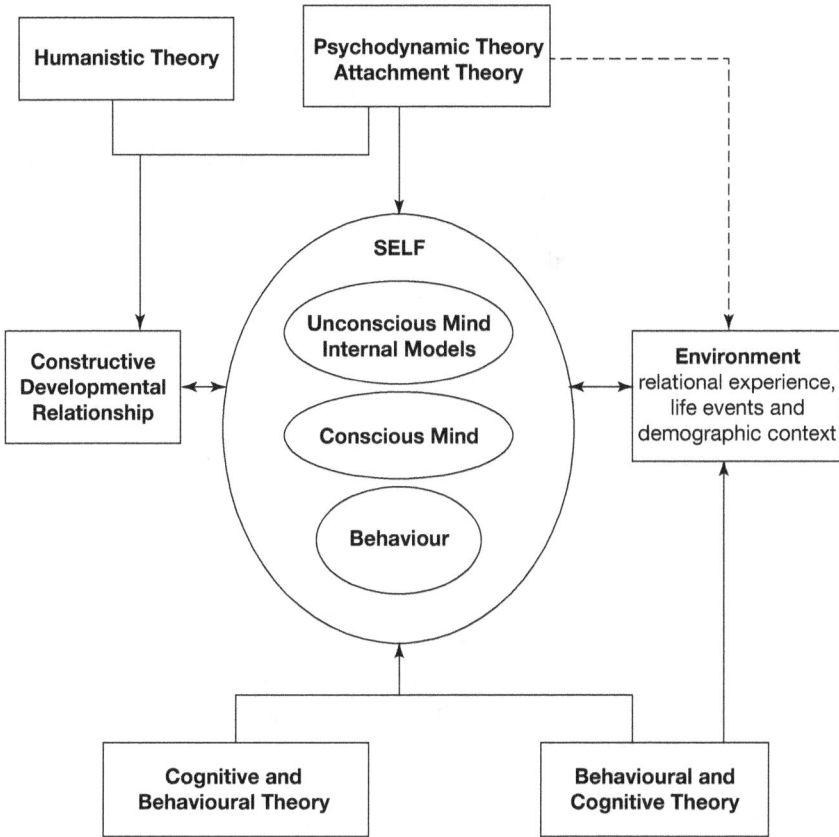

Figure 7   The Dialectical Integration of Approaches to Psychotherapy
Meta-Framework

relationship, and will then be structured under the process related subheadings used in Chapter 17. Since it is only feasible to mention a few selected aspects of each approach in this discussion, some readers may find it useful to re-visit Chapters 6-10 to support a broader-based depth in relation to each approach to be held in mind as well.

The Constructive Developmental Relationship: All therapy relationships should involve what we might refer to as a baseline constructive developmental relationship: a relationship that is sufficiently attuned, empathic, genuine and emotionally containing to be helpful within itself and to support a wide range of other therapeutic interventions, as discussed in Chapter 16. This relationship is valued by all of our major approaches to psychotherapy, and is particularly advised by humanistic, attachment and psychodynamic theory. As discussed in Chapter 16, it can of itself support reductions in unhelpful defences and the beneficial processes of development and change that enable our internal models to reflect more of our true rather than our defensively distorted false selves.

In addition to this baseline context, the nature, depth and complexity of the relationship and the work done within it by therapist and client, may reflect a more intensive, theoretically driven relational experience that carries greater potential to influence our internal models of self, others and relationships and to support our innate capacity for growth and development. This will be supported by aspects of psychodynamic, attachment and humanistic theories, and in such instances it will be important for the specific theories involved to be identified as making additional contributions to therapy process that are above and beyond baseline provision. Amongst other things this is likely to involve deeper experiences of emotional connection and security, increased opportunities for identification and internalization, a greater likelihood that helpful re-enactments will emerge as part of therapy process, and an overall increase in corrective emotional experience. All of these will provide greater opportunity for our innate capacities for growth and development to support our internal models in evolving towards our true rather than our defensively distorted false selves. From a cognitive and behavioural perspective, the constructive developmental relationship is particularly evident within Compassion Focused Therapy, Constructivist Psychotherapy and Functional Analytic Psychotherapy. It is also emphasized as a central part of Dialectical Behavior Therapy.

Unconscious Mind: Everything that happens in therapy, whatever the approach, will be available to unconscious mind, potentially influencing memory related structures, unconscious processes of learning and the nature of our unconscious internal models. In this respect every approach to psychotherapy will be generating experiences that can have a broad-based influence on those processes.

From a behavioural position, interventions that address the processes of classical and operant conditioning and our accumulated complex learning histories through attention to our overt behaviours, in effect influence underlying processes within unconscious mind, as do cognitive approaches that seek to achieve change in underlying unconscious schemas.

Psychodynamic theory directly addresses a wide range of unconscious processes that influence the nature of our unconscious internal models and their functioning, including the processes of unconscious defence, identification, internalization, projection, projective identification, transference and countertransference, as discussed in Chapter 8. It recognizes the unconscious impact of all aspects of the therapeutic relationship. From a more cognitive perspective, Constructivist Psychotherapy and Safran's work involving cognitive-interpersonal cycles overtly address unconscious processes relating to our internal models.

The Boundary Between Unconscious and Conscious Mind: Within all approaches to psychotherapy, the increased availability of unconscious material to conscious mind is an important aspect of therapy process, and is automatically supported by the emotional safety of the empathic and attuned therapeutic relationship. The relational aspect of therapy will contribute most strongly in this way within humanistic and psychodynamic/attachment related therapies.

Psychodynamic therapy specifically seeks to influence this boundary by allowing time and space for whatever comes to mind to be spoken about, and its attention to the functioning of defences plays a particularly important part in previously hidden thoughts, feelings and memories coming to conscious mind.

The boundary is also directly influenced within the cognitive and behavioural therapies. Structured identification of negative automatic thoughts brings material on the edge of conscious awareness to full conscious attention so that those thoughts can be articulated, catching our unhelpful unconscious internal models in action. The downward arrow technique supports access to unhelpful conditional assumptions, rules for living and core beliefs that are not immediately available to conscious awareness, and Mindfulness-Based Cognitive Therapy, Acceptance and Commitment Therapy, Behavioral Activation and Functional Analytic Therapy all support the accessing of thoughts and feelings that are similarly outside of conscious awareness. In all of these examples therapy is seeking to influence the boundary between unconscious and conscious mind.

Conscious Mind: All of our therapeutic approaches directly interact with our conscious thinking, feeling and ways of making sense of things that happen to us. They all have the capacity to influence conscious processes in ways that can feed back into unconscious mind and alter our unconscious internal models. The nature of these differing influences varies considerably across our major models. Any changes within conscious mind may also spontaneously influence the ways in which we behave; new and better outcomes may result, which can then feed back into both conscious and unconscious mind as well.

Within the cognitive and behavioural therapies, a wide range of therapeutic interventions directly address aspects of conscious mind and the relationship between cognition and emotion. Overt formulations set the scene and lead into active often structured processes designed to change unhelpful negative automatic thoughts, conditional beliefs and assumptions, rules for living, and underlying core beliefs and schemas in positive, constructive directions. A variety of strategies and therapeutic styles draw on discussion and logical thinking to explore, understand, appraise and challenge unhelpful conscious cognition, and to support alternative ways of thinking in a context of collaborative empiricism as discussed in Chapter 9.

From a behavioural position attention is often directly paid to the processes of conscious mind in ways that are framed and analysed by the principles of radical behaviourism and functional analysis, with anything a person thinks, feels, or imagines being categorized as behaviour.

Applied behaviour analysis and functional analysis influence our conscious understanding of ourselves and the world around us and bring the existence of unconscious processes of reinforcement into conscious awareness. They support us in thinking about the function our behaviours fulfil for us, what we have gained from them and what may have been avoided. The consequences of prior experiences of classical and operant conditioning may also now be understood and taken into consideration, and as our behaviour changes, all of its outcomes will be available for conscious mind to process. All of these experiences are likely to have significant impacts on our conscious thoughts, beliefs and emotions, all of which may contribute to changes within our unconscious internal models. They will be reflected in the processes of therapies such as Dialectical Behavior Therapy, Acceptance and Commitment Therapy, Behavioral Activation and Functional Analytic Psychotherapy, as discussed in Chapter 10.

Within psychodynamic therapy our past and current lives are explored with aspects of self, memories, emotion and relational experience coming to greater conscious awareness. All of these are thought about, discussed and understood at a conscious level, making sense of the present in terms of the past. Evidence and understanding emerge that that can offer new conscious learning about ourselves, others and our relationships. The involvement of conscious mind is an intrinsic part of every personal and interpersonal aspect of experience within therapy, with consequent, sometimes powerful effects on our conscious thoughts, feelings and beliefs as the work together unfolds. In addition, psychodynamic theory recognizes the benefits that reductions in internal anxiety can produce in relation to our overall capacities for constructive thinking, and our abilities to share those processes of thinking with each other. All will play crucial parts in the nature of evolving change in our unconscious internal models.

Much of the work done in therapies advised by attachment theory will reflect a similar context, with emphasis on the realities and unhelpful consequences of damaging relational experiences and respect for the felt validity of clients' recollections of the past. In providing empathic and attuned listening psychodynamic, attachment and humanistic/client-centred and experiential therapies will have powerful effects on the processes of conscious mind. In addition, Gestalt Therapy as an experiential approach includes the 'two-chair' technique, designed to integrate disparate aspects of unconscious internal models by working with conscious mind.

The Processing of Emotion: Emotion is intimately connected with the nature and functioning of our unconscious internal models. It will be a strong component of those therapy models that relate to self, others and relationships, and many of those relating to the outside world. It plays significant roles in the activation of our internal models and their subsequent influence on conscious mind and behaviour. Conscious processing of emotion within therapy may help to reduce the activation of unhelpful/damaging internal models, and contribute to their beneficial change. It may also increase the activation of models that function on a more constructive basis, and strengthen them.

Within psychodynamic therapy, time, space and understanding are provided in relation to all aspects of emotion, especially those that have been limited or hidden by defence related processes. Emotional containment within therapy is crucial to its secure experiencing and processing. Within the humanistic/client-centred and experiential therapies, the conscious experience of emotion and its processing are core aspects of the empathic attuned relationship and therapy process.

From an overall cognitive and behavioural position, attention to the processing of emotional experience and the importance of living with and living through distressing emotion is supported by Safran's work on cognitive-interpersonal cycles, Mindfulness-Based Cognitive Therapy, Compassion Focused Therapy, Acceptance and Commitment Therapy and Behavioral Activation. In addition, the experiencing and regulation of intense emotion is an important part of Dialectical Behavior Therapy.

Psychological Defences: Defence related processes are core components of our unconscious internal models. They also function at unconscious and conscious levels in ways that both contribute to the nature of those models and are influenced by them. They can have powerful effects on the nature of our consciously experienced emotions, cognitions and overt behaviours. In multiple ways changes in unhelpful defences can be essential to the processes of constructive change within our unconscious internal models.

Psychodynamic therapy provides us with considerable theoretical understanding in relation to our mechanisms of defence, taking them into account throughout therapy. Experiencing and living through previously hidden and avoided emotions, thoughts and memories can remove the need for unhelpful and distorting defences. Reductions in their functioning may also be supported by explicit interpretation, explanation and discussion, or they may be enabled to change without being mentioned at all. Psychodynamic, attachment and humanistic/client-centred theory all support aspects of therapeutic relating that naturally help to reduce them. In addition, attachment theory acknowledges the power of parental behaviour to have directly generated unhelpful defences that keep aspects of a damaging developmental past in their hidden place.

From within overall cognitive and behavioural positions, Safran's work in relation to unconscious processes and cognitive-interpersonal cycles addresses our defences in the form of security operations, and Mindfulness-Based Cognitive Therapy and Behavioral Activation explicitly work towards the experiencing of previously avoided aversive private events, so that they are less likely to fuel unhelpful avoidant, defence related behaviours.

Acceptance: Acceptance of our selves for who we are and of the realities of our current lives are both seen as contributing to the potential for constructive, beneficial changes within our unconscious internal models. Such acceptance is most powerfully supported in theory and practice by humanistic/client-centred theory, and will be part of the constructive developmental relationship across all approaches to therapy. It also holds a focused place within Compassion Focused Therapy, Mindfulness-Based Cognitive Therapy, Acceptance and Commitment Therapy and Dialectical Behavior Therapy.

Whilst the specific concept of acceptance is not particularly discussed in psychodynamic theory, therapy has the capacity to markedly influence it as an integrated part of process. This is reflected in the depth of attention given to the empathic understanding and acceptance provided within relational, attachment related and self-psychology perspectives, and the undefended access to and lived-with acceptance of previously avoided experience.

Overt Behaviour: Changes in our overt behaviours may relate to any aspect of our behaviour towards ourselves, others and the outside world. Beneficial consequences of those changed behaviours will feed back into conscious and unconscious mind, influencing maintenance and change processes within our unconscious internal models in constructive directions.

Behaviourally led approaches give specific and sometimes directive attention to changes in behaviour. The need for behavioural change is often assessed by functional analysis, and can emerge from detailed attention to clients' histories and current life situations. Skills training may be used to address self-management and coping skills; interpersonal skills including communication skills and assertiveness; the skills of emotion regulation; and problem-solving skills. Effective change leads to new and constructive behaviours with the potential for positive outcomes involving the self, others and relationships. Stage one of Dialectical Behavior Therapy involves a combination of all of these approaches to behavioural change.

The therapeutic benefit of changed behaviour is illustrated particularly clearly in relation to anxiety and avoidance. In any context facing anxiety that is unhelpfully associated with a stimulus, rather than continuing to avoid it, can enable a conditioned association to be brought to an end. To achieve this, we need to behave differently in some way, expose ourselves to the feared stimulus, and forego the negative reinforcement afforded by defence related avoidance. When effective, the feared object, person, situation or emotion is then no longer feared; we continue to behave differently in relation to it, and are free to develop further new behaviours. New opportunities may open up in our lives. The nature of our unconscious internal model of that stimulus has changed, maybe quite dramatically, and our internal model of self will have changed as well. It is also likely that our internal models of others, relationships and the outside world will change too, depending on the role that anxiety had played in our life, and the nature of the stimulus involved. Whole new realms of experience may be opened up to us because a particular anxiety or fear no longer limits our lives, and our unconscious internal models will grow and change accordingly. The most powerful part of this process may be behaving differently, facing and living with the awfulness of anxiety, rather than avoiding it.

Within the behaviourally led therapies these principles are particularly reflected within Acceptance and Commitment Therapy, in which conscious distressing emotions are lived with, at the same time as commitment is made to a range of potentially challenging but rewarding behavioural goals. Such changes in overt behaviours often involve new skills and abilities, and frequently bring with them experiences of success and achievement.

In behavioural terms the process by which beneficial outcomes feed back into changes within our unconscious internal models would equate with the concept of positive reinforcement. This theoretical context is reflected in Behavioral Activation's focus on establishing a diverse range of stable sources of positive reinforcement, which become part of new learning histories. Similarly, Acceptance and Commitment Therapy encourages the setting of behavioural goals that are consistent with people's values and likely to result in positive reinforcement. All can lead to significant changes in our unconscious internal models of ourselves and the world around us.

From humanistic, psychodynamic and attachment approaches, changes in behaviour are more likely to be left to unfold on a spontaneous basis, and may particularly involve changes in relational behaviours. As they unfold, they will be discussed from their particular therapeutic perspectives, which may influence the ways in which they evolve. Behaviour in relation to avoided and feared distressing emotion is a core aspect of therapy from these perspectives as defence related processes are worked with and enabled to change.

Within therapies that rely primarily on influencing cognitive processes there may be a somewhat similar assumption that behaviour will change as a consequence of changes in conscious cognition; however, overt behaviour will often be addressed directly as well. In addition, the behavioural experiments used in primarily cognitive approaches to gain evidence in relation to cognition, may also actively support behavioural change.

In all instances, if the outcomes of our changed behaviours are beneficial they will feed back into our unconscious models and influence them for the better.

Relational Experience: As discussed in this chapter and in Chapter 16, the overall experience of a constructive attuned and empathic developmental relationship will provide important and maybe crucial opportunities for growth promoting relational experiences and corrective emotional experiences influencing the evolution of less damaging internal models of self, others and relationships, and will be particularly supported by humanistic, psychodynamic and attachment theories.

In addition, specific aspects of clients' relational behaviours may directly reflect unhelpful unconscious internal models of self, others and relationships that distort current perception and have been affected by earlier damaging relational experiences. These are defined as transference-based responses within psychodynamic therapy, and as clinically relevant behavioural patterns within Functional Analytic Psychotherapy. Therapist responses that bring these processes in to conscious awareness with care and empathy, and recognize the connection with previous damaging relational experiences, support the potential for them to change. Corrective emotional experiences may also be involved if clients have anticipated a negativity that does not emerge, and together these processes can influence the feedback loops maintaining clients' unconscious internal models, changing them for the better. Such contexts are addressed in psychodynamic therapy as they emerge spontaneously within the therapeutic relationship. They are actively prompted within Functional Analytic Therapy, and responded to strategically according to the principles of operant conditioning. They may also be addressed within cognitive-interpersonal and constructivist approaches to cognitive and behavioural therapies.

Particular attention may also be paid to repeated problematic relational experiences and re-enactments that may evolve between therapist and client, just as they do in everyday life. These are understood to involve mutual experiences of unhelpful aspects of transference and countertransference, and projective identification. The recognition and resolution of such re-enactments can provide powerful corrective emotional experiences and aspects of conscious awareness that enable unconscious internal models to change in constructive and positive ways. New and positive relational experience emerges where previously only hurt, upset and shame may have prevailed. These processes are particularly supported by psychodynamic and attachment theories, and by the therapeutic work advocated within Safran's approach to cognitive-interpersonal cycles, from a cognitive and behavioural perspective.

In all of the above contexts, the beneficial nature of relational therapeutic processes will be augmented by clear and honest communication, and the capacities of both parties to mentalize, and appreciate the nature of minds that are separate from their own, as particularly discussed within attachment theory.

Therapy may also influence the nature of relational experiences within clients' everyday lives. Any changes that start to unfold within clients' internal models of self, others and relationships may prompt clients to behave differently within other relationships; if good outcomes emerge changes in unconscious internal models will be further enhanced. Behavioural approaches may directly support such changes in clients' relational behaviours. Experiences in therapy may foster the potential for repeated unhelpful relational patterns to be resolved in ways that provide corrective emotional experiences within clients' everyday worlds.

The Environment and Our Place in the Lifespan: The DIAP meta-framework fully recognizes the importance of the social, relational and practical environments we live in, and our place in the life span in relation to our psychological well-being and processes of change, as discussed in Chapters 11 and 12.

Behavioural theory is the main approach to focus on and advocate direct change in our environments and the nature of the world around us, where it is feasible for changes to be made, and whilst not included here as an approach to therapy, Community Psychology plays an important part in working to address the nature of unhelpful social and demographic environments (Kagan et al., 2020).

From a very different perspective, structured and straightforward cognitive approaches might focus on our beliefs and unhelpful thoughts about our environments and lifespan positions and their associated experiences, in the hope of altering our attitudes and behaviours in more helpful directions.

From a psychodynamic position our relational, social and work-related environments often constitute a major focus of discussion. This may also be the case from cognitive-behavioural perspectives that take our interpersonal contexts into account. Being able to think about and understand the roles that our environments can play, may make important contributions towards our capacities to be less critical and more accepting of ourselves. It may also support our potential to recognize the avenues towards constructive changes that might be feasible, and directly influence the nature of the physical and relational environments that surround us. In terms of unhelpful relational contexts, we may come to recognize more clearly when others are treating us in ways that are damaging, as well as our own capacities to behave in damaging ways towards other people. Such awareness may be the start of our potential to influence beneficial changes within those environments, and therapy may support us in trying to do so.

Our place in the lifespan involves significant processes of transition as we move through into adult life from childhood, and from adulthood on into older age. Opportunities for growth and development may present welcome but challenging psychological and emotional demands on us, or the lack of such opportunities face us with a sense of absence and loss. The ultimate decline in physical capacities whenever it comes to each of us in older age may be much mitigated by our own secure sense of self, our capacity to constructively adapt to our changing world place, and our supported and loved place amongst family and friends. Or it may be made all the harder by loss and absence in all these respects. Where beneficial changes in our environments are possible, they will play their part in supporting constructive change in our unconscious internal models of self, others, relationships and the outside world. In all contexts the nature of the relational and physical/practical world we live in will play crucial roles in the processes of change, adaptation and growth throughout the lifespan.

In the context of psychotherapy, we may make constructive changes, come to think and feel differently about ourselves and behave differently. Our unconscious internal models may change, but the consequences of those changes will be experienced in the most straightforward ways if the environment around us is able to respond well and engage positively with our changing ways of being.

Significantly, the world we currently live in, particularly our relational world, may support or actively limit the ways in which we are able to change, and significant aspects of those worlds may be out of our personal power to influence. Hard lessons may sometimes need to be learnt about the limits of psychotherapy to engender change.

Summary

Chapter 18 has discussed the Dialectical Integration of Approaches to Psychotherapy, DIAP meta-framework, and ways in which our five major approaches may influence the components of the UDM supporting change in the nature and functioning of our internal unconscious models of self, others, relationships and the outside world. Chapter 19 will consider the ways in which the mechanisms and processes associated with our different theoretical approaches may make mutual, synergistic contributions in practice, looking at the overall pragmatics of integrative practice, and discussing the importance of taking the current nature of our unconscious internal models into account.

The DIAP Meta-Framework in Practice: Dialectically Integrated Psychotherapy

19

Following the discussion of the DIAP meta-framework in Chapter 18, we will now consider the basis on which our five major approaches may make their integrative synergistic contributions within therapy practice, and discuss the overall pragmatics of theoretically integrated psychotherapy.

We will also look at the importance of developmental vulnerability in relation to the nature of our unconscious internal models and the long-term consequences of developmental environments that have failed and damaged us. The perspectives that Dialectically Integrated Psychotherapy may contribute in this context will be explored.

The Mutual, Synergistic Contributions of Different Therapy Approaches: Dialectically Integrated Psychotherapy

All of the overlapping and compatible mechanisms and processes associated with the major theoretical approaches included in the DIAP meta-framework may contribute to constructive change within individual experiences of psychotherapy. All provide their own routes towards changes in our unconscious internal models and all are potentially available to complement and support each other. This integration may sometimes only be appreciated after an experience of therapy has unfolded.

Therapists may deliberately influence these contributions by conscious intent, or they may have their effects as the result of naturally unfolding processes. They may be planned in advance in a formal and structured approach to integration, or they may be thought about on an individualized basis as therapy unfolds. They may also emerge as the result of serendipitous changes and events within the client's everyday world. They may not have been led by the therapist at all, or necessarily have been recognized as taking place, but they may all have been part of mutually synergistic beneficial processes of change; change that may not have taken place without them acting together. All of these possibilities are validated and supported by the principles of Dialectically Integrated Psychotherapy. The interventions guided by our different theoretical approaches may be applied within the same therapy experience, with the integrative processes of their associated mechanisms taking place in synergy, or they may be applied in relation to the same client within separate single model therapies, with these integrative processes taking place on a sequential basis.

Dialectically Integrated Psychotherapy primarily supports therapists' individualized decisions about interventions to be used on this integrative basis, rather than prescribing specific ways to achieve that integration. However, a few general points will be discussed here in relation to the mutual support that may be experienced across traditional cognitive behavioural and psychodynamic/attachment-based approaches.

The Benefit of Psychodynamic/Attachment-based Principles Within Cognitive Behavioural Therapies: As discussed in Chapter 16, our internal models follow a pathway of development from birth onwards, resulting in our own individual mix of early immature potentially pre-cognitive models and more mature models influenced by cognition, language and increasingly adult experience of self, others, relationships and the outside world. All of these models may be relatively more constructive or more damaging, largely depending on the nature of our early and later developmental relationships and life events, and be influenced to varying degrees by the functioning of defence related processes.

Taking these considerations into account, traditional cognitive behavioural interventions addressing conscious mind may be most straightforward in their effectiveness when we are working with unhelpful internal models which clearly function at a cognitive and linguistic level and are not unduly influenced by defence related processes. The situation may be different if we are dealing with significant proportions of immature non-cognitive, non-linguistic models and/or the significant functioning of psychological defences. Drawing on attachment-based and psychodynamic relational understanding may be particularly helpful in terms of non-linguistic aspects of communication and emotional connection, and will support the importance of emotion and meaning in this way at conscious and unconscious levels. These aspects of therapy may also be significantly supported by humanistic client-centred theory. In relation to defences, both psychodynamic and attachment theories directly support reductions in unhelpful defences, and drawing on them in this respect may, to greater or lesser extents, support the effectiveness of all cognitive and behavioural approaches. Traditional cognitively led interventions might prove actively unhelpful if they challenge thoughts and beliefs associated with significant defences that are currently an integrated part of psychological functioning, without taking those defences into account.

The Benefit of Cognitive Behavioural Principles Within Psychodynamic/Attachment-Based Therapies: Within psychodynamic and attachment related therapies, overt attention to aspects of unhelpful conscious cognition could be supportive of beneficial changes in our unconscious internal models; the value of directly addressing unhelpful beliefs about the self, others and relationships may be considerable. In some contexts, a direct focus on overt behaviour, what clients say and do within their daily lives and relationships, may be essential to the experience of different, beneficial outcomes and consequences, and to subsequent enduring changes in our internal models. In addition, the supportive and containing nature of structure and explanation may be helpful for a wide range of clients, particularly if it enables a greater sense of mutual collaboration and interpersonal equality than might otherwise exist.

The Overall Importance of the Nature of Our Unconscious Internal Models: The balance between immature and mature models, those that are damaging rather than constructive and the nature of their associated processes of defence can impact on the potential appropriateness and helpfulness of all our different therapeutic approaches. Any thoughts we have about the potential mix within each individual client may influence the judgements we make as therapists about the nature of therapy best suited to their needs, and advise our decisions about the use of theoretically integrative approaches. This becomes increasingly important when our unconscious internal models have been significantly influenced by the inadequate nature and quality of our developmental relationships, including experiences of deprivation, trauma and abuse. This context will be considered in more depth following the next section on the practicalities of integrative practice.

The Pragmatics of Dialectically Integrated Psychotherapy Practice

Whilst this work takes the fundamental position that at an intransitive level the compatible psychological processes and mechanisms associated with all of our differing major approaches to psychotherapy are able to function together in our minds in integrative and unified harmony, the same cannot be said in relation to the pragmatics of psychotherapy practice. Therapy practice has been developed so that therapists applying single-model approaches can directly influence the specific psychological mechanisms and processes deemed to be of causal relevance within each approach.

Thus client-centred therapy leaves sometimes almost total space for clients to express and explore themselves, with very little suggestion or guidance from the therapist, but with the support of sensitive, attuned understanding. Psychodynamic therapy will also allow time and space for process to unfold, working to create an environment in which aspects of unconscious mind will be free to enter consciousness and be talked about. Both of these therapeutic approaches have often been described as process oriented, allowing time and space for clients to take the lead and follow their own train of spontaneous thought, with varying degrees of therapist intervention in terms of empathic understanding, clarification and explanation or interpretation.

In contrast, cognitive and behavioural therapy approaches, and behaviourally led therapies may actively limit the opportunity for clients to pursue their own spontaneous thoughts, particularly in their more protocol-led and agenda directed formats. Since therapy aims to focus on particular aspects of thinking and/or behaviour that are seen to be problematic, it is structured so that these may be identified, clarified and addressed, whilst distractions are reduced. Sessions are often actively planned in advance, sometimes with a written agenda, and therapy may be guided by explicit and overt goals, with the content and nature of therapy sessions being designed to actively enable those goals to be achieved. At the same time, some space is given to listening, hearing and appreciating the nature and experience of clients' lives as part of a supportive therapeutic and collaborative relationship. In other contexts such as Constructivist Psychotherapy, cognitive approaches will be much more flexible and process oriented.

Aspects of these descriptions may appear rather stereotypical and realities will probably vary considerably. However, the distinctly different styles of therapy practice across our major approaches raises issues about the nature of practice that may most appropriately support the provision of a theoretically integrative psychotherapy experience. No issues arise if we provide these therapies separately and leave the integration to happen purely within the client's mind, but issues do exist when we seek to enable the mechanisms and processes of different approaches to complement each other within the same experience of therapy.

However therapy unfolds, it needs to evolve as a consistent and reliable experience between therapist and client; one which both can have faith in. Most therapists find themselves more drawn towards some theoretical perspectives and styles of being as therapists than others. As discussed earlier, we each have a theoretical or therapy home. Mine would be a psychodynamic and humanistic home, very much supported by attachment theory. For others their home is definitely a cognitive behavioural, rather more structured one. For others it is one that is supported by a formally defined integrative therapy such as Cognitive

Analytic Therapy: we all need a therapy home. Each of us as therapists work from the primary basis of our own theoretical home, where we feel most secure in relation to both therapy theory and the nature of practice.

Some changes will need to be made in our therapy home if we are going to work with processes and mechanisms that are helpfully considered from other theoretical perspectives. The nature and degree of change will depend on our starting point, and the judgements we make in relation to the feasibility of effective practice; from any perspective therapists may have concerns about the nature of these changes. For example, the highly structured nature of a classically protocol and agenda led cognitive behavioural therapy will need to become more flexible and process oriented when it seeks to accommodate the value of humanistic and psychodynamic listening, discovery and the mutual evolution of thinking, feeling and understanding; this may raise concerns regarding a loss of essential focus and action.

Similarly, the process oriented, unstructured listening and responding of humanistic and psychodynamic therapies needs to become more open to some use of structure and aspects of guidance when it seeks to benefit from cognitive and behavioural understanding and practice. From a psychodynamic position there may be concern that such changes may influence the nature of the transference relationship and the relational patterns and enactments that may evolve, and may limit the exploration and discovery of defences and hidden feelings.

However, rather than necessarily being a disadvantage, the experience of different styles of being within the therapeutic relationship may prove fruitful in terms of the range of transference, counter-transference and defence related experiences that may unfold. From a cognitive behavioural perspective, some of the structured control over the content of therapy sessions may be lost and process may evolve in less predictable ways. The benefits that emerge may lie in the increased opportunity for emotion and associated cognitions to emerge, for defences to be recognized and understood, and for the relived experiences of relational contexts to enable greater sense to be made of the cognitive-interpersonal cycles associated with damaging and unhelpful internal models of self and others.

The exact ways in which interventions are implemented when they are being carried out in an integrative therapeutic context may clearly vary compared with their potentially pure form in an exclusively single-model therapy. The crucial issue will be whether the nature of integrative therapy practice has then enabled important and necessary processes and mechanisms to unfold, in ways that would not have been possible otherwise. This, as with so much in psychology and psychotherapy, can never be proven, but as in other instances if the hoped-for benefits are gained, we hope and maybe assume that they have been.

Essentially in any theoretically integrated psychotherapy we are seeking a sufficiently middle path for elements of more than one theory to influence practice effectively at the same time, in ways that are compatible with each other and enable us to continue to feel comfortable and secure as therapists.

Many therapists who feel free to do so choose to practice from an integrative position, and this model is offered in support of their existing practice. For those wishing to work in a more integrative way the DIAP meta-framework may provide a useful rationale in support of their efforts. For them and for currently integrative therapists, it may also help to support an integrative analysis of therapy process.

The freedom of integrative practice is not always available since we are often faced with the constraints of evidence-based practice as implemented in the current contexts of state and insurance-based psychotherapy provision in England and the US. All of the factors at the heart of theoretically integrative practice cut across the overt requirements of logical positivism and empirically defined psychotherapy in clinical and research contexts. They fly in the face of strict protocol-led therapies and the belief that everyone can receive exactly the same psychological 'medicine'; they always have done. However, within each and every one of the protocol-led therapies provided by researchers and routine practitioners, whatever their stated single-model approach, the actual experience of psychotherapy is still likely to be influenced by processes and mechanisms that are defined by other approaches.

The principles of Dialectically Integrated Psychotherapy can support single-model therapists in getting the best they can from the overt model they are working with. They may find aspects of their own understanding endorsed by other approaches, and that understanding may be further illuminated. They may find out more about the constructive developmental relationship that they are building with their client, whatever their orientation. They may become more able to recognize when unhelpful defences are at play, and finds ways of helping them to change. They may think more about the importance of emotion and the significance of acceptance. They may be supported in recognizing the powerful self-perpetuating nature of unhelpful beliefs and automatic thoughts, and share that understanding with their clients. They may gain insight into ways in which a particular aspect of behaviour that is unhelpful may be understood in the context of its environment. They may think that bit more about the social, physical, cultural and political world their clients live in, and that bit more about their clients' gender, their sexuality and the place in the life-span from which they are currently living their lives.

They may be supported in finding ways of understanding and responding to difficult relational contexts between themselves and their clients; they may recognize when changes in overt behaviour may be an essential starting point, or crucial to further progress; and all therapists may be supported in thinking about themselves, who they are, their own personal place within the therapy relationship, their strengths and vulnerabilities, and the developmental backgrounds that have shaped them.

Developmental Vulnerability and Dialectically Integrated Psychotherapy

As the nature of our developmental environment becomes gradually less and less conducive to the development of the healthy more mature constructive unconscious internal models that enable us to thrive, the proportion of those models that are unhelpful and damaging to us will increase, as discussed in Chapter 16. As adults we are also likely to have a greater proportion of more immature and potentially pre-cognitive models than we might have done otherwise, with a greater proportion of those being unhelpful and damaging rather than constructive, and carrying with them the enduring influence of unfulfilled developmental relational needs. These models are likely to be more heavily influenced by unhelpful defences, and will include greater proportions of more immature and strongly distorting defences as the damaging nature of our developmental environment increases.

If we add in the experience of emotional deprivation, overt relational trauma, and physical and sexual abuse, that might have been present from infancy onwards, overall we are presented with a very wide potential continuum of unconscious internal models, in terms of their maturity versus immaturity, and constructive capacity versus unhelpful and damaging influences, as illustrated in Figure 5, p 178. The higher the proportion of immature potentially pre-cognitive, non-linguistic models, the greater becomes the overall therapeutic importance of non-verbal aspects of communication and connection; unhelpful immature models may not be amenable to influence by changes in conscious cognition if they exist at a pre-cognitive level.

As the overall proportion of damaging internal models increases, with greater proportions of immature compared with mature models, and increased prevalence of powerfully distorting immature defences, we move towards the territory of what we often refer to as personality disorder. The nature of disturbance becomes greater as the proportion of damaging immature models associated with immature defences rises. In routine therapy provision it tends to be found that single-model therapies are more limited in their helpfulness for clients diagnosed with a personality disorder. Their capacity to straightforwardly support constructive changes in unconscious internal models is reduced as we move across this continuum, and is accompanied by an increase in the potential benefit of theoretical integration. As in all contexts the effectiveness of any approach, single-model or integrative, will vary across individuals, and will be influenced by the therapeutic relationship.

The concept of basic trust is also relevant here. If our unconscious internal models have developed in the context of inadequate developmental relationships, the experience of attachment related trauma, emotional deprivation and a maturational environment that failed us, we may not have been able to experience what Erickson refers to as basic trust, as discussed in Chapter 12; a crucially important inner state associated with the first months of our lives. Basic trust means that we are in a position of existential security as an infant; without words or cognition of any sort we 'know' that when we are in distress someone will come to deal with that distress, when we need someone to be there, they will be there, when we need stimulation and pleasure through interaction and care, it will be provided. We come to trust the world around us and trust ourselves at a totally implicit level. When our infant world has not been like that, our internal models will reflect that state of affairs, and we can be left vulnerable, anxious and uncertain, at an emotional non-linguistic, pre-cognitive level in relation to our fundamental existential security, and the interpersonal security of our lives.

The nature of relating that might help to change our associated internal immature and pre-cognitive models and generate something of that trust for us, whatever our chronological age, lies within a caring relationship that includes emotionally attuned responsiveness, expressed through both linguistic and non-linguistic aspects of being that are genuine and reliable at a fundamental level; they may fluctuate but they never fundamentally fail. Aspects of psychodynamic object relations and self-psychology theories, attachment theory and humanistic client-centred theory are best positioned to help advise us in these respects. The therapeutic constructive developmental relationship may need to evolve in particularly sensitive and meaningful ways, and the relevance of non-verbal ways of being could matter at quite a profound level as significant proportions of pre-cognitive, non-linguistic internal models prevail.

If we are faced with high proportions of very damaged and immature unconscious internal models, that are intertwined with powerful immature defences, it may be that only limited change is feasible, and sometimes no significant fundamental change may be feasible at all. We may be dealing with a context of extreme pre-cognitive and cognitive distortions of internal and external experience, fragmentation, possibly dissociation, and the products of powerful immature defences. All of these factors make it very much harder for new relational experience and the current processing of our conscious and unconscious minds to help our internal models change, with the additional possibility that overwhelming emotion may destabilize a delicate internal psychic balance.

In some situations, it is important to deliberately moderate or avoid activation of problematic aspects of existing internal models, and focus primarily on providing opportunity for relatively more mature models to be developed and strengthened in constructive ways, which then become available for activation. This position is consistent with the use of what we often refer to as ego strengthening approaches and supportive psychotherapy, which minimize the challenges to fragile selves, accept limits to the changes that may be achieved, but still provide opportunities for growth and development.

In such situations the opportunity for emotional connection and containment, the discovery of one's own spontaneous thoughts and feelings, and the experience of being heard, listened to and understood remain important. Their value is added to by the potentially crucial ways in which transformative relational contexts advised by psychodynamic, attachment and client-centred theories can support the natural innate capacities for beneficial change, growth and development that exist in all of us.

Cognitive behavioural approaches that focus on changes in conscious cognition, behaviour and the role of the immediate environment make important contributions to the development of new models of self, others and relationships. They can also support the everyday active management of the impact of damaging unconscious internal models. It is in these contexts that we may need to let go of the hope for fundamental change within those models, while still appreciating the very real benefits of the routine ongoing use of prompts, encouragement and contingency management in minimizing their impact and supporting alternative conscious cognition and constructive helpful behaviours.

In order to illustrate aspects of potential fit between some of these thoughts and therapy practice, the protocols of Dialectical Behavior Therapy (Swales & Heard, 2009) will now be considered, in relation to Borderline Personality Disorder and the self-harming behaviour that may be associated with it.

Within stage one intense painful emotion and damaging impulsive behaviour is addressed by structured approaches that set a firm limit in relation to self-harm and aggression, while also providing an empathic, understanding approach that validates individuals in the suffering they have experienced and supports the mindful experience of and living with painful feelings. Skills-based learning supports the use of helpful strategies to support the regulation of intense emotion and interpersonal problem solving, helping to reduce the risk of harmful behaviours. This approach may reflect the ways in which a parent might accept, understand and contain the intense emotion of a young child, and set firm boundaries to protect them, alongside efforts to support what might be done to help a situation become better. If so, it might reflect ways in which good and caring parenting helps problematic immature internal models and unhelpful immature defences develop along a more constructive path. Caring, emotionally containing behaviour, and firm but not punishing limits may provide the necessary developmental environment for clients, just as it can in childhood.

Stage two then enables exploration and understanding of important unresolved personal and interpersonal experiences, taking care not to touch on contexts that may seriously destabilize the client. At times it may be crucial not to activate certain aspects of our damaging unconscious internal models, especially immature and potentially pre-cognitive ones. As well as putting the client directly at risk, the emotional and behavioural consequences may also risk feeding back into unconscious mind, strengthening those damaging internal models further.

Therapy in stage two supports a further path of development and change within unhelpful unconscious internal models of self, others and relationships involving both immature and more mature models, that takes advantage of a wider range of approaches from within the cognitive behavioural theoretical umbrella as well as psychodynamic and attachment related perspectives.

Summary

This chapter has discussed the capacity for the processes and mechanisms of our major therapeutic approaches to mutually support each other, and considered some of the issues involved in making decisions about the nature and style of integrative therapy practice. It has also discussed the therapeutic implications of the ways in which clients' unconscious internal models may have been be influenced by the quality of their developmental environments. Part 4 will provide a detailed example of individualized integrative psychotherapy which will be analysed and discussed in relation to the principles of Dialectically Integrated Psychotherapy.

Part 4

Dialectically Integrated Psychotherapy
in the Consulting Room

An Experience of Therapy: **20**
A Content Analysis of Integrative Process

Introduction

In Part 4 Dialectically Integrated Psychotherapy is brought to life through the retrospective analysis and discussion of an integrative therapy experience, drawing from my work with a client I am calling 'Becky'. She is married and has a young daughter. I am calling her husband 'Sebastian' and her little girl 'Julia'. Becky gave her signed consent for details from her therapy experience to be used in published material in ways that would help professionals get a picture of how problems were understood, what happened during therapy and what sort of changes took place. I explained that this would be done on an anonymous basis, her identity and the identity of others would be protected, and aspects of therapy would be described as they took place between us. This was discussed at the start of therapy and again at the end, when consent was given. The information sheet and consent form are provided in Appendix 2. Thomas-Anttila (2015) provides a thoughtful discussion of the tensions, complexities and dilemmas of confidentiality and consent involved in the publishing of therapy material in case reports.

When we meet, Becky is struggling to deal with her grief at losing her mum and dad, and experiences significant problems with anxiety and depression. Persistent mood-swings are with her every day, she feels too anxious to go out on her own, contact with people other than her husband Sebastian is really hard for her, and she rarely leaves the house. Her main focus is looking after Julia. Our work together describes an individualized, formulation led experience of therapy, and illustrates the typical nature of my approach to integrative practice. We meet at two-weekly intervals for a total of 27 sessions over 15 months. The benefits she gains are reflected in the Brief Symptom Inventory, BSI scores illustrated at the end of this chapter (Derogatis & Melisaratos, 1983).

Brief therapy experiences are often presented in case discussions as falling into the stages of beginning, middle and end to support considerations of process over time, and a similar practice has been adopted here. Therapy is divided into four stages, with the four assessment and formulation sessions being identified as stage one. The rest of therapy is divided into the post-assessment beginning of therapy, sessions 5-11; the middle, sessions 12-19; and the end, sessions 20-27. Whilst the nature of therapy certainly changes over time and reflects these stages, the exact point at which a boundary is set between one phase and another is to some extent rather arbitrary. I have chosen to place the boundary between the beginning and the middle at the point where we have largely identified and begun to work with most of the different themes in Becky's life that together contribute to her difficulties. The boundary between the middle and the end falls after core aspects of our work together have started to lead into significant progress.

In this chapter we consider the proportional contributions of the major theoretical approaches across the stages of therapy, and look at a brief summary of our work together. In Chapter 21 we will discuss the integrative processes of therapy that make their synergistic contributions to change within Becky's unconscious internal models of self, others, relationships and the outside world.

My therapeutic work with Becky reflects an integrative approach that relies heavily on process oriented, exploratory and relationally based practice, while also reflecting aspects of cognitive behavioural theories. Its humanistic, client-centred style sets the context for the phenomenological nature of my psychodynamic and attachment related interventions, and in this context cognitive behavioural principles are used in ways that can co-exist with and do not disrupt the primacy of those approaches.

The converse could equally be the case for a primarily cognitive behavioural therapy, supported by a secure empathic relationship, in which psychodynamic and attachment theories are drawn upon in ways that valuably contribute to change processes, but do not disrupt or distract from the primacy of a cognitive behavioural approach.

I work in ways that I hope will build an experience of human connection, acceptance and understanding between myself and my client, and may facilitate changes in the ways in which she or he experiences themselves, the world around them and their ways of existing within and relating to that world.

For any of us as therapists, the outcome of our therapeutic thinking and the nature of our responses to our clients will be uniquely our own, so that no two therapists would respond to any one client in exactly the same way, whatever theoretical positions they are working from. Differences will be most evident between therapists who are working from single-model positions that rely on very contrasting theory-based assumptions about practice. In other contexts, there will often be common ways of understanding and thinking about the options available to us, and maybe at times considerable similarity in the theoretical principles that underlie our functioning.

Practitioners may behave in similar ways within therapy, but describe themselves as being advised by different theoretical positions. Within my work I see myself as being guided by psychodynamic understanding in most of my responses addressing relational issues and unconscious processes. I draw on attachment theory when I experience it as having something different to add. Another therapist may see some of what I understand from the perspective of psychodynamic theory as reflecting their understanding gained from attachment theory. They might then describe a therapy that was phenomenologically similar to my work, as being more advised by an attachment theory approach than a psychodynamic one, whereas I would describe it the other way around.

This work is based on my personal understanding of theory and practice, my beliefs and assumptions about the validity of the theories involved, and ideas about the ways in which their associated processes and mechanisms make mutual and synergistic contributions to beneficial psychological change. The specifics of this content analysis of my sessions with Becky and my discussion of the integrative application of different theoretical perspectives are in various ways unique to me, and to the relationship between myself and Becky. They may at the same time echo the therapeutic work of a wide range of therapists who see themselves as integrative practitioners. They may also support the possibility that some degree of theoretical integration in keeping with the premises of the UDM and the DIAP meta-framework may be of benefit to single-model psychotherapy practitioners whatever their primary orientation.

The Therapeutic Application of Different Theoretical Approaches

Defining the Therapy Variables: Content is analysed here in relation to the application of our major theoretical approaches. The cognitively led and behaviourally led approaches to CBT, initially separated out for detailed theoretical consideration in Parts 2 and 3, are re-combined in this analysis, as we return to the routine world of therapy practice. As discussed in Chapter 18, all therapies whatever their theoretical orientation should include a baseline provision of the secure relational connection, acceptance and empathic attunement that can naturally enable growth and development and supports the effective application of other interventions. In addition, I make decisions in this analysis about the nature of interventions and responses that go beyond this baseline provision in terms of their frequency and depth, their psychological contexts, and the mechanisms and processes they are addressing; judging humanistic, psychodynamic and attachment theories to have been applied in more intensive and advanced ways compared with baseline provision; judgements that are reflected in the following data.

Quantitative Analysis of Theoretical Perspectives: This analysis involves the identification of the perspectives applied in each session of therapy across all 27 sessions and is shown as collated data in Appendix 3. Four category labels have been used: humanistic/client-centred theory (H), psychodynamic theory (P), attachment theory (A), cognitive behavioural theories (CB).

Therapy as a Whole: Within therapy as a whole all sessions were judged to have provided the integrated perspectives involved in the provision of a baseline constructive developmental relationship. Humanistic/client-centred theory is applied in ways that go beyond this baseline in 89% of my sessions with Becky, psychodynamic theory 87%, and attachment theory 54%. Cognitive behavioural theories are applied in 58%. On relatively rare occasions a session involves only one theoretical model, beyond the core basis of the constructive developmental relationship: two sessions in relation to humanistic/client-centred responding, and one relating to psychodynamic theory. All four psychotherapy models are drawn upon in a single session in a total of six sessions, and all of these are in the first half of therapy. The combined use of humanistic, psychodynamic and attachment theory is evident in eleven sessions. Although I see my work as being very strongly advised by psychodynamic theory, there are six sessions in which there are no specific contributions from psychodynamic or attachment perspectives. These sessions all primarily reflect humanistic/client-centred responding, with four also including cognitive behavioural interventions.

Across the Stages of Therapy: Becky's therapy sessions are categorized as assessment and formulation, beginning, middle and end supporting us in appreciating therapy process over time. Looking at the percentage of sessions including each approach at each stage of therapy provides a picture of the changes in theoretical approaches applied. This data is presented in Table 1 and Figure 8.

Table 1 Application of Theoretical Approaches Across Therapy

Stage of Therapy	Theoretical Approach			
	H	P	A	CB
Assessment and Formulation	100%	100%	75%	75%
Beginning	85%	71%	67%	71%
Middle	75%	75%	38%	75%
End	100%	75%	38%	0%

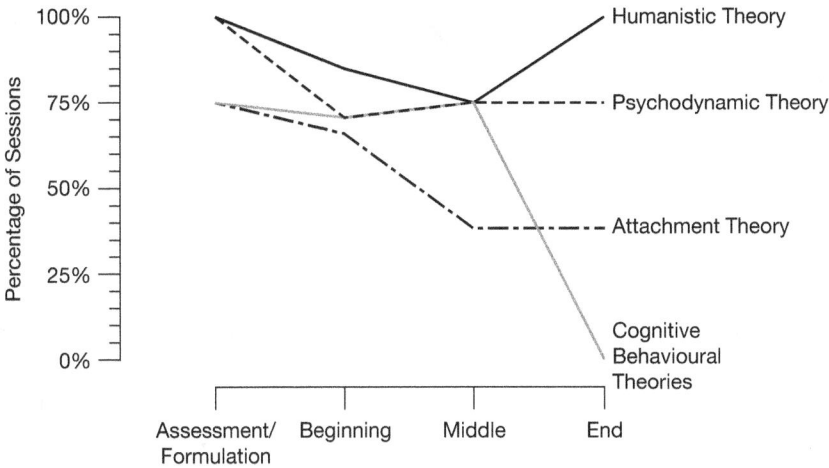

Figure 8 Application of Theoretical Approaches Across Therapy

The degree of integration across all therapeutic approaches is greatest at the start of therapy, and highest overall during assessment and formulation; however, this data may be distorted by the smaller number of sessions included in that stage of therapy. The contribution made by cognitive behavioural approaches remains strong until the end of the middle phase of therapy. Up until that point, cognitive behavioural theories are evident at similar frequencies to humanistic and psychodynamic perspectives. After this, they no longer directly influence my responses. Cognition and behaviour are still talked about but not in ways that have been guided by them. Use of psychodynamic and humanistic theories stay at a high level across therapy, whilst the frequency with which I specifically draw on attachment theory to advise my responses falls to roughly half its earlier level after the second stage of therapy, and stays constant to the end.

A Brief Summary of Therapy

Assessment reveals various aspects of Becky's life that have led to self-critical and negative beliefs about herself, and we talk a lot about her growing up, and her close and loving relationship with her parents. A cognitively based formulation is followed by the initially helpful use of a deep muscle relaxation CD as she thinks about her goals for change. Therapy discussions are largely exploratory looking at her grief for her mum and dad and understanding her self-protective defence related processes as they emerge. Her negativity towards herself is addressed from psychodynamic and cognitive perspectives. Behavioural progress is repeatedly followed by resurgences of her anxiety-based avoidance and her fears of my criticism. We start to understand more about what makes it so hard for her to change, however much she feels she wants to. Eventually we face core issues underlying this situation and from session 14 Becky becomes free to move forward. She makes decisions about behavioural change, her negative beliefs about herself continue to recede, and we share and understand her new experiences as they unfold. We work through the emotional complexities of her love for her parents and the nature of her grief, as Becky moves on in her life. As we approach the end of therapy, she is now confident in herself and more secure in her relationship with Sebastian. Negative comparisons with other people no longer plague her, and she is respectful of both their opinions and her own. She feels that she has nothing to be ashamed of. She seeks out contact with others and enjoys it, and can be assertive when she needs to stand up for herself; everyday life unfolds in a way that is so very different from before. She feels that she has got her old self back, and that it is even better than before. Finally, we experience the loss in our relationship coming to an end.

An Illustration of Change: Brief Symptom Inventory Data

Becky completes the Brief Symptom Inventory, BSI at the start of assessment and again when therapy ends. From an empirical perspective the pre- and post-therapy scores echo and support the progress Becky makes during therapy, as illustrated in Figure 9, which includes those sub-scales that I consider to have strong face

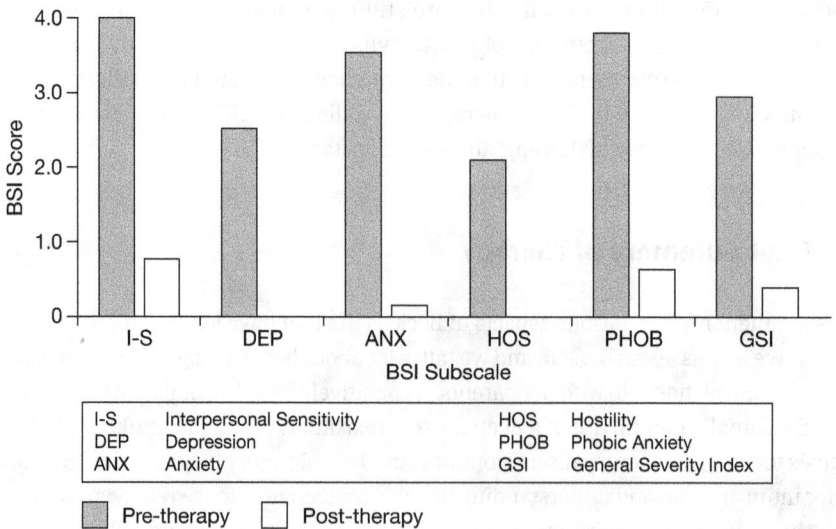

I-S	Interpersonal Sensitivity	HOS	Hostility
DEP	Depression	PHOB	Phobic Anxiety
ANX	Anxiety	GSI	General Severity Index

Pre-therapy   Post-therapy

Figure 9 Brief Symptom Inventory Scores Pre and Post Therapy

validity in relation to their constituent items. The post therapy scores very much echo the changes that Becky describes and that we experience directly within our relationship. Depression is now absent, anxiety almost so, and her unhelpful sensitivity to others very much reduced. The anger represented by the hostility sub-scale is absent too, and in her everyday life this is reflected in the anger that has now disappeared from her marital relationship. Finally, the considerable reduction in the phobic anxiety sub-scale reflects the major changes Becky has made in no longer avoiding daily life activities and involvement.

Summary

In this chapter we have looked at the proportions of different theoretical approaches reflected in my responses and the work done between Becky and myself across the 27 sessions of therapy. This analysis indicates a balanced contribution from humanistic, psychodynamic, attachment and cognitive behavioural approaches during assessment and the first stage of therapy, with many sessions being influenced by all of them. Subsequently there is a decrease in the extent to which attachment theory overtly advises my responses, and cognitive behavioural practice does not play a part in the last stage of therapy. Humanistic and psychodynamic theory continue to be reflected in practice for the majority of sessions throughout our work together. Chapter 21 will now look in some detail at the nature of Becky's unconscious internal models of self, others, relationships and the outside world, and the therapy processes that help them to change in beneficial directions.

An Experience of Therapy: Integrative Processes of Change in Unconscious Internal Models

21

Introduction

This chapter focuses on the nature of Becky's unconscious internal models of self, others, relationships and the outside world, exploring the processes that are likely to have influenced their development. It then looks at some of the key therapy processes supporting their constructive change, illustrating them by examples of the interactions between us.

All the assumptions we make about the nature of unconscious mind are inevitably hypothetical and products of our imaginations; they can never be observed and proven, but for the sake of narrative fluency I will write about them as if they have observable status, as if these hypotheses are facts. I will start by looking at Becky's earlier relational developmental context, the impact of significant life events and her resulting unconscious internal models of self, others, relationships and the outside world.

Within the Unifying Dialectical Model feedback processes maintain or change the nature of our unconscious internal models. In Chapter 17 therapeutic interventions influencing these feedback processes are discussed in terms of conscious and unconscious mind, the processing of emotion, psychological defences, acceptance, overt behaviour, relational experience and the innate capacity for growth and development. These subheadings are used here to structure an analysis of the therapy processes that enable Becky's unconscious internal models to change. The contributions of our major therapeutic approaches are identified, and their synergy is reflected in how intimately their different mechanisms of change relate to each other as interactions between Becky and myself proceed. The constructive developmental relationship, Becky's social and demographic environment and her place in the lifespan are also taken into account, as recognised within the DIAP meta-framework.

Finally, some focused attention is given to the changes in Becky's internal models of her parents and to her potential for change.

The Developmental Context of Becky's Unconscious Internal Models

Early Experience: The deep, sincere and genuine love and care, support and encouragement given to her by her parents during childhood gave Becky a core sense of being loved, and of others being loving towards her, with the nature of an intense loving relationship existing as an intrinsic part of her sense of self. Who she was, who she could become, and her capacity to grow and develop were in many ways believed in and supported by loving others, and grew as core aspects of her internal models of self. These contexts meant that Becky did not carry with her into adulthood an unhelpful proportion of damaging immature internal models accompanied by damaging immature defences, and the balance was more towards a mix of helpful and unhelpful more mature models largely involving more mature defences. However, this mix included significant unhelpful internal models of self, also influenced by aspects of her relationships with her parents, that could not be fully integrated into her evolving sense of a securely loved, capable self, and securely loving others.

In her educational world, a teacher at primary school underestimated her abilities, mistaking the impact of her difficulties in concentrating as low ability, and she was put in a low-ability sub-group. These damaging judgements of her persisted at secondary school, contributing to a sense that she was not worthy of other people's attention and undermining her potential to learn. She developed a strong and enduring belief that she was 'thick' and less capable than other people.

As well as loving and supporting her so much, a certain lack of confidence on her parents' part seems to have led them to overprotect Becky and not be as able as they would have liked to support her in ways that she needed at times. It may also have detracted from their capacity to be attuned and containing in relation to aspects of her emotional experiences when they were associated with problems or issues that they felt unable to face. Becky felt a need to protect them in some ways, and would avoid taking to them some of the things that troubled her most, such as her teachers' treatment of her at school. The responsibility for dealing with those issues in practical, psychological and emotional terms was left to her. At the same time, Becky's mum and dad were concerned that she may not be able to cope on her own as she grew up.

Defences naturally evolved within her, to protect the special closeness of the relationship with the mum and dad she loved so dearly and depended on so much. These defences contributed to the development of the more negative, unhelpful unconscious models of self and others that could not be securely integrated with her more constructive ones.

In many ways disappointment, frustration and maybe anger that could not be expressed towards others became directed towards herself. These more negative models involved inadequacy and dependence, a sense of inferiority in being 'thick' and not worthy of other people's attention and interest, and being the person responsible when other people let her down. In internal representation, and subsequently in her perceived external reality it became Becky, not her parents or teachers who were responsible for the unhelpful developmental experiences they played a part in. Aspects of her upbringing, including her mum and dad's tendencies to overprotect her, their difficulty in trusting her capacities to survive on her own, and in not supporting her at certain important junctures, remained hidden along with any negative emotions associated with them. Instead, only the good sides of her mum and dad prevailed, they were the perfect parents, and any negativity towards them was kept at bay. Her continued emotional dependence on her mum and dad, and their uncertainties about her capacities to be independent, disrupted important aspects of separation and individuation.

In this context, Becky's internal models were impeded in their development towards more integrated models of a securely loved and competent, separate and individuated self, one that could have inadequacies and make mistakes, had responsibilities but knew that others had them too, and models of others who could be trusted and would respond in the ways that she needed.

For a long time, her continued day-to-day experiences of her parents' love, advice and encouragement and the support and love of her friends, combined to minimize the overt influence of these problematic aspects of her internal models of self, others and relationships. In everyday life during her teens and early twenties, Becky experienced security and happiness in her social relationships, enjoyed her school life and then her job, loved socializing with her friends and looked forward to a married life in the future.

The Impact of Life Events: This balance between helpful and unhelpful unconscious internal models, related to and associated with each other, but not fully integrated, was adversely influenced by life events. The impact of a long-term boyfriend's unexpected abandonment undermined her unconscious sense of being securely lovable and gave a boost to her pre-existing but more latent models of herself as not being worthy of interest and attention, inadequate and the person who must be to blame. Her unconscious defences protecting her from negativity towards her parents automatically channelled things in this direction. To some degree she lost connection with the trust in others that was part of her more positive and constructive models of self, others and relationships, and it was replaced by a mistrust of other people's liking and love for her.

Despite her relationship with her husband Sebastian and the love between them, and alongside the birth of their daughter Julia, these latent internal models and the nature of her emotional connection with her mum and dad left her in a vulnerable place when they died. She struggled to cope with the reality and pain of her loss, and her defences came into play diverting any internal processes that may have involved negativity towards the parents she cherished and had relied on so much. The balance between Becky's constructive internal models of self and her negative, damaging ones became precarious, and the latter became predominant. It was now the turn of her constructive internal models to become more hidden and latent. This process was fuelled by the defences holding disappointment and anger at bay, and maintaining the intense emotional bond with her parents that her sense of psychological security relied on. Thus protecting her from an unbearable depth of loss, and the reality of a separation that she was not ready for or able to live with. Becky lost much of her capacity to securely experience herself as a loveable, competent, pretty and sociable woman. She was now far more powerfully influenced by guilt and self-blame, by her sense of being 'thick', and not worthy of attention or being cared for. Within her unconscious models, other people became manifestly more capable and competent than she was, were not the ones to be in the wrong, and their love for her could not truly be believed and trusted.

Changes in Becky's Unconscious Internal Models of Self, Others, Relationships and the Outside World

I will now discuss the nature of the processes that I believe influence helpful changes within Becky's unconscious internal models over the duration of therapy. We will look at the particular importance of changes within her unconscious internal models of her parents, and the overall changes within Becky's internal models of self, others and relationships.

The Constructive Developmental Relationship: Throughout therapy changes in Becky's unconscious internal models are influenced by the nature of the constructive developmental relationship as it grows between us. In addition to reflecting the parameters of its basic level of provision, the nature of our relating evolves in ways that enhance the complexity of empathic understanding, the nature of emotional connection and the opportunities for corrective emotional experience; therapeutic work that is supported by significant application of humanistic, psychodynamic, and attachment theoretical approaches.

Our relationship naturally helps to reduce defence related processes, enhancing connections across the boundary between unconscious and conscious mind. In conjunction with the space provided for her own thought processes to unfold, Becky is supported in allowing a wide range of experiences to come to mind, relating to her current life, her memories of past experiences, their detail and aspects of the emotions associated with them, many of which have been out of mind and not within her conscious awareness for a long time. Her experiences are heard, reflected, understood and validated in the context of an emotionally secure relationship involving genuine and open communication.

Within this genuinely lived relationship we have meaningful experiences that reflect her unconscious internal models of self, others and relationships in action between us, and work through the re-enactment related processes that they involve.

In terms of our core developmental theories, a relationship is experienced that helps to free developmental arrest and support Becky's innate potential for growth in moving her on from a defensively influenced, incongruent self to a more congruent, true self freed from the inhibiting consequences of conditions of worth.

In so many ways our relationship provides her with the foundational support of a secure base for growth, exploration and development. It constantly supports the potential for Becky's unconscious internal models to be influenced in beneficial ways, and provides the secure relational context for all of the work we do between us, and for all the work that Becky does outside of our therapy sessions.

Conscious and Unconscious Mind: All aspects of therapy automatically influence conscious and unconscious mind, and this particularly applies to the nature of the therapeutic relationship as discussed above. The boundary between them is influenced throughout therapy from the start of assessment onwards, as material that has been out of conscious mind and forgotten to lesser or greater degrees now becomes available to it. This section will particularly focus on those therapeutic interventions and processes that are guided and supported by psychodynamic and cognitive behavioural approaches.

As material comes to be experienced in Becky's conscious awareness, it becomes available to her spontaneous thinking, reasoning and creative processing, which is added to by the interpretations, explanations and understanding that I offer, reflecting psychodynamic, attachment and cognitive behavioural theories.

From a psychodynamic perspective I work to connect with underlying unconscious processes that may be affecting Becky's thoughts, feelings and behaviours and her unhelpful beliefs about herself, recognising the influences of transference and countertransference, working with unhelpful processes of unconscious defence and projective identification, and hopefully enabling helpful identification and internalisation. Unconscious process is constantly taken into account and is particularly reflected in the later section on psychological defences and the section on relational experiences.

Across therapy overall conscious experience is added to by the increased availability of emotion. Painful feelings become more available to be experienced within conscious mind and lived with, sometimes within our sessions, and often when Becky is on her own at home. Gradually, over time, more and more details of her emotional life emerge at a conscious level between us, particularly in relation to her mum and dad, and to the experiences associated with their dying.

From a cognitive behavioural perspective, cognitive approaches are used at times to directly influence Becky's processes of conscious cognition. A particular example early in therapy is my use of a cognitive style diagrammatic formulation in session 4 looking at the childhood origins of her underlying unhelpful core beliefs. This work between us leads on to interactions we will look at later in the section on psychological defences:

> I use the whiteboard to clarify early experiences that seem to have led to the lack of confidence that Becky has identified as the main problem. We look at her teachers attitudes towards her, and she also identifies not being able to play the one sport she was good at because it was taken off the curriculum at secondary school, and a difficult relationship with another girl at school. We write these on the whiteboard and add in the beliefs they seem to have led to, that she is 'thick' and in some ways not worth as much as other people. I talk about these beliefs as seeds, which were there but didn't grow too much at the time because a lot of other things were fine, and she got on alright. Becky asks why these things affect her now, and we add in the later impact of her boyfriend's abandonment, which she interpreted at the time as her fault, and made her feel that she wasn't attractive or worthy of anyone's interest.

At times the cognitive challenge of Socratic enquiry is used to directly influence Becky's conscious thought processes in relation to her unhelpful beliefs about herself and others. In session 5 I use a Socratic question that prompts an important brief and positive interaction between us about the negative comparisons she makes between herself and others, when she talks about some friends thinking differently to her in some respect:

> Becky says "but that doesn't make them a better person than I am does it" I reply "a very good question" and almost in unison we both say "no". Becky looks pleased with herself and I say "and you said that for yourself!" Just at the same time Becky gives me a small 'thumbs-up' sign and we both smile.

In session 10 Socratic discussion relates to her blaming herself for her teacher's treatment of her at primary school, and the strength of her associated beliefs:

> I ask Becky if she would feel the same about Julia if exactly the same happened to her, would she say it was her fault? Absolutely clearly Becky says no, not at all. I say she would expect the teacher to help Julia to learn to do what was needed, not undermine her, and Becky says yes, of course she would. I then reflect how hard it is for her not to automatically put the blame onto herself, and that her beliefs in these respects are very strong and hard to shift, and Becky agrees that they are.

I then tie in a psychodynamic intervention with this Socratic discussion and link the strength of these beliefs with her need to protect her mum and dad from criticism:

> I say it is as if we keep on chiselling away at those beliefs, and Becky nods. I then bring in her mum and dad and say that if our chiselling at these beliefs starts to involve seeing important things that her mum and dad couldn't do she might want us to stop chiselling altogether, and Becky says yes, she would.

In session 15 a cognitive behavioural approach is used to actively influence conscious cognition by guiding work on the whiteboard, using CBT understanding to validate her success and achievement when she drives herself to our session for the first time:

> I share with Becky my recognition of all the hard work she has done. I then review the ways in which anxiety symptoms are understood from a CBT perspective and we use the whiteboard to identify her own examples of escalating spirals of anxiety together. We then think about coping strategies, and recognise the ways in which recommended strategies are reflected in the ways she coped with driving here today, identifying why her efforts were successful. At the end of this work together Becky looks at the whiteboard and says, "well if you think about all that, I really did do a lot of work this morning!".

As Becky's behaviour begins to change in positive directions and she does more on her own, she starts to connect with lots of memories of what it was like being independent, what she used to do and how good it felt. As they become available to conscious mind, they feed into her capacities to build on her progress. All of Becky's conscious processes are available to feed back into unconscious mind, with the potential to influence her unhelpful internal models in constructive ways, and strengthen those helpful models of self, others and relationships that have become weakened, latent and inactive. As conscious mind then influences what Becky says and what she does, the outcomes of her behaviour will feed back to influence her unconscious internal models as well.

The Processing of Emotion: As the safety of the empathic therapeutic developmental relationship enables Becky's greater conscious awareness of emotion, it is supported by acceptance and emotional containment. A wide range of difficult emotions become acknowledged, talked about and more overtly experienced, including feelings of guilt, shame, sadness and fear. Sometimes they are experienced within therapy sessions, but often painful emotions are felt more openly when she is on her own, particularly her sadness and grief. Her self-blame, shame and guilt become increasingly apparent, and we come to know her very real fear of the unbearable impact of her parents' loss.

Emotions are often inextricably connected with defences, with the recognition and understanding of those defences helping hidden feelings to become more tolerable and more able to be known and experienced. As difficult emotions become known, experienced and survived in conscious mind, their nature evolves and over time their painful intensity can become reduced, and they may become transformed. Changes in unhelpful defences enable emotion to be known and expressed, and the therapeutically supported processing of painful emotions reduces their continuing power. As the nature of emotion changes, the nature of associated unconscious internal models changes as well. Changes in conscious cognition will also be part of these processes, and conscious cognition will also influence felt emotion. Changes in behaviour towards self and others will be in the mix as well, within sessions between us and with other people in her everyday world.

Positive emotions emerge for Becky as well as difficult and painful ones; they are similarly recognized, accepted and validated, with their frequency increasing through the second half of therapy as Becky starts to make significant progress. They support the processes of positive reinforcement that help to maintain beneficial changes in behaviour, and become core aspects of her emerging, and re-activated constructive internal models of self and others.

In many ways the supportive processing of emotion plays a particularly central and interactive role in the capacity of her unconscious internal models to change in constructive directions.

Psychological Defences: Psychological defences play a crucial part in Becky's difficulties and the nature of the therapy that we experience together. They are apparent in multiple respects: they are experienced within her relationship with Sebastian; they constitute a key factor in the maintenance of the bond with the parents she has lost, and her avoidance of a grief she feels she cannot bear; they protect her from recognizing anything at all that is negative or disappointing in relation to her mum and dad; they play powerful roles in her self-deprecation, self-blame and lack of confidence; and ultimately they interfere with and block her capacity to change in the ways she knows she needs to.

Early in therapy in session 4 her defences are triggered by the cognitive formulation that we share together, as discussed above in the section on conscious and unconscious mind, and she pulls back from its meaning and significance:

> After a few moments silence Becky's says she thinks she is wasting my time, she has never thought of it like this before, other people have had really difficult times at home and she didn't, so she must be weak to have let these things affect her. I acknowledge that what I have written down is hard for her to see. I ask if she would like me to wipe the whiteboard clean, she does. I clean the whiteboard and then find myself thinking about the process that has taken place between us. I say that I wonder if she is concerned about what I might think of her. She says how hard it is that someone else knows these things about her, and I say maybe she is afraid I will think the same of her as she thinks about herself.

In this context the most important aspect of responding is that I recognize her upset. In attachment terms it is crucial that I am sensitive and attuned to what is happening within her, and modify how I relate to her in ways that take that into account, hopefully not forcing her to experience more than she is able to manage. I accept her need to protect herself, and offer her a way we might understand and think about it.

In session 7 I think with Becky about the ways in which she deals with different emotions, exploring the defences that may be associated with them, as we talk about issues of trust in her relationships and the patterns of interaction that can emerge at times between her and Sebastian:

> I reflect that Becky can express her anger in this situation but may hide her feelings of hurt, and I ask if it is sometimes easier to be angry with Sebastian than to show her upset and sadness. She recognises that this can be true.

In session 8 after initially benefitting from the relaxation CD, then using it less, Becky has stopped using it altogether, and work on her other goals seems to have reduced as well. I understand this as a process of defence and offer an interpretation:

> I say that although she very much feels she wants to be different, it may be very difficult for her to let changes happen. If she becomes more confident, closer to other people and more involved with them, it may mean that she loses some of her bond with her parents, which is something she very much doesn't want to happen. Becky listens quietly; she seems to understand and doesn't disagree

with what I am saying. She moves on to talk more about the months before her
mum died.

This particular work relating to her defences was followed two sessions later by my reference to our chiselling away at her unhelpful beliefs, and Becky agreeing that she would want that to stop if doing so touched on anything her parents couldn't do. These interventions all involve core aspects of defence that function together to maintain her existing internal models of her parents and the strength of emotional connection and inter-dependence between her and them. It seems impossible for her internal models of self to change in a constructive direction without destabilizing her current models of her parents. This situation reflects aspects of insecure attachment, within an overall context of truly supportive love and care.

The dominance of her own negative models of self helps to protect her positive models of her parents, preventing their feared and unbearable destruction. Their limitations and human failures are negated, with blame and responsibility falling on Becky; accompanied by her intense sense of dependence on them and a parallel negation of her own capabilities.

In session 14 after making further progress in going out with Sebastian and Julia to places she had been avoiding, and deciding to focus on further behavioural changes, Becky's progress has gone into reverse. This powerful emergence of defence related process is responded to and resolved in a way that involves key relational experience between the two of us, and will be discussed later in that section.

In session 18 we start to look at the defence related link between blaming herself rather than someone else, and the avoidance of angry feelings:

Becky tells me that a nurse had treated her in an off-hand way at a routine hospital
appointment; it made her feel guilty that she was wasting her time. Then another
nurse said "don't worry about her, she's like that with everyone". This had helped
Becky to recognize she wasn't wasting their time and she had started to feel a bit
angry about how she had been treated. We look at the way her beliefs about herself
often lay with what other people thought about her, and I say to Becky that blaming
herself may also protect her from feeling angry. She seems to see a lot of sense and
meaning in these thoughts.

In session 20 we have been able to move beyond her defences in relation to difficult feelings about her parents, sharing anger, as well as hurt and deep sadness about her mum's death:

Becky talks again about her mum's illness. Her mum hid her problems from
everyone, no one knew about them until too late. I say that Becky is angry with her

mum for not getting the medical help she needed, and Becky says yes, she is. I go on to say that, in a way her mum let her down by not being able to take care of herself. This is very hard for Becky to hear, she says that she is not pleased I said that, and I recognize the sense of anger within her. I say maybe she is feeling angry with me. She is, and I say "because it feels like I have criticized your mum" and Becky says "yes". After a few minutes silence, she talks about a newly married friend who had been uncertain about accepting some preventive medical treatment, until Becky challenged her to think about her husband. Afterwards her friend was so grateful Becky had said what she did. I say to Becky, with sadness that her friend would have risked letting down someone she loved by not getting the care she needed, just like her mum. Becky has been looking at me, our eye-contact very clear through all of these interactions between us and at the end she simply says, yes.

All of the defences we work with together play crucial roles in relation to changes in Becky's internal models of self, others, relationships and the outside world.

Acceptance: My acceptance and understanding of Becky help to support her in starting to accept and live with the realities of her life, who she is, what she thinks and feels, what has affected her in the past and what continues to do so, and the realities of her current relationships. Starting to see some of these realities is a shock for her, and her defence related processes naturally come into play. We work through them, and my acceptance of the nature of those processes with all their ups and downs, supports Becky in living with their realities too. I also accept the reality of all of the precious love and care that her parents gave her. None of that is taken away by coming to know the things they were not able to do so well, their human frailties. These are realities that Becky becomes able to accept too. Accepting the nature and experience of painful emotions, and living with them is a large part of these processes, and is importantly supported by empathic attunement and emotional containment. I accept her vulnerabilities and her strengths and capacities. Supported by all of the processes of therapy Becky becomes more accepting, trusting and valuing of herself.

Overt Behaviour: Behaviour, its consequences, and the functioning of Becky's conscious and unconscious mind are all in such mutual and constant interaction that it is probably impossible to clearly define a primary starting point for overall processes of change. Changes in conscious cognition and in unconscious internal models can be the origins of behavioural change, and behavioural change can be the starting point for consequent changes in cognition and in unconscious internal models. It is also hard to imagine that some initial change within those models is not involved for an individual to make the decision to act differently in the first place. By whatever path they emerge, Becky's changing ways of being and behaving, and their outcomes all play essential and central roles in the changes within her internal models of self, others, relationships, and the outside world; the two are inseparable.

Behavioural change is directly addressed within therapy. In session 5 we bring in deep muscle relaxation, using it at home results in helpful conversations with Sebastian, and it is directly helpful in reducing anxiety and tension. In session 7 we discuss anxiety management from a cognitive behavioural perspective, and in session 11 we talk more about the basis of graded exposure and goal setting. Becky wants to set her goals for herself, and the decision to behave differently is always left up to her. She starts to make some progress and in session 13 we decide she will make a record of things she currently avoids doing, and her further goals for change.

Towards the end of session 14 I use a behaviourally advised discussion about how she may prepare for the mother and toddler group she has decided to attend for the first time the next day:

> I then look with Becky at how she might prepare for doing this tomorrow, to help reduce any risks of opting out, and Becky decides she could put her clothes out tonight, be more organised and decrease the risk of using being in a rush as an excuse not to go. In responding to her uncertainty about talking to other mothers, I ask her what she thought people might talk about, and she comes up with ideas about babies, children, relationships and holidays.

From a rather different perspective we also address some aspects of Becky's relational behaviour with Julia and in session 19 explore the possible need for Becky to set some boundaries and limits, a discussion that reflects a more psychodynamic way of thinking:

> Becky says that she and Sebastian have started to think about when they might have another baby. She wonders what the impact might be on her relationship with Julia, and says that if she has two children to look after she won't be able to spoil her any more. I ask what might be important about that, and would there be anything valuable about that happening? Becky says no, that is what she is there for, to spoil Julia and give her everything she wants and needs. I ask her if there is anything that matters about Julia feeling she can always have everything she wants? Becky turns away from me, and rather quickly says, yes that did need to change, as she grew up Julia would need to learn she couldn't always have everything she wanted. I say she did know, but didn't want to hear me say it, and Becky says yes. I reflect how hard it is for her to be part of helping Julia to learn that, because it will sometimes involve her having to deny Julia something she wants to have or wants to do. Later Becky says that Julia still sleeps with Becky and Sebastian at night rather than in her own room.

These are issues that Becky takes on board, and as she starts to set some limits on Julia, she says that Julia gradually becomes more settled too. When Julia starts to sleep in her own room overnight Becky says she feels quite sad about that, and I empathise with the sense of loss that this separation involves.

These discussions are all advised by psychodynamic understanding, touching on issues of symbiosis, separation and individuation. As well as focusing on Julia, they are also significant in terms of the relationship between me and Becky. Just as she needs to start setting some limits and boundaries for Julia, facing her with experiences of optimal frustration, I am doing something similar in relation to Becky by raising these issues with her.

Within our sessions overall Becky's behaviour in relation to her life activities and relationships, are always a topic of our conversations. Up to session 14 the nature of behaviour is often discussed explicitly, and often with the implication that doing things differently could be beneficial, as well as some discussions about specific goals for change. Becky's behaviour changes markedly in constructive directions after session 14; she decides to drive herself to our sessions, starts going to the mother and toddler group, she talks to people more, becomes more assertive and makes progress in many everyday contexts over the rest of our time together. All of these experiences are responded to with empathic and attuned discussion and validation, with particular examples being provided in sessions 18 and 25. In session 18 we look at Becky's abilities in supporting Julia in facing her fears:

> *Recently Julia has started to feel fearful of men who are strangers to her. Becky has helped her when men she doesn't know have come to the mother and toddler group by telling her what the man is doing, supporting her in being involved in what is happening, and resisting the temptation to fuss. The same thing happened elsewhere and a friend dealt with it by taking Julia out of the room. Becky says she explained to her friend that she would have preferred her to keep Julia in the room and help her to discover there was nothing to be afraid of. I support and validate her knowing what needed to be done to help Julia face her fears, and in being assertive about it.*

Not only has Becky become able to face her fears herself, she has also become able to support her daughter to do so too, and be assertive in asking other people to support Julia in the same way.

In session 25 Becky talks about her experience of a door-to-door sales person:

> *Becky shares another important experience. She opened the door to a salesperson from one of the power companies who was quite forceful and persuaded her to change from her existing provider, giving her hardly any time to ask questions or to think. She had felt quite pressurized, and afterwards felt very unhappy about*

the decision. She decided to phone and cancel the arrangement, and did so. We share some smiles as we reflect on the progress here - in the past she wouldn't have opened the door! And even more through opening the door, and experiencing dubious sales tactics, she had the valuable opportunity to think about how she would deal differently with any similar situations in the future. We both recognize that a lot of people would have done exactly as she did, and a lot may not have been so assertive and got themselves out of the agreement: Becky stood up for herself.

Overall, all of very varied positive and constructive personal, relational and social outcomes of her changed behaviours feed into and extensively support her emerging positive unconscious internal models of self, others, relationships and the outside world.

Relational Experience: Relational experience within therapy is crucial throughout, with my thinking and responding being advised by psychodynamic and attachment theories, in the overall context of the attuned, empathic relationship. The start of session 5 reflects something of this attuned relationship between us and the containing style of therapy; ever-present aspects of our being together:

Becky arrives looking particularly attractive and wearing a bit more make-up, which makes me think she is feeling better. I ask her where she wants to start and expect her to say something positive, instead she says she feels really tired, hadn't felt like making the effort to come, and put some make-up on to help her get out of the house. I reflect that she'd just like to curl up and go to sleep; the make-up on the outside doesn't mean she is feeling alright on the inside. I then think about our previous session when we shared the formulation on the whiteboard that was so challenging for her. I say we did a lot of work together last time we met. Becky agrees, saying she'd had a lot to think about. I say how shocked she had been when we wrote things on the whiteboard, and Becky says yes, and it had all come from her, she hadn't realized those memories still mattered so much.

Fuelled by her unconscious internal models, Becky's conscious belief that she is 'thick', gets things wrong, and that other people, especially authority figures are much more capable than her and will judge her badly, repeatedly leads her to be truly fearful of my annoyance, disappointment, criticism and rejection, particularly when she has not engaged in planned behavioural activities and changes. At the start of session 8 she is powerfully convinced I will be annoyed with her:

Becky hasn't used her relaxation CD at all and is very condemning of herself for not managing something she sees as helpful and easy to do. She is absolutely sure I am going to be angry and send her away, feeling she is wasting my time. Her fear is palpable and she is on the verge of leaving the room. I say that I think it will be good if she can stay. I tell her I am not annoyed, but it feels as if things are stuck for us. I say I know she feels sure that I must be annoyed with her and think it isn't worth my seeing her again, and that this is a strong belief.

This interaction is followed by the interpretation of defence discussed in the earlier section on psychological defences, as I share the understanding that her need to maintain her close connection with her parents may make it very hard for her to change. In saying this, I am expressing acceptance, understanding and care rather than the anger and rejection she was expecting. Repeatedly she discovers that my anticipated negative and critical feelings towards her simply do not exist: I am not judgemental or annoyed with her. Each process and discovery represents a corrective emotional experience, and new learning about who people can be in their relationships with her, who she is and who she can be with them.

Our relationship brings the realities of her unhelpful underlying internal models into current active awareness, and they become intimately alive within and between her and me, involving processes of re-enactment between us. In session 4 my own confusion contributes to a mistake that Becky blames on herself, and I am able to recognize and take responsibility for my part within a problematic re-enacted relational process, at the same time as recognizing her tendency to blame herself rather than others. This interaction takes place immediately after we have discovered how painful it is for her to see her self-critical beliefs and their potential origins on the whiteboard, as discussed in the section on conscious and unconscious mind:

I now find myself thinking of the difficult start to the session when I was confused about which therapy session this was. I ask Becky about her reaction to my error, and she says she would never question me if she thought I was wrong, because she is 'thick' and I am the professional. As we discuss this, we realize that we had both contributed to the error. We also realize that this experience has quite powerfully illustrated an important theme in her life: Becky tends to see herself as at fault rather than other people. I clarify that she puts herself down automatically, even when others are at fault, and that this has happened here between us.

My place as a professional who she would always assume to be better than her makes this a particularly important experience as we share responsibility for a mistake from a basis of equality.

On other occasions experience between us involves her anger towards me, as in session 20 discussed in the section on psychological defences, when she feels that I am being critical of her mum. I am able to recognize, understand and live with it, without feeling annoyed in return, when it would probably have never felt possible for her to express anger and disappointment to her parents or her teachers; another corrective emotional experience.

The significance and emotional importance of our relationship particularly emerges in relation to Becky's need of me and her feelings about my loss when therapy ends. The following extracts touch on these themes, and reflect the progress that evolves as we live through contexts of needed dependence, growth and development, separation and loss, starting with session 12 as we approach our therapy review:

> We now have three meetings before we review therapy and decide about further contact, and I mention this to Becky. She says I am her lifeline at moment and she doesn't know how she would cope without our meetings.

As we start to move towards the end of therapy in session 21, we make an overt connection between her feelings when her mum and dad died and her sense of abandonment and loss within our relationship:

> I interpret something of her possible feelings towards her mum and dad when each of them died. Maybe it felt as if mum and dad both abandoned her when they died, and this involved some sense of anger towards them, and it feels like that with me now as well. Becky thinks about this and then says yes it does feel like that, and as if I am a surrogate mum and dad rolled into one.

In our final session we touch on this again:

> I say to Becky that maybe it feels a bit as if I am abandoning her as it did when her parents died. Becky agrees, it really does feel a bit like that, although it isn't the same at all, it does feel a bit like it did, especially when her dad died; as if she is being left to cope with everything on her own, but she says she feels excited about this as well as scared.

Taking us back again to earlier stages of therapy, in session 12 I make a brief but important connection between our relationship and the difficulties Becky experiences when Julia refuses to eat, a context that was significant between her and her mum when she was little. In this context I see a possible parallel between Becky not being able to following through on ideas we have shared about making changes in her life, and her not eating for her mum:

> Becky has been feeling tearful and upset, experiencing painful and sad memories of her mum. Her battles with Julia over food and eating have been getting worse. She feels she is playing her up, and knows she needs to be steadier and calmer

about it, but finds that impossible. If Julia eats well, she feels fine and happy, but if she doesn't eat, everything feels wrong. Logically she knows Julia is healthy, there is no risk to her if she doesn't eat at some meal times; she is well and healthy. I ask who she is getting Julia to eat for, and Becky says it is for herself, to decrease her anxiety. We talk together a lot about the connections between this experience and how Becky's mum was with her, how much she needed her mum to be calm and steady in dealing with her refusal to eat, and how hard it is for Becky to do this herself with Julia. I make a connection with the two of us, saying that I wasn't able to force her to take food that didn't seem right for her either, a comment that makes Becky smile.

The nature of re-enactment between us is particularly important in session 14. It is in this session that we discover Becky has pulled back from positive behavioural change, and progress has gone into reverse. My understanding of this situation draws on the possible meaning of 'feeding' and being 'fed' within our relationship discussed above, and is particularly influenced by psychodynamic understanding:

Becky has recorded many repeated examples of avoiding people, not answering the phone, or the door, not going into the garden if people are outside next door, and asking Sebastian or a friend to do her shopping for her. Her avoidance, and requests for reassurance, have all increased, and there have been no thoughts on her part about goals related to change or the steps she might take towards them. We seem to be at an impasse, Becky's avoidant way of being has returned and escalated. I tell her that I think we have reached crunch time. I talk to her calmly, gently but seriously. I say that we are coming up to our review point and that I can offer her twelve more sessions, but after that our work together will end whether anything has changed or not. I say that I will not punish her if she doesn't change, that I hope she will, but I will be alright if she doesn't, it won't hurt me. I say with sadness that however much she tries to spoil her life her mum and dad won't come back, they are never coming back, they can't; they are not alive any more. I also say that when we do end our time together after our further twelve sessions, our ending may feel a bit like losing her parents all over again.

This withdrawal from progress has brought the issue of feeding and accepting food or not that she has described between herself and her mother as a child into my mind. I think of the process between us as symbolically relating to her taking my therapeutic 'food' and throwing it onto the floor. I am firm and I set limits, but my caring about her is never in doubt. I am open and direct with her, saying that I think it is crunch time. I also say we can work together for a full second set of sessions. At the same time, I set an absolute limit to our time together, and I also say that whatever she does, her mum and dad are never coming back. I am firm, but I am not punishing; I never stop understanding or accepting how things are for her. I do not make my care for her conditional; making changes or not is her decision. I hope she does change, but I am not anxious about it, and if she doesn't, I can live with it, I will survive. Neither my well-being nor her being cared for are conditional on what she chooses to do. I believe that Becky really does know that this is the case. Part of the value she later placed on what I said was that she finally knew that I wanted her to change. This was not what I had actually said, but it was what I felt - it did matter to me, and Becky comes to know that, free of any pressure to change for my personal benefit or need.

These interactions have an effect on both Becky and myself, and free up both our capacities to think differently. I find myself shifting to a more behavioural way of responding:

It then comes to my mind to talk to Becky about the things she is avoiding doing and I ask whether some of these things are actually things she could do if she wanted to and really made the effort. To my surprise Becky seems very clear, there is no doubt within her mind that there are; for the first time she tells me that Sebastian drives here her, bringing Julia with them. But she can drive, it is something she enjoys, and she knows that if she really decided to, she could do it for herself. She says she will drive here next time, and she is determined to go to the mother and toddler group tomorrow.

We have managed to step into a different place between us, one from which active behavioural change is able to proceed:

Becky says she knew she did need to do these things for herself, not for her mum and dad. She says she looked at their picture one evening recently when she was upset, and told them that she knew she deserved it for herself. I say, yes, not for her parents and what they would think, or for Sebastian, or even for Julia, but for her. Later as we reach the end of the session the mood between us has changed from seriousness and sadness, to enthusiasm and laughter. We joke with each other, and Becky looks at me very directly. There seems to be no sense of her hiding in shame from me, or anything that points towards her fears of my negative judgement, or her earlier self-blame, self-criticism or helplessness.

As well as drawing strongly on psychodynamic understanding, my work in this session reflects the crucial importance of maintaining the secure attachment relationship between us, and the core humanistic principles of genuineness and acceptance. In a very meaningful way Becky discovers that she can be totally separate from me, not responsible for my well-being or my security. And again, I have not been annoyed with her. She knows that she will be cared about, whatever happens. Within this overall corrective emotional experience we have together been able to experience her strength and her underlying capacities to change.

My relationship with Becky with its echoes of her relationship with her parents, and our opportunity to live through some very significant developmental experiences in a different way remains important throughout the rest of our time together, and is reflected in our saying goodbye. We are able to become separate, in support of her more individuated self, in which the love and care her parents gave her will always sustain her on a more secure basis than before. In session 26, after a longer gap between sessions than usual Becky talks about the forthcoming ending:

> *Becky tells me that she now feels this is the right time for us to be ending. Fortuitously she has now had the opportunity to experience being able to feel different and better on her own for several weeks without seeing me. If we had been able to continue, she thinks it would have become a habit, and she would have wanted to see me for ever. We both think it will feel sad to say goodbye, a sadness that Becky feels in touch with as I say the word.*

In session 27 we say goodbye:

> *Becky shares her mixed emotions. I hear her, and in my own way feel them too. In those last moments of ending, I don't avoid acknowledging her anxiety, and say that maybe she is more anxious because she has changed so much, if she hadn't, she might have felt less anxious about saying goodbye, there might have been less to lose. Becky says yes, that is exactly how it feels. I don't avoid acknowledging that she will miss me. It is clear that as much as anyone can be she is ready and excited to go, but that does not take sadness and uncertainty away. I say that maybe a little bit of her still believes that the things she does now are because of me, and our ending may be the only way she can find out differently, Becky nods in response to both. As the moment comes to say goodbye, I say that I will live on in her mind and she will live on in mine.*

All of the relational experiences discussed in this section have significant, and sometimes powerful effects on her unconscious internal models of self, others and relationships and their associated defences.

Environment and Place in the Lifespan: It is primarily Becky's social environment that is of crucial importance to Becky and the progress she makes during therapy. Within her marriage and her friendships, she experiences outcomes in relation to her changed behaviours that support the constructive changes taking place in her internal models. In her relationship with Sebastian he listens and cares about her experiences and always plays his part in sharing childcare. As she works to deal differently with her relational insecurity and anger, he does nothing to maintain the mutual upset that used to unfold between them. He moves on as well.

Within the mother and toddler group, she discovers women who are interested in her and her daughter, and understanding of her experiences; her opening up to them is responded to by warmth and caring. Her closest friends stay constant throughout Becky's struggles, and prove to be people who can change their minds about their own attitudes in response to Becky's assertiveness.

These experiences within her relationships create positive supportive feedback loops that maintain the changes taking place in Becky's unconscious internal models of self, others and relationships, and provide fertile ground for their further development.

In terms of a broad range of demographic variables, Becky's life context does not particularly restrict the potential for positive consequences to unfold as her capacities to behave differently evolve. She is not restricted in what she can do and who she can be by economic or social factors, or by any negative stereotypes associated with ethnicity, sexuality or age, and gender does not seem to present a particular issue either.

Throughout therapy we are in many ways working together on aspects of Becky's lifespan transitions, particularly in terms of her separation and individuation from her mum and dad. Her unconscious internal models change in ways that are consistent with this transition. Something of the relationship between us and the way we work together helps Becky to move beyond her difficulties involving the classic Eriksonian issues of autonomy, shame and guilt that have held back her development, and plagued her so much since her parents' deaths, and again her internal models change accordingly. Similarly, her sense of self as an adult, partner and parent in her relationships with Sebastian, Julia and her friends become stronger.

My hearing, recognizing, and validating all of these experiences also supports their spontaneous capacity to foster and strengthen the changed constructive internal models that are taking their needed place within unconscious mind.

Innate Capacity for Growth and Development: In all of the above contexts the changes that evolve for Becky take place in intimate interaction with her innate potential for growth and development, which is particularly supported by the relationship between us.

Unconscious Internal Models of her Parents

Becky's unconscious internal models of her parents and her relationship with them change. Her mum and dad are now fallible, and in some ways more vulnerable people, rather than perfect; she knows of her disappointment and anger towards them, but none of the precious love and care between them is lost, and she discovers that she can survive her grief. Her unconscious internal models of her parents have changed, as has her model of herself, and of the relationship between her and them. Maybe we could say that an internal secure attachment has now been able to evolve. As we move towards the end of our relationship, we understand the parallels between losing me and losing her mum and dad. I provide tacit, implicit faith in her capacity to survive without me, but at the same time recognize that the loss matters to her. In surviving this loss without the need for defences to protect against unbearable emotions, Becky is further able to discover her separate independent strength.

Becky's Potential to Change

The potential for any individual to change depends on their own psychological nature and the nature of their environment. For Becky there are ways of thinking about her potential to change that have implications for understanding the nature of the therapy that was able to help her, and the relevance of the environmental context of her life.

Whilst there are aspects of Becky's relational experiences with her mum and dad that contribute to her vulnerability to psychological distress, she has experienced secure and reliable love, care and support. That she was loved and valued was in no doubt, and trauma and abuse have been absent from her life. She also knows how to do all the things she currently doesn't do, and she has a loved child, good friends and a husband who loves her. All of these adults, it turns out, have the capacity to change as well. Becky also experiences a secure life context in terms of her financial security. Her overall environment is able to play an active, positive and constructive part in her processes of change.

In terms of her unconscious internal models of self, others and relationships, whilst those models do not initially seem to be fully integrated, they are not severely fragmented either, or affected by dissociation. They are relatively accessible to conscious mind, and not overly disturbing in their effects on conscious emotion, or current relational experience, which is affected but in containable ways that can be understood and lived with to beneficial effect; overall a manageable mix of constructive and damaging mature internal models, without the influence of damaging immature defences or damaging immature models.

These considerations of the nature of self and Becky's social and demographic world reflect the psychodynamic concept of ego strength and the psychosocial factors commonly quoted as important indicators of suitability for psychotherapy. They do so in ways that take the nature of unconscious internal models and the active contribution of social and relational environments into account.

The initial fragmentation within Becky's unconscious internal models keeps her strengthened negative models of self, others and relationships quite separate from her positive models, that are lying latent in the background; the person she used to know herself as being. This fragmentation is tied up with her defence related, self-protective responses to the loss of her parents, with the seeds of her negative models lying with her early school experiences and her parents' struggles with their own confidence, in themselves and in her abilities to cope and survive on her own.

Relational issues loom large in this context, as does Becky's vulnerability to feeling guilty, responsible, inadequate, and fearful of others' criticisms, anger and condemnation. In this situation my natural tendency to take a largely relational approach advised by psychodynamic, attachment and humanistic theory, whilst remaining overtly cognizant of the benefits of cognitive behavioural understanding probably suits the nature of Becky's potential for change.

I validate and add to her pre-existing appreciation of CBT based anxiety management, discuss and value behavioural change, but do not get directly involved in goal setting or apply structured cognitive approaches towards addressing unhelpful thoughts and beliefs.

As change starts to unfold, Becky gradually reconnects with her positive internal models of self and then draws upon her pre-existing social and practical knowledge, skills and abilities within a social and relational world that is receptive and positively responsive towards her. The impact of her negative models recedes, and her positive models grow and develop further, hopefully now securely integrated within unconscious mind.

In her own words, Becky's self becomes even better than before.

Summary

This chapter has given detailed attention to Becky's unconscious internal models of self, others, relationships and the outside world. It has looked at their early and more recent development, the ways in which the components and processes of the Unifying Dialectical Model and the DIAP meta-framework are reflected in their constructive change during therapy, and the role that their developmental nature plays in the potential for those changes to take place.

In Part 5 I will discuss Dialectically Integrated Psychotherapy in the context of the aims and principles of psychotherapy integration, and compare it with a range of other approaches, before considering its implications for theory development, and psychotherapy research, practice and training. Finally, I will summarize the work that has been done in carrying out this dialectical study of theoretical integration, and provide some reflective thoughts on the unfolding processes that led to the final outcome.

Part 5

Discussion, Summary and Reflections

Dialectically Integrated Psychotherapy and the Aims and Principles of Psychotherapy Integration

22

This chapter will consider the current work on Dialectically Integrated Psychotherapy in relation to the overall principles and aims of psychotherapy integration. We will also look at its relationship to the categories of theoretical, technical and common factors integration, particularly in terms of commonalities, and compatible and incompatible differences. These discussions will reflect the key premises of critical realism and will assume that all effective approaches to psychotherapy integration relate to the functioning of the same integrated substrate of the intransitive human mind.

Whilst the current work sits soundly within the theoretical approach to integration, it supports and is not inconsistent with integration that is primarily led by technical considerations rather than theoretical ones. It is also supportive of components of therapy deemed to be important by therapists working from a common factors perspective.

Dialectically Integrated Psychotherapy is at odds with those common factors approaches that reject the validity of our differing theoretical approaches and their direct contribution to therapeutic change. For example, whilst acknowledging the value of the range of new learning experiences that the application of different theoretical approaches can provide, Frank and Frank (1991, 2004) position those theories within their general concept of myths and rituals. They seem to recognise their value but dismiss their contribution at the same time. A similar position is adopted by Wampold and Imel (2015), who see the mechanisms and processes described by our theories as playing no direct part in the remediation of psychological problems, and the effectiveness of psychotherapy. Wampold (2019) sees the value of theory as lying in its capacity to guide, support and structure therapy provision, but not in its ability to provide potentially valid understanding of human psychological functioning. Dialectically Integrated Psychotherapy clearly considers otherwise, but is not incompatible with his views on the contributions made by theory in the above respects, or of the value of other common factors within psychotherapy. His position on the validity of theory and his rejection of the possibility of theoretical integration on philosophical grounds, are both incompatible with this work.

The term common factors is problematic, with factors that are a particular focus of one psychotherapy approach sometimes being deemed to be non-specific common factors in relation to all approaches. The term is also used to refer to factors that are judged to exist in common across different therapies, with this commonality or overlap being used as a reason to reclassify them as non-specific common factors and to give them much reduced status in theoretical terms. The approach may then assume that theoretical approaches to psychotherapy should be based on psychological constructs and variables that are unique to each of them. On this basis, Frank and Frank, and Wampold and Imel reject and dismiss the validity of both cognitive therapy and psychodynamic therapy theory because they are both deemed to engender changes in the same psychological variables.

The valuing of theoretical triangulation in this work takes the completely opposite approach. Overlap and commonality of psychological constructs across different theoretical approaches is seen to strengthen the theoretical validity of those constructs. Using the compatible contributions of the differing perspectives to define them on an integrative basis increases the depth and complexity of our understanding. In terms of practice, the different therapies provide mutually supportive pathways of change in relation to the same construct.

At the same time as demonstrating incompatible difference in relation to the value of theory within human psychology, Dialectically Integrated Psychotherapy is fundamentally supportive of the vital importance of the therapeutic relationship which in most instances stands as a central pillar of common factors approaches. The relevance and validity of different theoretical positions is powerfully asserted in relation to the range of understanding of that relationship provided by humanistic, psychodynamic and attachment theories, and supported by the research associated with each of them. It recognises that common change processes are evident across approaches, but sees them as being achieved by differing routes and internal mechanisms that have the potential to complement each other.

Various authors discuss the aims of theoretical integration in psychotherapy and the factors that should characterize it. In a particularly thorough paper, Wachtel (2010) refers to the value of a common language, the need to generate generic concepts, and the importance of paying attention to both the higher-level construct nature of the 'woods' and the specific nature of the 'trees' within them. Lebow (2002) and Beitman and Manring (2009) both discuss the crucial importance of developing frameworks in which the concepts used by differing approaches are joined and connected to each other with internal consistency, so that core processes are seen as functioning as a cohesive whole. Similarly, Safran and Inck (1995) refer to the need for concepts to be integrated at an explanatory level across theoretical orientations, although they also believe our different theories are fundamentally incommensurable, and that it would be impossible to integrate them without losing the unique insights that each provide.

These principles and hopes for the future are reflected in the current work. The integrative definition of the five core psychological constructs in Chapter 16 is in keeping with the recommendations made by both Wachtel and Safran and Inck, and draws directly on psychodynamic, attachment, and cognitive and behavioural theories. The more generic term internal models is used instead of the potentially narrower concept of schemas, with the construct incorporating the characteristics of cognitive schemas alongside other attributes understood from more psychodynamic, attachment and behavioural perspectives, integrating them at an explanatory level. In doing so I have looked at both the 'woods' of the five core psychological constructs and 'trees' of theoretical detail associated with each major therapeutic approach. In relation to the 'trees', the language of their parent theories has been used for mechanisms and processes such as defence, identification, and classical and operant conditioning, which retain their theory specific labels and nature as they function alongside each other in synchrony.

The Unifying Dialectical Model and the DIAP meta-framework are consistent with Beitman and Manring's reference to the need for frameworks that provide internal consistency across theoretical approaches, describing the synergistic functioning of our integratively defined core constructs within the human mind, and the ways in which the procedures of our individual therapy approaches may each influence beneficial change processes within the UDM in mutually supportive and complementary ways.

A further crucial aspect of theoretical integration reflected strongly in this work has been the adoption of a 'both/and' inclusiveness in relation to theoretical understanding, a position particularly supported by Lebow (2002), as opposed to the 'either/or' decision making of the more traditional binary position. In the terms of Feixas and Botella (2004), a dialectical approach has been taken in which the differing beliefs of our range of major theoretical approaches have not been seen as absolute objective realities, but ones that can be open to dialectic process and mutually constructive dialogue.

This work addresses the core aims of integration defined by Wachtel (1997, 2010) in desegregating and breaking down the limiting boundaries of individual approaches through close attention to their theoretical underpinnings, without excessive allegiance to particular theories, or the denial of others. It has done so by taking down the boundaries of our five major theoretical approaches and focusing on their associated mechanisms and processes as stand-alone entities. Doing so has by-passed the limiting impact of the diverse natures of therapy practice across approaches and their associated world views. In all respects it has adopted the position of epistemological pluralism that is essential to the breaking down of barriers, and is crucially supported by critical realism.

Dialectically Integrated Psychotherapy also subscribes to the importance given by Wachtel (2010) to avoiding the creation of yet another therapeutic approach. In this work the Unifying Dialectical Model and the DIAP meta-framework are designed instead to support multiple, potentially individualized approaches towards integration in terms of psychotherapy practice. They do not support the possibility that a grand theory of therapy practice could be created, but do support the proposition that a grand unified theory of human psychological functioning, reflecting the nature of our theoretically integrative human mind, does actually underlie who we are and how we live our human lives, at an intransitive level, even if that unified theory is so grand that we may never be able to articulate it.

The Unifying Dialectical Model is described as a unifying model; it is an example of the ways in which the contributions that each of our major models of psychotherapy make towards understanding the functioning of our human mind, might be integrated and seen to function together in a unified way. Many more elements and processes could no doubt be added, and all would need to be functionally compatible with each other. Having been established on a theoretically integrative basis, human functioning as defined by the Unifying Dialectical Model is in a position to be influenced by the pragmatics of all our different and effective practical approaches to psychotherapy.

In a *Journal of Psychotherapy Integration* special issue on unification, Magnavita (2008) and Anchin (2008) discuss the essential parameters of a unified theory. Magnavita considers that such a theory of human psychology should identify essential functions, structures and processes common to all human systems, domains and areas of psychology; take a meta-theoretical perspective that can relate to all current paradigms; see the human personality system as the central organizing system of human adaptation and functioning; and draw on multiple paradigms of knowledge that together deepen understanding. In similar vein, Anchin (2008) emphasises the importance of commonalities; the dialectical process of developing bridging theories across disparate concepts and principles, and the valuing of methodological pluralism. Within Dialectically Integrated Psychotherapy the key place ascribed to the personality system by Magnavita is fulfilled by the self in the Unifying Dialectical Model with a central role being given to our unconscious internal models of self, others, relationships and the outside world. This psychological system interacts with relational, social and environmental domains, and demonstrates an overall consistency with these authors' positions in relation to the parameters of theoretical unification

(Magnavita & Anchin, 2014).

The perspective taken here on the world views and epistemologies of individual psychotherapy approaches is one that is consistent with the work of Austen (2000), Feixas and Botella (2004) and Wachtel (2010) as much as it is consistent with the tenets of critical realism. All of these authors believe in the transitive nature of our current knowledge, and Hollanders (2000) refers to the rejection of theoretical pluralism as the denial of the basic truth of the existence of a single world. The so-called world views of psychotherapy theory that can generate impermeable barriers between theoretical perspectives only do so because they have been reified to the status of absolute realities, and have been assumed to impose a similarly absolute requirement of epistemological compatibility on the integration of theoretical perspectives. Within the harmonious, unified functioning of our human mind, such barriers are non-existent.

Summary

In this chapter we have taken Dialectically Integrated Psychotherapy and the nature of the analytical processes undertaken to develop it, out into the wider world, and discussed it in relation to the aims and principles of psychotherapy integration. We have seen that it is consistent with key examples of the literature in these respects and supportive of hopes and aims within the field. Chapter 23 will now compare core features of Dialectically Integrated Psychotherapy with a range of other approaches to psychotherapy integration.

Comparing Dialectically Integrated Psychotherapy with other Approaches to Psychotherapy Integration

23

From a position advised by critical realism and a belief in the existence of an intransitive human mind, valid approaches towards psychotherapy integration would be expected to demonstrate theoretical overlaps and compatible differences when compared with each other. In this Chapter the following core characteristics of the Unifying Dialectical Model and the Dialectical Integration of Approaches to Psychotherapy, DIAP meta-framework will provide the basis for examining areas of congruence and difference between Dialectically Integrated Psychotherapy and a range of integrative models reflecting the categories of theoretical, technical and common factors integration:

- the importance of conscious and unconscious mind
- unconscious internal models of self, others, relationships and the outside world
- psychological defences
- feedback loops involving unconscious internal models, conscious mind, overt behaviours and their outcomes
- the importance of emotion within processes of change
- relational, psychosocial, demographic and cultural environments
- the constructive developmental relationship

The Importance of Both Conscious and Unconscious Mind

Theoretical Integration: As expected, the strongest support for the importance of both conscious and unconscious mind within integrated approaches to psychotherapy comes from those that draw on psychodynamic theory. Wachtel (1977, 1997) and Wachtel et al. (2005) support the existence and functioning of unconscious mind and associated internal structures, particularly the need for reduction in unhelpful unconscious defences, and describe a particular focus on working with the unhelpful relational and behavioural vicious cycles associated with conscious mind. In his more recent work (Wachtel, 2014), Wachtel places more emphasis on the integrative value of working with both conscious and unconscious processes, with therapy process involving the merging mutual influences of psychodynamic and behavioural theories. Stricker (2010) discusses the constant interactions between behaviour, conscious and unconscious mind, giving balanced and overt recognition to unconscious processes. Within Cognitive Analytic Therapy Ryle (1994b) makes very clear his fundamental understanding of the interaction between conscious and unconscious mind, and the need for unhelpful relational patterns fuelled by unconscious processes to become known and recognised within conscious awareness. From the practical perspective within therapy, however, Ryle's advised focus often seems to lie largely with pragmatic therapeutic attention to conscious mind, overt behaviour and specific types of relational patterns (Ryle, 1975, 1995a) and Ryle and Kerr (2020). Dialectically Integrated Psychotherapy is consistent with all of these positions.

From a rather more cognitive perspective, Power (2010) describes Emotion-Focused Cognitive Therapy, an integrative approach that is based on the Schematic Propositional, Analogical and Associative Representational System, SPAARS model (Power & Dalgleish, 2008). This work recognizes the powerful place of emotion within human experience and processes of change, and acknowledges the existence of unconscious/hidden processes. Theory focuses almost exclusively on the existence and primary power of conscious control, and therapy process is defined largely in terms of an educational/training stance. Whilst working very much at a level of conscious influence and control, the SPAARS model does allows for important unconscious contributions via the associative system. It recognises the fundamental importance of changing unconscious structures, the existence of unconscious emotion and the importance of the unconscious being made conscious, principles that are consistent with Dialectically Integrated Psychotherapy.

In contrast, Barnard and Teasdale (1991) and Teasdale and Barnard (1993) make no reference to the conscious or unconscious status of their Interacting Cognitive Subsystems approach but describe systems that would be consistent with aspects of both.

Technical Integration: Within the discussions of Multimodal Therapy provided by Lazarus (1958, 1997, 2005) and Palmer (2000) we find a recognition of the importance of conscious cognition, as well as unconscious and hidden affect, with attention being given to reduced defences in enabling hidden feelings to be experienced, recognizing the importance of both conscious and unconscious mind.

Common Factors Integration: Wampold and Imel (2015) take the potentially integrative position that both cognitive and psychodynamic therapies influence underlying schemas and conscious cognition, involve exposure to previously avoided experience and lead to genuine increases in psychological well-being. This position, and the Frank and Frank (1991, 2004) belief in an underlying assumptive world, could be seen to support the importance of unconscious as well as conscious mind, in keeping with Dialectically Integrated Psychotherapy. However, in both instances the related theories and their associated psychological constructs are dismissed because they are not model specific. For all therapies it is deemed to be the engagement in any trusted, healing therapeutic activity and subsequent general health promoting behaviours, that are responsible for constructive change, with improvements in psychological wellbeing emerging via an increase in clients' conscious expectations that they will be able to act effectively within their lives.

Unconscious Internal Models of Self, Others, Relationships and the Outside World

Theoretical Integration: Concepts equivalent to Dialectically Integrated Psychotherapy's unconscious internal models often appear as the central organising concept within approaches to theoretical integration, reflected in the terminology of the main theoretical approach that influences each of them. They are particularly evident in the integrative positions of Connors (2011); Fonagy (1989); Frank (1990); Greenberg (2004); Horowitz (1994); Murphy and Gilbert (2000); Ryle (1975, 1994a, 1995a); Safran and Inck (1995); and Wachtel (1977, 1997, 2014). They have an important place in Assimilative Integration grounded in psychodynamic relational theory (Stricker, 2010; Stricker& Gold, 2002); and are echoed within two key theoretically integrated models of human psychological functioning developed from cognitive starting points, Interacting Cognitive Subsystems, ICS (Barnard & Teasdale, 1991; Teasdale & Barnard, 1993) and the Schematic, Propositional, Analogical and Associative Representational System, SPAARS approach (Power & Dalgleish, 2008).

Horowitz (1994) and Murphy and Gilbert (2000) from psychodynamic/ relational positions and Safran and Inck (1995) from a more cognitive background, all consider the disconfirmation of dysfunctional schemas to be the common theoretical mechanism of change that underlies the benefit achieved by any effective therapy. Connors (2011) discusses psychoanalytic object relations and cognitive therapy perspectives, seeing them both as intersecting with attachment theory in relation to the importance of internalized representations or schemas, a position very much reflected within Dialectically Integrated Psychotherapy.

Stricker (2010) and Wachtel (1977, 1997, 2014) endorse the central place of unconscious internal models, primarily relating to the concepts of inner worlds and working models as they would be defined within attachment/ psychodynamic relational approaches to therapy. Frank (1990) believes that more of the complex unconscious phenomena elaborated by object relations theory should be incorporated into the integrative models of the inner representational world defined by approaches such as Wachtel's cyclical psychodynamics, a context that has been addressed within Dialectically Integrated Psychotherapy.

Ryle (1975, 1994a, 1995a) describes thoughts, actions and consequences as constituting procedural sequences, that result in repeated patterns of relational reciprocal role procedures, RRPs relating to an underlying repertoire of reciprocal roles, relational positions between self and others. RRPs are defined as aim-directed patterns of interaction that are associated with emotions, cognitions and memories, and are often unconscious and resistant to change (Ryle & Kerr, 2020).

Together these are seen as constituting a Procedural Sequence Object Relations Model, PSORM, relating to aspects of being and functioning at a conscious level and at levels that are outside conscious awareness. This system is reflective of both the cognitive concept of schemas and the psychodynamic concept of an inner world of object relations (Ryle, 1995b). The focus of Cognitive Analytic Therapy is on the modification of unhelpful RRPs that involve polarised 'either/or' behavioural dilemmas within interpersonal relationships. From a somewhat similar position, Frank (1990) supports the integrative central place of cognitive schemas and the inner world of object relations, but sees them as separate, co-existing phenomena, rather than part of the same underlying construct as is assumed within Ryle's theoretical position and is argued for in Dialectically Integrated Psychotherapy.

Greenberg (2004) in Emotion Focused Therapy also supports the existence of underlying models as central to human psychological functioning and processes of change, but defines them as schemas organised on the basis of different human emotions. Emotion schemas are assumed to exist in relation to each major type of human emotion, and are influenced by separate cognitive schemas. Therapy aims to transform maladaptive schemas drawing on humanistic and cognitive behavioural theoretical perspectives, in an experiential therapy process that focuses on emotion, and in its description seems to very much echo psychodynamic practice. From other integrative positions, including Dialectically Integrated Psychotherapy, cognitive schemas and emotion schemas would be seen as part of a single phenomenon, with cognition and emotion intimately bound up with each other.

Within Barnard and Teasdale's Interacting Cognitive Subsystems approach (Barnard & Teasdale, 1991; Teasdale & Barnard, 1993), developed from an essentially information processing position, the construct with the clearest equivalence to the unconscious internal models of Dialectically Integrated Psychotherapy would be the implicational subsystem, although the conscious or unconscious nature of subsystem processing is not explicitly discussed. The implicational subsystem is described as drawing on schematic models of experience that are influenced by developmental events from birth onwards, are particularly influenced by body state and sensory experience, and play a primary role in the experience of emotion.

The propositional subsystem carries out core functions related to the recognition of objects, their nature and their meaning, and feeds into the implicational subsystem. Subsystems may not share all available information, which is seen as explaining our capacity to experience emotion without conscious awareness of its origins. This would imply the capacity for the implicational subsystem to function at an unconscious level. The propositional subsystem is described as providing our awareness of semantics, and the experience of knowing, which would imply that it particularly functions at a conscious level. An absence of sharing between propositional and implicational systems is also seen as providing an explanation for our capacity to talk about an emotionally significant event without feeling the emotion.

Finally, in relation to depression, Barnard and Teasdale (1991) and Teasdale and Barnard (1993) echo Beck's cognitive triad in referring to the development of unhelpful schemas that maintain the depressive themes of negativity towards the self, the world around us and the future, which are synthesized in the implicational subsystem.

The unconscious internal models of Dialectically Integrated Psychotherapy would seem to relate to the combined equivalent of the unconscious implicational subsystem and unconscious aspects of the propositional subsystem.

Within the SPAARS model (Power & Dalgleish, 2008) the situation is rather more divergent and less compatible with Dialectically Integrated Psychotherapy. This approach does discuss the importance of unconscious and conscious experience; however, the schematic model system primarily relating to meaning is defined as a conscious high-level system, as is the propositional system comprising beliefs, ideas, and concepts, and the analogical system that conveys subtle, sensory information via multiple modalities such as facial expression. Within Dialectically Integrated Psychotherapy these systems would be seen as reflecting aspects of both unconscious and conscious mind. The associative system is the only unconscious system within the SPAARS model. It is described as carrying the influences of early interactions with attachment figures, and as having the capacity to bypass the conscious schematic model system, and would be consistent with the concept of unconscious internal models.

Unique contributions of Dialectically Integrated Psychotherapy lie in the ways in which unconscious internal models are defined and conceptualized, and the ways in which the processes involved in their constructive change are discussed. Both draw on integrative understanding derived from psychodynamic, attachment, cognitive and behavioural, and humanistic theories, with their conceptualization including basic aspects of cognitive science that extends them beyond the self, others and relationships.

Technical Integration: From the perspective of technical integration little attention is given to underlying theoretical constructs in general. However, occasional mention is made to aspects of therapy that may reflect the relevance of unconscious internal models, for example Beutler et al. (2005) refer to relational patterns that underlie client vulnerability, and discuss the importance of therapists not colluding with these patterns in their relationships with clients.

Common Factors Integration: From their non-specific common factors perspective, Frank and Frank (1991, 2004) refer to the assumptive world, describing the aim of psychotherapy as helping people to feel and function better by encouraging appropriate changes in their assumptive worlds, and through these changes, transforming the meanings of experience to more favourable ones. The concept of an assumptive world is consistent with the nature of unconscious internal models. It is via such modifications in our assumptive worlds that Frank and Frank see the psychotherapeutic benefits of re-moralization as being achieved. However, since the concept of an assumptive world is recognised as existing within more than one theoretical approach, it is dismissed as theoretically irrelevant because it is not limited to a single-model of therapy. Similarly, Wampold and Imel (2015) dismiss the relevance of schemas as psychological constructs, as discussed earlier.

Psychological Defences

Theoretical Integration: Austen (2000) and Brown (2015) both see the construct of psychological defence as being recognised across various approaches to psychotherapy integration, often expressed as warded off or avoided/inhibited experience or behaviours, with the therapeutic benefits of exposure to avoided experience either outside or within the self, reflecting the reduction of unhelpful defences. Brown (2015) particularly discusses exposure to anxiety, uncomfortable thoughts, feelings and situations as a process that is common to many, if not all approaches to therapy.

In this context Power and Dalgleish (2008), in their discussions of the SPAARS model, choose the terms cognitive-behavioural avoidance and cognitive inhibition when referring to avoided objects, situations, and feelings that are experienced as aversive. Power (2010) in further describing the related practice of Emotion-Focused Cognitive Therapy, uses the term repressive coping style when referring to aversive emotion that becomes hidden from overt experience and expression, and Greenberg (2004) from an experiential perspective refers to hidden core pain. All of these positions are consistent with the concept of psychological defence.

Cognitive Analytic Psychotherapy encompasses the concept of defence within the pragmatic, goal related concept of snags, a term that is also described as an anagram for subtle negative aspects of goals (Ryle,1975, 1995a; Ryle and Kerr, 2020). Snags refer to the ways in which appropriate goals may be abandoned because they are believed to be dangerous to the self or others in some respect, or disallowed. In this context behaviour that might otherwise follow through in a constructive manner becomes diverted off track because of a process that is motivated by some internal anxiety or fear of negative consequences for self or others: a context consistent with the nature of psychological defences.

Wachtel (1977, 1997) was directly influenced by the early integrative thinking of Dollard and Miller (1950) in recognizing the equivalence between behavioural negative reinforcement and the psychodynamic concept of defence, and seeing the experience of exposure to avoided stimuli, internal or external, as a therapeutic process in common across behavioural and psychodynamic therapies. Wachtel (1977, 1997) includes active interventions in the form of behaviour therapy methods in his cyclical psychodynamics approach to theoretical integration on this basis, to support the reduction in unhelpful defences that are also being addressed from a psychodynamic perspective. Murphy and Gilbert (2000) in an integrative approach influenced by psychodynamic relational theory, humanistic, behavioural and cognitive approaches, recognise the pervasive influence of systems of defence. From their perspective these systems protect us from the pain associated with early needs that parents were unable to respond to, resulting in the suppression of forbidden needs. Associated therapeutic reductions in the power of these systems of defence enables the expression of underlying feelings.

Barnard and Teasdale (1991) consider the context in which people talk about events associated with powerful emotions, but do not express or experience emotion at the time. This context is referred to as cold cognition, rather than hot cognition where the emotion is felt as well. This situation is seen as a problem for conventional cognitive therapy theory, with the Interacting Cognitive Subsystems approach offering the explanation that the propositional subsystem can function without contribution from the implicational subsystem, and thus separate cognition and affect in this way: a process equivalent to the functioning of psychological defences.

All of the theoretically integrative approaches discussed above directly or indirectly support the concept of psychological defence, in ways that are not inconsistent with their importance within Dialectically Integrated Psychotherapy.

Technical Integration: In relation to unconscious and conscious mind, Lazarus (1997, 2005) discusses the therapeutic process of bridging between immediately conscious mind and experiences of avoided emotion that are currently outside that awareness. He explicitly embraces a definition of defence as the avoidance of pain, discomfort, anxiety, guilt and shame. In addition, Beutler et al. (2005) in their approach to Systematic Treatment Selection recognize the relevance of hidden affect, and draw on the explanatory concept of associated coping styles in ways that are consistent with the functioning of defence related processes. Their support of the therapeutic value of exposure to avoided experience, would be consistent with the broad-based concept of psychological defence and the associated behavioural principle of negative reinforcement.

Common Factors Integration: Within the literature drawn upon in this work, defences and their related processes do not generally receive particular consideration within common factors approaches to integration. However, Wampold and Imel (2015) in discussing their Contextual Model describe both cognitive therapy and psychodynamic therapy as involving exposure to previously avoided experience, potentially recognising the concept.

Feedback loops Involving Unconscious Internal Models, Conscious Mind, Overt Behaviours and their Outcomes

Theoretical Integration: Albeniz and Holmes (1996) and Murphy and Gilbert (2000) particularly endorse cyclical processes and feedback loops as central themes within theoretical integration in psychotherapy. The approach to integration and relational psychotherapy described by Murphy and Gilbert has maintenance feedback loops in relation to unconscious core interpersonal schemas at its heart. They argue for the importance of understanding unhelpful relational patterns and vicious cycles, and the expression of underlying feelings and needs, with attention to outdated irrational beliefs and overt behaviour, processes that are very reflective of Dialectically Integrated Psychotherapy.

Wachtel (1977, 1997) and Wachtel et al. (2005) are amongst the early practitioners from a psychodynamic perspective to explicitly articulate the importance of complex feedback processes, involving the consequences of our behaviour and actions in terms of the responses we receive from other people. These recursive cycles are seen as playing a crucial part in maintaining our unconscious representations of self, others and relationships. Their identification led Wachtel (1977) to include interventions such as assertiveness training and direct behavioural attention to interpersonal relating, within his cyclical psychodynamic approach to therapy. Later work has evolved to sit within and alongside more recent relational developments within psychodynamic and psychoanalytic psychotherapy (Wachtel, 1997, 2014; Wachtel et al., 2005). Whilst Wachtel and others refer primarily to unhelpful vicious cycles, it is also important to recognise, as Dialectically Integrated Psychotherapy does, that exactly the same maintenance processes apply to helpful and constructive models of self, others, relationships and the outside world.

Stricker (2010) similarly endorses the existence of cyclical mutually interactive maintenance and change processes involving conscious and unconscious experience and overt behaviour, defining unconscious experience, conscious experience and behaviour as the tiers of a triangular model of human functioning, the Three Tier Model of Personality. Within his assimilative approach to theoretical integration, he argues for direct therapeutic attention to conscious experience, cognition and overt behaviour alongside work addressing unconscious processes, in ways that are consistent with psychodynamic relational theory.

Frank (1990) articulates a position that bears considerable similarity to Wachtel's work, emphasizing overt attention to unhelpful client behaviours that are part of the self-perpetuating transactional relational patterns of vicious cycles. In aiming to pay greater attention to the complex unconscious processes described by psychoanalytic theory, Frank (1990) sees them as exerting powerful intra-psychic influences within these circular processes through the continual re-internalization and consolidation of earlier unconscious relational configurations. All of these descriptions are consistent with the ways in which circular maintenance processes are considered and discussed within Dialectically Integrated Psychotherapy.

Ryle (1975, 1995a) and Ryle and Kerr (2020) consider the existence of maintenance loops and vicious cycles within the concept of traps in which the consequences of behaviour are seen to confirm underlying beliefs associated with relational reciprocal roles. The consequences of overt relational behaviour influence conscious mind (accessible beliefs), and unconscious mind (the motivations underlying reciprocal role procedures, RRPs and less accessible beliefs). Behaviours and consequences that are consistent with existing RRPs will act to maintain them. This approach to circular relational maintenance processes, and the interactive importance of behaviour, conscious and unconscious mind is again consistent with the principles of Dialectically Integrated Psychotherapy.

Within the largely cognitively framed Interacting Cognitive Subsystems model, Barnard and Teasdale (1991) and Teasdale and Barnard (1993) discuss the importance of maintenance feedback loops whereby both internal and external experience feed through the sensory and propositional codes into the implicational code. They also discuss the importance of positively influencing these feedback loops in the treatment of depression by focusing on changes in depressogenic schemas generated by the implicational system.

Again from a largely cognitive perspective, Power and Dalgleish (2008) and Power (2010) in their SPAARS model consider the interactive importance of emotion, behaviour, cognition and conscious and unconscious mind. They emphasize the potential for processes of re-learning to change cognitive structures in ways that result in more constructive views of life contexts that have previously been sources of distress, emphasizing the importance of emotion, and the transformation of meaning in these respects. They seem, however, to pay less attention to the relevance of circular feedback maintenance loops compared with other approaches.

Technical Integration: Lazarus (1958, 1997, 2005) does not consider issues of circularity and feedback loops within Multimodal Therapy, but does strongly recognize the importance of concurrently addressing behavioural, conscious cognitive and unconscious/hidden experience within therapy. Whilst the interactive capacity of these factors to work together towards constructive change is clearly implied, no theoretical basis for this is provided, and the validity and value of theoretical integration is soundly dismissed.

Common Factors Integration: Within the literature drawn upon in this work, circular processes, maintenance feedback loops, and related processes do not receive particular consideration within common factors approaches.

The Importance of Emotion Within Processes of Change

Theoretical Integration: Although emotion plays a centrally important role within psychodynamic theory and practice in so many respects, it is not necessarily particularly highlighted within theoretically integrative approaches to psychotherapy that are led by psychodynamic and relational perspectives such as those proposed by Horowitz (1994), Stricker (2010), Wachtel (1977, 1997) and Wachtel et al., (2005). Emphasis may be placed on repeated relational patterns, re-enactments, corrective emotional experience, the importance of the therapeutic alliance, emotional climate, the heightening of affective experience, the importance of defences and overall opportunities for new learning, but with less reference to the experiential importance of human emotion for clients and therapists, or the particular part it plays in the transformational processes of change. In comparison, Dialectically Integrated Psychotherapy gives a much clearer place to the particular importance of emotion.

Several integrative approaches give primary theoretical place to emotion. Greenberg (2004) emphasizes its importance from the experiential/humanistic position where it has traditionally been recognized, and Power (2010) does so from a cognitive behavioural perspective. Both are defined as emotion-focused therapies. Having proposed the existence of emotion schemes (the equivalent of schemas) Greenberg (1994) and Timulak and Pascual-Leone (2015) see them as the principal targets of therapeutic intervention within Emotion Focused Therapy.

Maladaptive emotion schemes, originating within early unhelpful developmental relationships and associated with experiences of fear and shame, are activated in therapy, understood and validated, and changed via the experience of new interpersonal relating. These processes incorporate aspects of psychodynamic and cognitive behavioural theoretical positions, with an overt aim of transforming maladaptive emotion into healthy emotional responses, in an approach that is defined as emotion coaching.

The approach includes reference to the importance of hidden core pain, the existence of resultant problematic secondary feelings, and the importance of accessing the core pain to help transform them; a position that is consistent with the functioning of unhelpful defences, their associated emotions and the therapy related processes that help them to change. The core processes related to Emotion Focused Therapy are reflected within Dialectically Integrated Psychotherapy, which adopts a broader-based position regarding the importance of emotion in conjunction with other aspects of change processes.

From his cognitively led position, Power (2010) supports the need for secondary emotion to give way to the experience of underlying primary emotions and major worries within Emotion Focused Cognitive Therapy. This can involve the experience of emotion which may feel overwhelming, and needs the support of therapy to enable it to be held in awareness. This is referred to as addressing the problem category of too much emotion. Emotion that is hidden, but without the problematic expression of secondary emotion, is described as resulting from a repressive coping style and allocated to a problem category labelled too little emotion. This is considered to be particularly associated with somatic symptoms, and to be dealt with by making connections between the two, often in the context of discovering unexpressed and hidden anger. All of these positions are consistent with the importance of emotion and defence related processes, and the processes addressed within Dialectically Integrated Psychotherapy.

Barnard and Teasdale (1991) give considerable theoretical attention to the ways in which emotion may be generated and its relation to cognition and the existence of affect-related schemas, within the Interacting Cognitive Subsystems approach; however, the place of human emotional experiences within processes of change seems to be unclear.

Overall, Dialectically Integrated Psychotherapy aims to reflect a balanced position that fully recognizes the powerful and integrated core place of emotion within our human psychological functioning, but does not particularly set it apart in terms of its status as being the primary indicator of difficulty or focus for change. The psychological constructs of emotion and cognition are given equal importance at conscious and unconscious levels, together with defences and behaviours, with all of them relating to our unconscious internal models. Feeling, thinking and being are all integrated with each other. Alongside them, the transformative opportunity to experience secure emotional connection with another human being within a containing, genuine and safe relationship that enables and supports the experience of emotion, is recognized as being crucial to the beneficial experience of therapy.

Technical Integration: From a pragmatic perspective, Lazarus (1958, 1997, 2005) clearly recognizes the importance of feelings and emotions being accepted and understood within Multimodal Therapy, including those associated with memories of painful experiences, and the existence of defensive reactions against such pain.

Common Factors Integration: Burns and Nolen-Hoeksema (1992) and Castonguay et al. (1996) support the broad-based importance of emotional connection and associated therapeutic empathy as a common factor across different therapeutic approaches, validating the overall importance of felt emotion.

Relational, Psychosocial, Demographic and Cultural Environments

Theoretical Integration: The approaches to theoretical integration in psychotherapy discussed above tend to pay attention to our environments largely in terms of our past and current relational environments, and the ways in which other people in our lives help to maintain unhelpful aspects of our internal models and associated beliefs. Wachtel (1977, 1997) and Wachtel et al., (2005) refer to the unhelpful contributions of others as their cooperation in the maintenance of our internal structures from the perspective of cyclical psychodynamics. In similar vein, Castonguay et al. (2005) recognize the importance of the quality of interpersonal relationships, and reflect the contribution that other people might make, within their approach to cognitive-behavioural assimilative integration. For Ryle (1975, 1995a) and Ryle and Kerr (2020), these relational contexts are recognized and worked with in the form of reciprocal role relationships and associated traps and snags, with the focus lying primarily with the client's contribution to problematic relational experiences. Whilst Teasdale and Barnard (1993) acknowledge the importance of our past developmental experiences, neither they nor Power (2010) seem to overtly address the current relational or broader based contexts of our lives. Overall, the impact on people's lives and psychological functioning of their wider psychosocial, relational, demographic and cultural environments seem generally to be ignored.

Dialectically Integrated Psychotherapy gives full place to the importance of both past and current relational environments in all our lives, recognizing the potentially positive and damaging consequences of them both, and the ways in which our current relational environment may both support and hinder change. It also takes the wider social, demographic and cultural environments into account. That we may experience powerful limits to our capacity to alter an unhelpful environment for the better is clearly recognized, as is the potential for the environment to be the primary cause of distress at times rather than the individual.

Technical Integration: Within Multimodal Therapy (Lazarus, 1958, 1997, 2005; Palmer, 2000) attention is paid to the ways in which others' behaviour towards us may maintain problematic patterns of being. This is generally defined as relational collusion on their part, a theme that is also echoed by Beutler et al. (2005) from a similar technically integrative perspective. In both instances the therapeutic focus seems to attend primarily to changes within individual clients, rather than acknowledge the potentially adverse nature of the relational environment. Again, the wider psychosocial, relational, demographic and cultural environments seem not to be attended to.

Common Factors Integration: Wampold and Imel (2015) consider culture and context to be inextricable parts of all aspects of psychotherapy. However, little reference to specific social, demographic or cultural factors seems to be made within their Contextual Model, as is the case for the other common factors approaches considered in this work.

The Importance of the Constructive Developmental Relationship

As a core concept within Dialectically Integrated Psychotherapy the term constructive developmental relationship has been adopted to refer to therapists' ways of relating to clients that, of themselves, foster psychological growth and development, and are supported by humanistic, attachment, and psychodynamic theories. This was done to highlight the developmental and facilitative functions of these particular ways of relating within the therapeutic relationship, at the same time as recognizing the everyday ubiquity of their importance within the broad range of human experience across the life span.

Theoretical Integration: Within the range of models discussed here several authors acknowledge, but do not particularly emphasize, the importance of empathy, acceptance, emotional warmth and security within the therapeutic relationship (Horowitz, 1994; Power & Dalgleish, 2008; Stricker, 2010; Wachtel, 1977, 1997; Wachtel et al., 2005). Power & Dalgleish (2008), however, expressly minimize the contribution made by this relationship to the processes of change. Whilst recognizing the importance of a sense of safety within an essentially positive therapeutic relationship, associated reductions in defences and the importance of repeated relational patterns, Ryle (1995a) and Ryle and Kerr (2020) do not appear to particularly discuss the importance of the empathic and emotionally attuned relationship in its own right within Cognitive Analytic Therapy. Little if any attention appears to be paid to it by Barnard and Teasdale (1991) and Teasdale and Barnard (1993) from a cognitive, information processing perspective. Castonguay et al. (2005) discuss the importance of new/corrective interpersonal experiences and the value of emotional experience within therapy, alongside more traditional cognitive-behavioural interventions, and refer to the importance of the therapeutic alliance, but make no reference to the empathic, attuned nature of the therapeutic relationship. Similarly, Safran and Inck (1995) consider the potential for different therapy approaches to mutually support constructive changes in dysfunctional schemas, with no mention of the empathic relationship.

Greenberg (2004) and Murphy and Gilbert (2000), however, both give a strong explicit place to the capacity for empathy, acceptance and validation within therapy to support the experience of emotion, new relational experience and associated processes of psychological change, growth and development.

Overall, it seems that some authors pay little or no attention to the empathic, attuned relationship within their theoretically integrative approaches. Others may acknowledge the value of emotional warmth in therapy, and support the importance of new relational experience, the emergence of painful previously hidden emotions, the value of emotional containment and the crucial contribution of corrective emotional experience, but not necessarily address in any depth, the empathic, validating and emotionally attuned therapeutic relationship, defined here as the constructive developmental relationship, or acknowledge its heritage within humanistic, attachment and psychodynamic theories.

Technical Integration: Beutler et al. (2005) clearly recognize the healing factors within the therapeutic relationship and recommend the use of interventions that will support and enhance those qualities of relating, whilst Multimodal Therapy (Lazarus, 2005; Palmer, 2000) values the capacity of empathy, acceptance and unconditional positive regard to support the educational function of the therapeutic relationship.

Common Factors Integration: From a broad based, largely common factors approach, O'Brien and Houston (2000) consider the nature and quality of the relationship between therapist and client to be the most important therapeutic variable predicting beneficial outcome across differing approaches to psychotherapy. This importance is seen to relate to the ways in which the therapeutic relationship fulfils the developmental needs of the client. In these respects, their work is consistent with the importance attributed here to the constructive developmental relationship. Their work valuably discusses the crucial importance of therapists' intuitive connection with the subjective uniqueness of each client in these respects.

Parloff (1986) in his discussion of Frank's non-specific common factors (Frank & Frank, 1991, 2004), somewhat similarly endorses the relationship as having a particular and unique corrective value across all therapeutic approaches. In addition, Burns and Nolen-Hoeksma (1992) identify therapeutic empathy and warmth as the characteristic most reliably associated with positive outcomes for cognitive behavioural approaches to depression, seeing empathy as a factor in common across all therapies.

Wampold and Imel (2015) in their Contextual Model describe the therapeutic relationship as the bedrock of psychotherapy effectiveness, making reference to the work of Bowlby and recognizing the importance of empathy. Similarly to Dialectically Integrated Psychotherapy, they clearly recognize the contributions that clients make to the nature of the relationship. In terms of theoretical understanding, the relationship is seen as important in this way because it is judged to be a powerful source of the increase in positive expectations and the re-moralization that are deemed to be the direct causes of improved well-being.

Overall common factors approaches to psychotherapy integration generally give a core place to the constructive developmental relationship, but not necessarily in a way that supports the nature and depth of its contributions, or acknowledge and value the range of theoretical approaches that support it.

Summary

In this Chapter we have considered a range of approaches to psychotherapy integration and discussed ways in which their premises compare with core aspects of Dialectically Integrated Psychotherapy. Greatest similarity is found regarding concepts relating to unconscious internal models, psychological defences, and feedback loops. There is variable mutual recognition of the importance of emotion, and the distinctive value of the constructive developmental relationship.

Within these comparisons, Dialectically Integrated Psychotherapy uniquely considers the constant mutual interaction between unconscious and conscious mind and the balanced importance of both, and gives comprehensive attention to the roles played by our social, relational, cultural and demographic environments. It is also the only approach to provide theoretically integrative descriptions of core psychological constructs that have been supported by theoretical triangulation. This unique contribution is of particular relevance in relation to our unconscious internal models of self, others, relationships and the outside world.

Chapter 24 will consider the practical implications of Dialectically Integrated Psychotherapy and its philosophical base in relation to theory development, research, clinical practice and training.

Implications for Theory, Research and Practice

24

This chapter explores the implications of Dialectically Integrated Psychotherapy and its philosophical base in relation to theory development, research, clinical practice and training.

A Changed Approach to the Development of Psychotherapy Theory

If the premises of Dialectically Integrated Psychotherapy and the critical realism that supports it, were accepted within our psychotherapeutic academic communities they would considerably influence our attitudes towards the theories of human psychology underlying therapeutic practice, and the ways in which we approach theory development.

We would expect to find theoretical overlap between all of our approaches, and would value compatible differences. We would be challenged to develop aspects of theory that illuminate the mutual functioning and complementarity of their differing mechanisms and processes. We would also face up to the existence of incompatible differences, accept that they needed to be resolved, and accept the reality that in some instances treasured aspects of theory may be wrong and ill-founded, or in need of modification. A transparent dialectical approach would become routine.

We would no longer see competition between different theoretical approaches. Overlaps and the existence of core constructs would be acknowledged and believed in. We would expect outcome research to show the on-average equivalence of efficacy that is so commonly demonstrated across our therapeutic approaches (Wampold & Imel, 2015) and we would fully accept Rosenzweig's 1936 'dodo-bird' conclusion that all our therapeutic approaches have won and all must have prizes (Rosenzweig, 1936/2002).

Different approaches would remain separate and each of them would be truly valued for their recognition of particular core constructs, their contribution to our understanding of those constructs, and the roles their mechanisms and processes play in the overall functioning of our unified human mind. Theory would be expected to advise practice in potentially integrated ways, supporting the capacity for different mechanisms and processes to mutually enhance common aspects of change. The inter-relationships between the concepts of our different theoretical approaches would become a commonplace focus of theory development, and associated research.

The principles of Dialectically Integrated Psychotherapy would enhance the status and relevance of theory in the practice of psychotherapy. In recent years the increased focus on efficacy and effectiveness of psychotherapy has pushed theory somewhat into the shadows. Instrumentalism and pragmatism have held particular sway, with the danger that how change, growth and development take place within us is not as important. At the extreme, all that may matter in a primarily evidence-based practice world is that therapy is seen to work. Less attention is paid to the nature of our psychological mechanisms and processes and the ways in which they function. Dialectically Integrated Psychotherapy would support theory remaining in the forefront, guiding what we do from a single-model perspective, and helping us make routine decisions enhancing integrative practice through the dialectically advised application of more than one perspective.

In order to reach this situation at any truly meaningful level within our organisations and institutions, the validity of the core principles of critical realism as discussed in this work need to be accepted. Doing so would not exclude the value of empiricism and logical positivism, but would strengthen the position of a broader range of epistemologies that would complement each other. It would also encourage empirical research to direct its focus towards the study of variables associated with multiple theoretical positions within the same study, and in relation to differing aspects of the same core psychological construct.

Implications for Psychotherapy Research

In a therapeutic and scientific world advised by the principles of critical realism, and the fundamental acceptance of the unified functioning of the human mind, the relationship between practice and research would remain similar to its present form, but also be different in significant ways. The value of evidence in support of therapy practice and efficacy would remain and empiricism and logical positivism would have their place, but they would no longer retain supremacy.

If the transitive nature of current knowledge, the importance of unconscious and hard-to-measure variables, the theoretically integrative functioning of the human mind, and the highly interactive and complex nature of the processes involved in psychological change were comprehensively accepted, it would always be understood that empiricism led by logical positivism could only ever address part of the overall picture. That part would be important, but in no way conclusive and would not be expected to necessarily be totally reliable and reproducible.

Current evidence-based practice research approaches would continue to provide support for manual based single-model therapies, including those that function on a formally integrative basis such as Cognitive Analytic Therapy, Schema Therapy and Dialectical Behavior Therapy, and outcomes in terms of symptom reduction would always be evaluated. But at the same time the fuller naturally integrative context of the processes and mechanisms involved in change would be taken into account, plus the potential for single-model therapy practice to beneficially reflect aspects of other theoretical models, as supported by DIAP meta-framework.

A particular context presents itself in relation to individualized process oriented integrative therapies in which interventions and process are adapted to the perceived needs of the client, are formulation led and unfold in ways that cannot be anticipated in advance. There are no problems in measuring symptom outcomes and process related variables across theoretical perspectives in these instances, or in undertaking observational studies on that basis. The issue lies in the acceptability or not, of a research methodology that does not define in advance how a therapist should behave.

This is where the dominance of empiricism and logical positivism that adheres to the belief that the future can be predicted with certainty really comes under challenge. Our acceptance of the validity of formulation and process led theoretically integrative psychotherapy practice will depend on us letting go of this often-unrealistic belief.

Approaches could be developed to support current process and outcome research being carried out on an integrative basis, incorporating process variables associated with a broader range of theoretical approaches, alongside those relating to a primary single-model. From an observational perspective, research recordings of therapy sessions may be analysed on the basis of other models as well as the primary single-model under study. Such an approach would involve a shift in the criteria used to select process and outcome measures, and challenge us to explore appropriate measures/indicators of psychological constructs that are hard to identify and quantify, such as therapist attunement and empathic connection, and the functioning of conscious and unconscious defences. This challenge particularly relates to those variables associated with unconscious mind. The principles of Dialectically Integrated Psychotherapy would usefully support such research.

Fresh and creative attention would be given to the identification of our hard-to-measure variables, and may usefully include re-visiting projective techniques and other methodologies previously used to explore the processes of unconscious mind. In some instances, we would need to be more accepting of identification and counts of frequency, rather than aiming for higher levels of measurement, supporting the increased status of qualitative research methodologies when they are appropriate to the variables under study.

Within this more flexible and integrative research ethos, the selective use of case-study research would have an important place, analysing repeated measures of symptomatology and psychological variables associated with integrative processes of change, in relation to the work done between therapist and client. This approach to case-study research is illustrated by my earlier research using the Brief Symptom Inventory, BSI and the Dysfunctional Attitudes Scale, DAS (Oliver & Baumgart, 1985) on a regular basis throughout therapy to assess symptom change and cognitions/beliefs, with the Object Relations Test, ORT (Phillipson, 1955) being used pre- and post-therapy to reflect changes in unconscious processes, particularly defences (Hingley, 1995, 2001).

The separation between evaluative applied research and pure research that investigates the existence and nature of psychological mechanisms and processes, would be reduced and each would more routinely feed into the other. Attention to how our mind works, and how change comes about, would be just as important as whether a therapy works or not.

Implications for Psychotherapy Practice

Single-Model Practice: The implications for therapy practice vary depending on the organisational context of therapy provision. From the position taken in this work, the independent value of our differing practical approaches to therapy is retained, since each is directing therapeutic attention in their own specific ways towards sub-sets of processes and mechanisms that lead towards beneficial change. However, elements of any therapy and its associated assumptions may come to be modified and improved if we see ourselves as having greater freedom to explore the premises of other approaches, accept their validity and use their perspectives to enhance our own theory and practice.

If the approach advocated by Dialectically Integrated Psychotherapy was adopted, a broader range of therapeutic principles might be more easily available to us, whatever single or integrative model we were applying. We may be supported in more routinely giving thought to the demographic and relational environment of our clients' lives, and their place in the life span; in thinking more about the importance of behaviour; in accepting the continuing and constant roles played by both conscious and unconscious mind; in being aware of the power of defences; thinking about the importance of emotion and in giving full recognition to the crucial role played by the developmental constructive relationship between ourselves and our clients. The nature of maintenance and change within unconscious internal models of self, others, relationships and the outside world would be used as a constructive avenue of connection between our own approach and other helpful approaches to theoretical understanding.

The approach taken here towards the constructive developmental relationship, and its integrative definition may encourage all therapists to draw more on a range of theories and literature that can support the helpful growth promoting relationships they build with all the people who come to see them. It may be in this respect that it would be easiest for any single-model therapy approach to acknowledge and draw more on other theoretical perspectives, since virtually all of our approaches accept that the relationship plays a significant part in supporting beneficial therapeutic outcomes.

In all respects this book overwhelmingly supports the importance of the therapeutic relationship and integrates the contributions of different but overlapping theoretical perspectives in supporting our practice in this respect. It seems so unfortunate at times when humanistic, attachment and psychodynamic theory become invisible in this respect, and are not necessarily acknowledged or referenced in the therapeutic literature in support of that relationship. Every approach to therapy has something to learn from those sources of knowledge and practice, whatever the nature of their evidence-based therapy protocols.

In the UK I believe it would be beneficial for the organisational and governmental systems involved in the implementation of evidence based practice and the delivery of the Improving Access to Psychological Therapies, IAPT initiative (Clark, 2012, 2018; National Collaborating Centre for Menta Health, 2019), plus the academic and research institutions that support them, to open their collective minds to the philosophical, academic, research and therapeutic positions discussed in this work.

Integrative Practice: Dialectically Integrated Psychotherapy provides support to those practitioners who wish to argue for the value of a more integrative approach to their therapeutic work within contexts that may not currently recognise its value and validity. In other contexts where organisations or independent practitioners do not adhere to the tight empirical requirements of evidence based practice, whilst still respecting the need for therapy to have a demonstrated capacity to help people, therapists will be more free to work in overtly integrative ways, drawing on different therapeutic approaches that each in their own right are supported by evidence of their efficacy.

It is in these contexts that Dialectically Integrated Psychotherapy may have most to offer. For those therapists who routinely practice in ways that are advised by more than one model, maybe drawing on psychodynamic, attachment, humanistic and cognitive behavioural approaches in similar ways to myself, I see this book as making transparent and overt the underlying beliefs and decision making that may be taking place in their minds as they integrate these models seamlessly on an everyday basis. For them nothing here may be new, but I hope that those therapists will feel supported by the integrative descriptions of core constructs, the principles of the Unifying Dialectical Model and the DIAP meta-framework, and the ways in which the arguments in support of integrative practice have been made.

For those therapists who are newly interested in practicing in more theoretically integrative ways, Dialectically Integrated Psychotherapy provides an overall framework to support their endeavours. Different therapeutic approaches may be integrated on the theoretically coherent basis of their mutually supportive capacities to lead to helpful changes in the nature of unconscious internal models of self, others, relationships and the outside world. Therapists will also be supported in thinking about the practical nature of any resultant integrative approach to therapy. Are the interventions associated with the approaches compatible with each other? If aspects of incompatibility exist, could they be modified, whilst still retaining potential therapeutic influence? Does one model of therapy, and its associated therapeutic style, hold primary place? Is the resultant therapy coherent in a way that holds together and makes sense for both therapists and clients?

Working through a rationale for integrative therapy in this way, even if such thinking takes place after the event rather than in advance, can provide practitioners with stronger ground to argue for their integrative approach with other professionals if necessary. It may also provide a starting point for developing rationales to explain the basis of therapy to prospective clients. If research looking at process and outcomes within integrative therapies develops as discussed above, it would be increasingly able to support therapists' thinking and decision making in all of these respects.

The Overall Context of Psychotherapy and its Limitations: This work makes explicit the belief that within psychotherapy the mechanisms and processes associated with a range of theoretical perspectives are likely to be automatically playing their part, in addition to the specific interventions that the therapist is making. This will also be the case in the world outside the therapy room. The totality of the processes and psychological mechanisms involved in therapy and any associated beneficial change will reflect far more than the specific interventions we have chosen to make as therapists. This does not diminish the role that our interventions play, or our capacity to have influence in sometimes hugely supportive and facilitative ways, but the context of people's lives and their own personal capacities and potential for growth and development will always play their own significant part.

This work supports us in recognising the very understandable but also disappointing and sometimes painful limitations to the impact that therapy may be able to have. Dialectically Integrated Psychotherapy supports four factors as playing important parts in those limitations:

- the initial nature of the client's unconscious internal models in terms of their immaturity versus maturity and their damaging versus constructive characteristics
- the similarly based nature of their psychological defences
- the mutual contributions of therapist and client to the quality of the therapeutic developmental relationship
- the relational and demographic nature of the world the client lives in

These factors mutually influence each other, and some or all of them may work against the possibility of therapeutic progress, or set significant limits on the gains that may be made.

It is important that all concerned with public service provision from government levels down are aware of the reality of these limitations, not least because doing so may support realistic expectations being set for everyone involved. Similarly, independent and private practitioners need to bear these issues in mind, and Dialectically Integrated Psychotherapy may support all concerned in this respect.

Implications for Psychotherapy Training

Single-Model Psychotherapy Training: The nature of psychotherapy training would be affected and influenced by all of the above considerations in relation to theory, research and the nature of therapy practice. Each single-model approach to psychotherapy would overtly position itself as an equal member of a community of validated and valued approaches to therapy. Individual therapeutic identities would not be sacrificed, but theoretical overlaps and the underlying reality of their associated processes and mechanisms existing as part of a unified, intransitive human mind would be recognised. The core psychological constructs identified by theoretical triangulation across therapies, and their integrative theoretical definitions would be acknowledged, alongside the in-depth theoretical and practical study of a specific single-model approach. Psychotherapists and other professionals in training would be encouraged to identify similarities between the psychological constructs and processes of different approaches, and the particular unique contributions made by the one they are specialising in.

It would also be appreciated that within every single-model approach, the variables associated with other theoretical approaches may also influence aspects of practice, the client's experience of therapy and their processes of change. Practitioners in training would be encouraged to read about the theories that could particularly support and enhance their single-model approach, and learn to develop effective ways of incorporating that awareness into practice.

The research literature would always constitute a central and integrated aspect of training, draw from a range of epistemologies, and be presented in a way that engenders a non-competitive ethos as well as overall critical appraisal. Research in support of core constructs and key psychological mechanisms and processes would be a particular focus of attention.

Since the importance of the therapeutic relationship is recognised within virtually all approaches to psychotherapy, it is in relation to the constructive developmental relationship that teaching and training influenced by theoretically unifying principles might most likely become established within single-model training courses. In this context, increased theoretical attention would be paid to humanistic, attachment theory and the relational aspects of psychodynamic theory whatever the single-model orientation. Such attention would be founded on a clear recognition that the relationship always makes its own constructive contributions to processes of change, as well as supporting the use of other interventions.

All of the possibilities discussed so far in relation to single-model training carry with them the implied acceptance of the validity of critical realism as the underlying philosophical basis of psychotherapy theory, research and therapy practice. The overt recognition and acceptance of this philosophical base would be likely to vary. I believe it to be implicit within the acceptance of the unifying position discussed in this book, but elements of this position may come to be accepted without critical realism being adopted or acknowledged. In instances where critical realism was recognised, it could also be an explicit part of the training curriculum.

Training relating to Improving Access to Psychological Therapies, IAPT, in the UK would more fully acknowledge the importance of theory and become more flexible in recognising the ways in which the practice of any one single-model therapy may be enhanced by other theoretical approaches, particularly in the context of the therapeutic relationship. It would also usefully explore ways in which integrative psychotherapy may be supported from an evidence-based practice position.

Integrative Psychotherapy Training: Some therapeutic training currently takes place on an integrative basis, allowing for the separate application of a range of single-model approaches, and for the provision of theoretically integrative therapies that draw on more than one model. Some theoretically integrative therapies such as Cognitive Analytic Therapy have become the equivalent of single-models and their training courses address them as such. All such training courses function currently in the context of the prevailing paradigm reflecting largely empiricist and logical positivist philosophical positions, sometimes emphasizing a constructivist or otherwise post-modern epistemology. For them I believe that Bhaskar's critical realism offers an improved and more secure philosophical base. The principles of Dialectically Integrated Psychotherapy support the ways in which psychotherapy integration may be justified, explained and translated into practice. I believe it has the potential to significantly influence psychotherapy training in these respects.

In the event of any greater acceptance of theoretically integrative psychotherapy practice within evidence-based state provision in the UK and the US, more training courses might move in an integrative direction. Those that currently provide teaching and training across a range of single-model approaches and value the provision of formulation-led theoretically integrated therapy tailored to the needs of individual clients would be more fully supported in doing so. They would be further supported in the attention they pay to the benefits of the constructive developmental relationship and the crucial importance of the relational, demographic and lifespan environments of clients' lives.

The research component of any training programme could provide the ideal opportunity to pursue research in support of integrative psychotherapy practice, as discussed earlier in this chapter. Ideally such research would be established as routine on-going research within training organisations, so that psychotherapists and other professionals in training would have the option to become involved in areas of ongoing projects and extend their remit. Such research would be of value to the practice of psychotherapy as a whole, and of particular value to individual training courses in supporting their integrative identity.

Summary

This chapter looks at the implications of Dialectically Integrated Psychotherapy and its underlying assumptions in relation to theory development, psychotherapy research, practice, and training. If its principles were to be accepted, attention to theory would be enhanced on a cooperative, dialectical basis across our theoretical perspectives, and research would function with similar flexibility across a range of epistemologies. Dialectically Integrated Psychotherapy supports the continued valuing of our current single-model therapies, offering a greater freedom for their current procedures to be enhanced by a wider range of theoretical knowledge, particularly in relation to the constructive developmental relationship. It fundamentally supports integrative therapy provision overall, and if accepted could influence the nature of psychotherapy training in all of the above respects.

Some Reflections on Process and Outcome

25

We have now reached the end of this exploration of psychotherapy theory, having travelled through the new territory of Roy Bhaskar's critical realism and taken a radical and comprehensive approach to epistemological pluralism and dialectical analysis; in some respects boundaries have been broken, and accepted rules have not always been obeyed.

Working on relatively detailed descriptions of our five major therapeutic approaches, I lowered the boundaries between them and made their overlaps and similarities explicit. It is in the detail that we discover the range of similarities that exist between them. When I found clear commonality across constructs, I judged the approaches involved to be referring to the same entity, and gave two of the most strongly supported and important constructs new, theory-neutral names to emphasize that situation.

Since I had now decided that these core constructs did represent the same entities, I was able to bring together the different ideas about each of them provided by the five approaches, when they were compatible with each other. I accepted the limit of reality; we do not have more than one human mind, and aspects of theory about that mind that cannot logically co-exist have to change in some way, or be abandoned. These positions set me free to re-define and describe these important psychological phenomena and processes in more fully comprehensive ways, incorporating compatible ideas from across our five different perspectives; a fundamental integration of theory. This process intrinsically and repeatedly involved the resolution of incompatibility that is central to dialectical process.

From that theoretically integrated starting point I developed the Unifying Dialectical Model of human psychological functioning; a complex interactive system in which feedback processes involving unconscious and conscious mind, our behaviour and the world around us, maintain our unconscious internal models of self, others, relationships and the outside world, or change them. All of our five major approaches, in their varying ways, can influence the processes within the UDM that help these models to change in beneficial ways. This potential is illustrated and described by the Dialectical Integration of Approaches to Psychotherapy, DIAP meta-framework. This is Dialectically Integrated Psychotherapy.

At the start of the book I talked about Joan, my client when I was a trainee, and my mistake of not having listened to her story, having given her a pre-prepared one of my own about how CBT can help us understand anxiety. We looked at the ways in which different theoretical approaches helped us think about what happened and about her response to me. They all had validity, some of them overlapped, some were more unique, and there seemed no problem in imagining that they could all have a role to play in advising how I might have responded to Joan, and be used alongside each other in complementary ways.

Maybe this represents the place that all of us start from; an implicit knowing that our different theoretical approaches can be integrated with each other. I imagine that many of us have an implicit theoretically integrative and unifying model in our heads. If we are working from a single-model perspective, and seek out alternative approaches to help us when things get stuck in therapy, or when aspects of client difficulty and processes of change don't fit with what we have been doing effectively so far, the answers we find make theoretical sense to us. If they work in practice, they must have become integrated together in the client's mind with the other things we were doing. An integrative, unifying system must be in there.

In this study I have been working to articulate that implicit model, and to give it explicit substance. I have always believed in it, and in my teaching in 1992 I first put together a version of the diagram that became the starting point for the DIAP meta-framework. In that early diagram I presented the major approaches as mutually influencing the nature of underlying schemas via the processes of conscious versus unconscious mind: at the time this seemed enough. In my discussions with trainees, we comfortably talked together in a general way about overlap and similarity, useful difference and complementarity. That seemed straightforward at the time; implicitly we all knew what we meant.

After starting work on this book, wishing to contribute something that would support broad based integrative psychotherapy practice on this basis, I discovered that it was not straightforward at all. After the chapters on the five major approaches were written and I began to write about their mutual influences on a central entity of mind, I discovered that I was facing a black hole. The term schemas could not be used in discussions involving psychodynamic theory because it did not relate to psychodynamic mechanisms or the specific characteristics of the inner world of object relations; similarly it did not relate strongly enough to the nature of therapy process influencing the internal working models of attachment theory, or connect with the concepts of behaviourally-led theories. I needed an alternative representation of this central entity within our human mind, and a way of defining the common and complementary pathways by which our different therapeutic approaches might influence it.

A belief in the importance of philosophy has always mattered to me, and I had started the book by overviewing a range of epistemologies and looking at the problems with logical positivism. By sheer good fortune I came across reference to Bhaskar's critical realism, and discovered that his work, as conveyed by Andrew Collier, was remarkably similar to the ways I already viewed the world, and psychotherapy theory. Overlaps and similarities were valued and to be looked for, incompatible differences were to be overcome, and compatible differences used creatively to carry us forward by dialectic process; and Bhaskar believed that scientists could be talking about the same thing, but either not realize it or not be prepared to believe it.

Encouraged by Bhaskar, I decided that I needed to draw on the specific details of the five theoretical approaches I had written about, and undertook the content analysis discussed in Chapter 15, so that I could more systematically identify what they had in common. This led to the identification of eleven aspects of significant overlap. Where these overlaps involved psychological constructs, I took the step of judging them to be referring to the same psychological entity. This led to the identification of the five core psychological constructs. One of these was based on the similarity between the schemas of cognitive therapy theory, the inner world of object relations of psychodynamic theory, the internal working model of attachment theory, and the complex learning history of behavioural theory. I gave this construct the theory-neutral name unconscious internal models of self, others, relationships and the outside world. The black hole still was not fully filled, but I did now have an integrative construct that could be influenced by the mechanisms and processes discussed within each of our therapeutic approaches: our unconscious internal models.

Once these five core constructs had been identified, it became obvious that the next step was to define them on an integrative basis. Our theories, their similarities and their compatible differences again came into their own as I drew on them to think about the nature of our unconscious internal models, their development, the ways in which they influence our behaviour and the processes that maintain and change them. The Unifying Dialectical Model, with our unconscious internal models at its heart, emerged out of this work. The scene was now set for our different therapeutic approaches to each influence our unconscious internal models via the processes of the Unifying Dialectical Model, and the model came to sit at the centre of the Dialectical Integration of Approaches to Psychotherapy, DIAP meta-framework. Together they became Dialectically Integrated Psychotherapy.

This work provided me with an opportunity to stand up for humanistic client-centred theory and practice, alongside psychodynamic and attachment theories in the irreplaceable contributions they all make towards our appreciation of the life-long importance of the love and care that is supported by attuned empathic relating, within therapy and elsewhere in all our lives. The term constructive developmental relationship is rather unwieldy, but for me it was essential for a neutral term to exist that all three theoretical approaches could be part of, and that applied beyond the therapeutic relationship; I didn't manage to find a better alternative.

The crucial interactive role of our relational, psychosocial, demographic and cultural environments emerged even more strongly as the work progressed, potentially contributing to the nature of individual psychological problems, and facilitating or limiting the ways in which our internal models may change in constructive directions. For every client all of their current life experiences play a part in the context of therapeutic change. Each client and each therapist makes their unique contribution to the mutually created nature of the constructive developmental relationship, and overall clients' relational and social worlds are likely to be the most important aspects of their environment that contribute to therapeutic progress. Sometimes the environment may also be entirely responsible for the problem.

In a recent article, Marvin Goldfried has talked about the obstacles faced by psychotherapy in its continuing efforts to find consensus. He sees our current scientific stage of development as pre-paradigmatic, because we have no agreed-upon core of knowledge. He makes the point that the different theory-based languages of our competing paradigms make it hard to translate between them, which prevents us from learning about similarities and points of complementarity across orientations. In this situation it is hard for us to build theory on the foundations of past contributions, and we keep on trying to invent something new, but quite often end up reflecting earlier contributions in new language (Goldfried, 2019).

Goldfried's suggested solutions have focused on the pragmatics of therapy, and the empirical nature of change related processes, such as corrective emotional experiences and reality testing, that may enable stable and long-term changes in expectations, feelings and behaviour; all of which are consistent with the changes in unconscious internal models discussed in Dialectically Integrated Psychotherapy. Goldfried's thoughts lean towards a common factors-based approach to integration, in which theory is not dismissed, but put to the sidelines because it cannot be resolved.

In this work I have addressed the issues of competing paradigms and the problems of theory-based language. I have done my best to translate between them, to develop some common language, and to foster the common use of some theory specific theoretical terminology. Dialectically Integrated Psychotherapy has addressed the issues of similarity and overlap, from a position of epistemological pluralism, and has celebrated the amazing wealth of theoretical understanding available to us across our five major models. They have all been brought together within integrative core psychological constructs, common constituents of change processes, and a model of the functioning of the human mind that supports all of them in feeding into unique experiences of psychotherapy and processes of change.

Dialectically Integrated Psychotherapy has been examined in terms of its relationship to a selection of other key approaches to psychotherapy integration, and it is compatible with most of those considered. In various instances its core components are echoed within other approaches, although often expressed in diverse terminologies. The one inevitable exception to compatibility clearly lies with those common factor approaches that choose to dismiss the relevance and importance of the complex psychological concepts, mechanisms and processes functioning within the human mind, and the potential validity of the theories that address them.

Whichever way it unfolds, I believe it is only comprehensive theoretically integrative approaches to the nature of our human mind such as this, that recognize its complex, compatible and unified functioning from a position of epistemological pluralism, that will support consensus across our accepted, validated and valued approaches, and enable human psychology and psychotherapy to move beyond the current pre-paradigmatic position that Goldfried has so eloquently clarified.

The T S Eliot epigraph at the start of this book has echoes for me. A colleague said it came to her mind, when I was talking about my experience of doing this work. My exploration of theory has brought me back to where I started from, it is essentially the same place but also so very different; in some ways I do now see it for the first time.

In relation to the human mind we will never cease in our exploring.

Appendix 1

Elements of Theory Identified Across the Major Approaches to Psychotherapy

Attachment Theory

n=19

- acceptance by parents and others
- empathic attunement: emotional availability, reading infants' feeling state, cooperation and equality, 'psychic human membership'
- concepts of secure and insecure attachment; categories of attachment in childhood and adulthood
- attachment security and secure base supporting healthy development and exploration
- reciprocal connectedness
- innate human capacity for growth
- defensive exclusion of emotions and own needs
- importance of psychological security of parents
- benefits of reduced need for defences
- need for psychological survival in childhood situation of total dependence
- importance of non-verbal communication
- internal working models; unconscious stereotypes
- importance of relational experiences and re-enactments in therapy

- open communication helps to revise and update internal working models
- capacity to recognise existence of separate minds within self and others
- recovery of lost emotional life and sense of real self
- reorganisation of models of self and others
- impact of separation and loss; grief processes
- attuned, empathic therapeutic relationship

Humanistic and Experiential Theory

n= 14

- acceptance by others especially parents & unconditional positive regard
- self-acceptance
- conditions of worth leading to incongruence and defensive exclusion of experience from conscious awareness
- actualising tendency, human potential and organismic valuing
- benefit of high functioning parents
- importance of parents' capacity for genuineness
- therapeutic relationship involving empathy, genuineness, unconditional positive regard, psychological contact and capacity to read other's feeling states
- undistorted development of self
- reduced functioning of defences
- need for psychological survival and value of defences
- importance of non-verbal communication
- re-organization of self
- relevance of power and control; importance of empowerment of individual, their freedom to make own choices
- relationship between people can be coloured by past relationships

Psychodynamic Theory

n= 28

- importance of unconscious mind
- symbolism & primary process thinking
- central importance of emotion
- psychological defences and associated intra-psychic conflict
- living with painful emotions, memories and current realities

- inner world of object relations
- importance of past experiences especially in early relationships
- transference & countertransference
- identification
- internalisation
- projective identification
- parallel process
- re-enactments
- emotional containment
- empathic mirroring and emotionally attuned care
- self-selfobject relationship
- optimal frustration
- basic trust
- developmental arrest
- development of self: symbiosis, separation, individuation
- basic fault
- separation anxiety
- distortions of self-development, 'true' & 'false' self
- ego-strength
- intrapsychic and interpersonal boundaries
- life instinct/libido/life-force
- pleasure principle
- reality principle

Cognitive and Behavioural Theory

n=19

- conscious cognition influences thoughts, feelings and emotions, and vice versa
- importance of negative automatic thoughts, functioning just outside of conscious awareness
- people interpret and actively construct their perceptions
- schemas: unconscious memory related structures influenced by childhood and life experiences, associated with core beliefs, attributions & automatic thoughts
- patterns of relational behaviour influenced by schemas & emerging in other relationships
- behaviour therapy used when needed
- behavioural experiments to test conditional beliefs and rules for living
- affect and cognition inseparable within schemas

- avoidance of internal emotion via 'security operations' leading to distortions of schemas of self and others and influencing schema maintenance
- damaging impact of unmet emotional needs in childhood and persistence of younger selves and associated schemas in adulthood
- aspects of personal difficulties seen as fulfilling a function involving unconscious self-protective processes linked with hidden emotional truths
- impact of powerful emotion in generating distortions of cognition
- avoidance and escape from unbearable suffering
- developmental impact of invalidating environments
- the importance of validation
- benefit of painful hidden experience becoming known and lived with as defensive strategies are reduced
- the value of cognitive coping skills, such as cognitive defusion
- value of acceptance, living with the reality of current life experience with compassion towards self
- empathic therapeutic relationship

Behavioural and Cognitive Theory

n=20

- classical conditioning and related process of habituation
- operant conditioning: positive and negative reinforcement, punishment, and extinction; schedules of reinforcement
- interactive importance of both classical and operant conditioning
- accumulation of complex learning histories based on past experiences of reinforcement over lifespan
- safety behaviours
- a focus on changes in behaviour and associated environmental contingencies
- influence of learned logical relational rules on the making of inference and judgement in relation to ourselves and the world around us
- functional analysis, applied behaviour analysis & chain analysis identifying patterns of reinforcement and function of behaviour
- behaviour seen as including cognition, affect and range of private experiences
- relevance of behavioural skills deficits
- emotional/experiential avoidance, the avoidance of distressing and aversive private events, emotional experiences, feelings, sensations & distress that people may not be aware
- value of undefended contact with previously avoided emotional experience
- the value of behavioural coping skills

- human values (personal 'states of affairs' people want to experience) as basis of enduring positive reinforcement
- benefit & need for experience of stable sources of positive reinforcement
- repeated experiences of punishment, and subsequent learned helplessness
- the principle of secondary gain
- importance of relational processes and operant conditioning
- value of acceptance of distress and pain
- non-judgemental empathic, understanding and accepting therapeutic relationship

Appendix 2

Client Consent Form

Consent to Information Being Used in Journal Articles and Other Publications to Help Improve the Knowledge of Professional Staff

Please read the following information carefully. It is asking you to give consent to information about you being used to help increase the knowledge which professionals share amongst themselves. It is very important that you think carefully about this, and only give your consent if you are sure that you are happy about information about you being used in this way. Please ask the psychologist who is working with you any questions you wish to ask. Your decision will not affect the treatment you receive in any way, now or in the future.

Professional staff working with people with psychological problems find it helpful to be able to read about examples of clients' problems and the work which psychologists have done with them in professional journals and other publications. When the information that clients have shared during their contact with psychologists is used in this way the client's personal details are changed so that no one would be able to identify them.

There are two ways in which information might be used:

1. As a brief example of a type of problem.
2. As a more detailed example of a type of problem. The problem and the work done by the client and the psychologist are described more fully. This helps the professionals who read about it to get a clearer picture of how the problems were understood, what happened during therapy, and what sort of changes took place.

If you are happy for information about you to be used in either of these ways, please fill in the consent sections below. You will need to fill in a consent section for each of the two ways in which information might be used.

CONSENT FOR INFORMATION BEING USED IN JOURNAL ARTICLES OR OTHER PROFESSIONAL PUBLICATIONS

1. I have read the information above and give my consent for information about me to be used anonymously in brief examples of psychological problems in journal articles or other professional publications.

    SIGNATURE: DATE:

    NAME:

    (Please print in capital letters)

2. I have read the information above and give my consent for information about me to be used anonymously in more detailed descriptions of psychological problems and the work done together by clients and psychologists in journal articles or other professional publications.

    SIGNATURE: DATE:

    NAME:

    (Please print in capital letters)

Appendix 3

Application of Major Theoretical Approaches Across Sessions

Session													
1	2	3	4	5	6	7	8	9	10	11	12	13	14
H	H	H	H	H	H	H	H		H	H		H	H
P	P	P	P	P	P		P	P	P		P	P	P
A		A	A		A		A	A	A			A	A
	CB	CB	CB	CB	CB	CB			CB	CB		CB	CB

Session												
15	16	17	18	19	20	21	22	23	24	25	26	27
H	H	H	H		H	H	H	H	H	H	H	H
	P		P	P	P	P		P	P	P		P
				A	A	A						A
CB		CB	CB	CB								
S				S								

H	Humanistic theory	CB	Cognitive Behavioural theory
P	Psychodynamic theory	S	Focus on social environment
A	Attachment theory		

References

Ainsworth, M. D. S., Blehar, M. C., Waters, E., & Wall, S. (1978). *Patterns of attachment: A psychological study of the strange situation.* Erlbaum.

Albeniz, A., & Holmes, J. (1996). Psychotherapy integration: Its implications for psychiatry. *British Journal of Psychiatry, 169*(5), 563-570. https://doi.org/10.1192/bjp.169.5.563

Alderson, P. (2021). *Critical realism for health and illness research. A practical introduction.* Bristol University Press.

Anchin, J. C. (2008). Pursuing a unifying paradigm for psychotherapy: Tasks, dialectical considerations, and biosocial systems metatheory. *Journal of Psychotherapy Integration, 18*(3), 310-349. https://doi.org/10.1037/a0013557

Austen, C. (2000). Integrated eclecticism: A therapeutic synthesis. In S. Palmer & R. Woolfe (Eds.), *Integrative and eclectic counselling and psychotherapy* (pp. 127-140). Sage Publications.

Axelrod, S., McElrath, K. K., & Wine, B. (2012). Applied behavior analysis: Autism and beyond. *Behavioral Interventions, 27,* 1-15. https://doi.org/10.1002/bin.1335

Baer, D. M., Wolf, M. M., & Risley, T. R. (1968). Some current dimensions of applied behavior analysis. *Journal of Applied Behavior Analysis, 1,* 91-97. https://doi.org/10.1901/jaba.1968.1-91

Bakan, D. (1966). *The duality of human existence.* Rand McNally.

Balint, M. (1968). *The basic fault.* Routledge.

Baltes, P. B., & Baltes, M. M. (1990) Psychological perspectives on successful aging: The model of selective optimization and compensation. In P. B. Baltes & M. M. Baltes (Eds.), *Successful aging: Perspectives from the behavioral sciences* (pp. 1-34). Lawrence Erlbaum.

Baltes, P. B., & Smith, J. (2003). New frontiers in the future of aging: From successful aging of the young old to the dilemmas of the fourth age. *Gerontology, 49*(2), 123-135. https://doi.org/10.1159/000067946

Bandura, A. (1977). *Social learning theory.* Prentice Hall.

Bandura, A. (1997). *Self-efficacy theory: The exercise of control.* W H Freeman/Times Books/Henry Holt.

Barnard, P. J., & Teasdale, J. D. (1991). Interacting cognitive subsystems: A systemic approach to cognitive-affective interaction and change. *Cognition and Emotion, 5*(1), 1-39. https://doi.org/10/1080/02699939108411021

Barrett-Lennard, G. T. (1998). *Carl Rogers' helping system. Journey & substance.* Sage Publications.

Bartholomew, K., & Horowitz, L. M. (1991). Attachment styles among young adults: A test of a four-category model. *Journal of Personality and Social Psychology, 61*(2), 226-244. https://doi.org/10.1037//0022-3514.61.2.226

Bartlett, F. C. (1932). *Remembering: A study in experimental and social psychology.* Cambridge University Press.

Bateman, A., Brown, D., & Pedder, J. (2010). *Introduction to psychotherapy: An outline of psychodynamic principles and practice* (4th ed.). Routledge.

Beck, A. T. (1999). Cognitive aspects of personality disorders and their relation to syndromal disorders: A psychoevolutionary approach. In C. R. Cloninger (Ed.), *Personality and psychopathology* (pp. 411-429). American Psychiatric Press.

Beck, A. T., Rush, A. J., Shaw, B. F., & Emery, G. (1979). *Cognitive therapy of depression.* Guilford Press.

Beck, A. T., Ward, C. H., Mendelson, M., Mock, J., & Erbaugh, J. (1961). An inventory for measuring depression. *Archives of General psychiatry, 4*(6), 561-571. https://doi.org/10.1001/archpsyc.1961.01710120031004

Beck, J. S. (2011). *Cognitive behaviour therapy: Basics and beyond* (2nd ed.). Guilford Press.

Becker, E. (1973). *The denial of death.* The Free Press.

Beitman, B. D., & Manring, J. (2009). Theory and practice of psychotherapy integration. In G. O. Gabbard (Ed.), *Textbook of psychotherapeutic treatments* (pp. 705-726). American Psychiatric Publishing.

Bem, S. L. (1974). The measurement of androgeny. *Journal of Consulting and Clinical Psychology, 42*(2), 155-162. https://doi.org/10.1037/h0036215

Bem, S. L. (1975). Sex role adaptability: One consequence of psychological androgeny. *Journal of Personality and Social Psychology, 31*(4), 634-643. https://doi.org/10.1037/h0077098

Beutler, L. E., Consoli, A. J., & Lane, G. (2005). Systematic treatment selection and prescriptive psychotherapy: An integrative eclectic approach. In J. C. Norcross & M. R. Goldfried (Eds.), *Handbook of psychotherapy integration* (2nd ed., pp. 121-143). Oxford University Press.

Bhaskar, R. (2015). *The possibility of naturalism. A philosophical critique of the contemporary human sciences* (4th ed.). Routledge.

Bhaskar, R. (2016). *Enlightened common sense: The philosophy of critical realism.* Routledge

Bhaskar, R. (2017). *The order of natural necessity: A kind of introduction to critical realism.* (Gary Hawke, Ed.).

Bidell, M. P. (2016). Mind our professional gaps: Competent lesbian, gay, bisexual, and transgender mental health services. *Counselling Psychology Review, 31*(1), 67-76.

Bion, W. (1984). *Elements of psychoanalysis.* Karnac Books. (Original work published 1963)

Bjork, D. W. (1997). *B F Skinner: A life.* American Psychological Association. https://doi.org/10.1037/10130-000

Blackburn, I. M., & Davidson, K. (1995). *Cognitive therapy for depression and anxiety.* Wiley.

Blackburn, I. M., & Twaddle, V. (2011). *Cognitive therapy in action: A practitioners casebook.* Souvenir Press.

Blair, K. L., & Holmberg, D. (2008). Perceived social network support and well-being in same-sex versus mixed-sex romantic relationships. *Journal of Social and Personal Relationships, 25* (5), 769-791. https://doi.org/10.1177/026540750809665

Bohart, A. C. (2007). The actualizing person. In M. Cooper, M. O'Hara, P. F. Schmid, & G. Wyatt (Eds.), *The handbook of person-centred psychotherapy and counselling* (pp. 47-63). Palgrave Macmillan.

Bowlby, J. (1988). *A secure base: clinical applications of attachment theory.* Routledge.

Bozarth, J. D. (1998). *Person-centred therapy: A revolutionary paradigm.* PCCS Books.

Bozarth, J. D., & Motomasa, N. (2005). Searching for the core: The interface of client-centred principles with other therapies. In S. Joseph, & R. Worsley (Eds.), *Person-centred psychopathology: A positive psychology of mental health* (pp. 293-309). PCCS Books.

Brewin, C. R. (2014). *Cognitive foundations of clinical psychology* (pp. 13-30). Psychology Press. (Original work published 1988)

Brofenbrenner, U. (1979). *The ecology of human development. Experiments by nature and design.* Harvard University Press.

Brofenbrenner, U. (Ed.). (2005). *Making human beings human: Bioecological perspectives on human development.* Sage Publications.

Brown, J. A. C. (1961). *Freud and the post-Freudians.* Penguin Press.

Brown, J. (2015). Specific techniques vs common factors? Psychotherapy integration and its role in ethical practice. *American Journal of Psychotherapy, 69* (3), 301-316.

Brown, G. W., Bifulco, A., & Harris, T. O. (1987). Life events, vulnerability and the onset of depression: Some refinements. *British Journal of Psychiatry, 150,* 30-42. https://doi.org/10.1192/bjp.150.1.30

Brown, G. W., & Harris, T. O. (2011) *The social origins of depression: A study of psychiatric disorder in women.* Routledge. (Original work published 1978)

Burns, D. D. (1980). *Feeling good: The new mood therapy.* Signet.

Burns, D. D., & Nolen-Heoksema, S. (1992). Therapeutic empathy and recovery from depression in cognitive-behaviour therapy: A structural equation model. *Journal of Consulting and Clinical Psychology, 60,* 441-449.

Carlson, R. (1971). Sex differences in ego functioning: Exploratory studies of agency and communion. *Journal of Consulting and Clinical Psychology, 37* (2), 267-277. https://doi.org/10.1037/h0031947

Casement, P. (2014). *On learning from the patient* (classic ed.). Routledge. (Original work published 1985)

Castonguay, L. G., Goldfried, M. R., Wiser, S., Raue, P. J., & Hayes, A. M. (1996). Predicting the effect of cognitive therapy for depression: A study of unique and common factors. *Journal of Consulting and Clinical Psychology, 64*(3), 497-504. https://doi.org/10.1037/0022-006X.64.3.497

Castonguay, L. G., Newman, M. G., Borkovec, T. D., Holtforth, M. G., & Maramba, G. G. (2005). *Cognitive behavioral assimilative integration.* In J. C. Norcross & M. R.

Goldfried (Eds.), *Handbook of psychotherapy integration* (2nd ed. pp. 241-260). Oxford University Press.

Clark, D. M. (2012). The English improving access to psychological therapies (IAPT) program. History and progress. In R. K. McHugh & D. H. Barlow (Eds.), *Dissemination and implementation of evidence-based psychological interventions* (pp. 61-77). Oxford University Press.

Clark, D. M. (2018). Realizing the mass public benefit of evidence-based psychological therapies: the IAPT program. *Annual Review of Clinical Psychology, 14,* 159-183. https://doi.org/10.1146/annurev-clinpsy-050817-084833

Clark-Carter, D. (2007). Effect size and statistical power in psychological research. *The Irish Journal of Psychology, 28*(1-2), 3-12. https://doi.org/10.1080/03033910.2007.10446244

Clarke, G. S. (2006). *Personal relations theory. Fairbairn, Macmurry and Suttie.* Routledge.

Clarkson, P., & Cavicchia, S. (2013). *Gestalt counselling in action.* Sage Publications.

Cleary, P. D., & Mechanic, D. (1983). Sex differences in psychological distress among married people. *Journal of Health and Social Behaviour, 24*(2), 111-121. https://doi.org/10.2307/2136638

Collier, A. (1994). *Critical realism. An introduction to Roy Bhaskar's philosophy.* Verso.

Connors, M. E. (2011). Attachment theory: A "secure base" for psychotherapy integration. *Journal of Psychotherapy Integration, 21* (3), 348-362. https://doi.org/10.1037/a0025460

Crane, R. (2009). *Mindfulness-based cognitive therapy.* Routledge.

Craske, M. G. (2003). *Origins of phobias and anxiety disorders: Why more women than men?* Elsevier.

Cumming, E., & Henry, W. (1961). *Growing old: The process of disengagement.* Basic Books.

Curwen, B., Palmer, S., & Ruddell, P. (2018). *Cognitive behaviour therapy* (2nd ed.). Sage Publications.

Dana, D. (2018). *The polyvagal theory in therapy. Engaging the rhythm of regulation.* W. W. Norton.

deCarvalho, R. J. (1999). Otto Rank, the Rankian circle in Philadelphia, and the origins of Carl Rogers' person-centred psychotherapy. *History of Psychology, 2* (2), 132-148. https://doi.org/10.1037/1093-4510.2.2.132

Deklyen, M., & Greenberg, M. T. (2016). Attachment and psychopathology in childhood. In J. Cassidy & P. R. Shaver (Eds.), *Handbook of Attachment. Theory, research and clinical applications* (3rd ed., pp. 639-666). Guilford Press. https://doi.org/10.1002/imhj.21730

Derogatis, L.R., & Melisaratos, N. (1983). The Brief Symptom Inventory: an introductory report. *Psychological Medicine, 13,* 595-605. https://doi.org/10.1017/S0033291700004801

DeYoung, P. A. (2015). *Relational psychotherapy. A primer* (2nd ed.). Routledge.

Dollard, J., & Miller, N. E. (1950). *Personality and psychotherapy.* McGraw-Hill.

Egan, G. (2017). *The skilled helper. A problem management and opportunity development approach to helping* (9th ed.). Brooks/Cole.

Eichenbaum, L., & Orbach, S. (1983). *Understanding women: A feminist psychoanalytic approach.* Basic Books.

Elliott, R., & Greenberg, L. (2007). The essence of process-experiential/emotion-focused therapy. *American Journal of Psychotherapy, 61*(3), 241-254. https://doi.org/10.1176/appi.psychotherapy.2007.61.3.241

Englar-Carlson, M., & Stevens, M. A. (Eds.). (2006). *In the room with men: A casebook of therapeutic change.* American Psychological Association.

Erickson, E. H. (1980). *Identity and the life cycle.* W. W. Norton. (Original work published 1959)

Erikson, E. H., & Erikson, J. M. (1998). *The life cycle completed.* W.W. Norton. (Original work published 1982)

Fairbairn, W. R. D. (1952). Schizoid factors in the personality. In *Psychoanalytic studies of the personality.* Routledge. (Original work published 1940)

Fairbairn, W. R. D. (1958). On the nature and aims of psycho-analytic treatment. *International Journal of Psychoanalysis, 39*(5), 374-385.

Feixas, G., & Botella, L. (2004). Psychotherapy integration: Reflections and contributions from a constructivist epistemology. *Journal of Psychotherapy Integration, 14*(2), 192-222. https://doi.org/10.1037/1053-0479.14.2.192

Ferster, C. B. (1973). A functional analysis of depression. *American Psychologist, 28*(10), 857-870. https://doi.org/10.1037/h0035605

Fivush, R., Brotman, M. A., Buckner, J., & Goodman, S. (2000). Gender differences in parent-child emotion narratives. *Sex Roles, 42,* 233-253. https://doi.org/10.1023/A:1007091207068

Flaxman, P. E., Blackledge, J. T., & Bond, F. W. (2011). *Acceptance and commitment therapy.* Routledge.

Flew, A. (1984). *A dictionary of philosophy.* Pan Books.

Fonagy, P. (1989). On the integration of cognitive-behaviour theory with psychoanalysis. *British Journal of Psychotherapy, 5*(4), 557-563. https://doi.org/10.1111/j.1752-0118.1989.tb01114.x

Fonagy, P., & Bateman, A. W. (2007). Mentalizing and borderline personality disorder. *Journal of Mental Health, 16*(1), 83-101. https://doi.org/10.1080/09638230601182045

Fonagy, P., & Target, M. (1996). Playing with reality: I. Theory of mind and the normal development of psychic reality. *The International Journal of Psychoanalysis, 77*(2), 217-233.

Fonagy, P., & Target, M. (2006). The mentalization-focused approach to self pathology. *Journal of Personality Disorder, 20*(6), 544-576. https://doi.org/10.1521/pedi.2006.20.6.544

Fonagy, P., Gergely, G., & Target, M. (2008). Psychoanalytic constructs and attachment theory and research. In J. Cassidy & P. R. Shaver (Eds.), *Handbook of attachment: Theory, research and clinical applications* (pp. 783-809). Guilford Press.

Frank, K. A. (1990). Action techniques in psychoanalysis. *Contemporary Psychoanalysis, 26,* 732-756. https://doi.org/10.1080/00107530.1990.10746688

Frank, J. D., & Frank, J. B. (1991). *Persuasion & healing. A comparative study of psychotherapy* (3rd ed.). John Hopkins Press.

Frank, J. D., & Frank, J. (2004). Therapeutic components shared by all psychotherapies. In A. Freeman, M. J. Mahoney, P. Devito & D. Martin (Eds.), *Cognition and psychotherapy* (2nd ed., pp. 45-78). Springer Publishing.

Frawley O'Dea, M.G., & Sarnat, J.E. (2001). *The supervisory relationship. A contemporary psychodynamic approach.* Guilford Press.

Frederickson, J. (1999). *Psychodynamic Psychotherapy. Learning to listen from multiple perspectives.* Routledge.

Freeman, A., & Martin, D. M. (2004). A psychosocial approach for conceptualizing schematic development. In A. Freeman, M. J. Mahoney, P. Devito & D. Martin (Eds.), *Cognition and psychotherapy* (2nd ed., pp. 221-255). Springer Publishing.

Freud, S. (1977). *On sexuality.* The Pelican Freud Library, Vol 7. Penguin Books. (Original work published 1905-1931)

Freud, S. (1979). *On psychopathology.* The Pelican Freud Library, Vol 10. Penguin Press. (Original work published 1895-1926)

Freud, S. (1984). *On metapsychology.* The Pelican Freud Library, Vol 11. Penguin Press. (Original work published 1911-1940)

Fromm, E. S. (2013) *The art of loving.* Open Road Media. (Original work published 1956)

Gantt, E. E., Lindstrom, J. P., & Williams, R. N. (2016). The generality of theory and the specificity of social behavior: Contrasting experimental and hermeneutic social science. *Journal for the Theory of Social Behaviour, 47* (2), 130-152. https://doi.org/10.1111/jtsb.12111

Gendlin, E.T. (1996). *Focusing-oriented psychotherapy. A manual of the experiential method.* Guilford Press.

Gilbert, P. (2010). *Compassion focused therapy: Distinctive features.* Routledge.

Gilbert, P., & Irons, C. (2005). Focused therapies and compassionate mind training for shame and self-attacking. In P. Gilbert (Ed.), *Compassion. Conceptualisations, research and use in psychotherapy* (pp. 263-325). Routledge.

Goldberg, D. P., & Huxley, P. (1992) *Common mental disorders: A bio-social model.* Tavistock/Routledge.

Goldfried, M. R. (2019). Obtaining consensus in psychotherapy: What holds us back. *American Psychologist, 74(4), 484-496.* https://doi.org/10.1037/amp0000365

Goodman, S. H., & Lusby, C. M. (2014). Early adverse experiences and depression. In I. H. Gotlib & C. L. Hammen (Eds.), *Handbook of Depression,* (3rd ed., pp.220-239). Guilford Press.

Gotlib, I. H., & Hammen, C. L. (1992a). The social functioning of depressed persons: I. Life events, social support, and interpersonal behavior. In I. N. Gotlib & C. L. Hammen, *Psychological aspects of depression. Toward a cognitive-interpersonal integration* (pp. 141-165). Wiley.

Gotlib, I. H., & Hammen, C. L. (1992b). The social functioning of depressed persons: II. Marital and family relationships. In I. N. Gotlib & C. L. Hammen, *Psychological aspects of depression. Toward a cognitive-interpersonal integration* (pp. 166-192). Wiley.

Gove, W., & Tudor, J. F. (1973). Adult sex roles and mental illness. *American Journal of Sociology, 78*(4), 812-835. https://doi.org/10.1086/225404

Green, J., & Goldwyn, R. (2002). Attachment disorganization and psychopathology: New findings in attachment research and their potential implications for developmental psychopathology in childhood. *Journal of Child Psychology and Psychiatry, 33*(7), 835-846. https://doi.org/10.1111/1469-7610.00102

Greenberg, L. S. (2004). Emotion-focused therapy. *Clinical Psychology and Psychotherapy, 11,* 3-16. https://doi.org/10.1002/cpp.388

Greenberg, L. S. (2011). *Theories of psychotherapy. Emotion-focused therapy.* American Psychological Association.

Greenberg, L. S., & Safran, J. D. (1987). *Emotion in psychotherapy: Affect, cognition and the process of change* (pp. 13-72). Guilford Press.

Greenberger, D., & Padesky, C. A. (2015). *Mind over mood. A cognitive therapy treatment manual for clients* (2nd ed.). Guilford Press.

Guidano, V. F. (1991). *The self in process: A developmental approach to psychotherapy and therapy.* Guilford Press.

Haliburn, J. (2017). *An integrated approach to short-term dynamic interpersonal psychotherapy.* Karnac.

Hammen, C. L., & Shih, J. (2014). Depression and interpersonal processes. In I. H. Gotlib & C. L. Hammen (Eds.), *Handbook of Depression,* (3rd ed., pp. 277-295). Guilford Press.

Hammen, C. L., Brennan, P. A., & LeBroque, R. (2011). Youth depression and early childrearing: Stress generation and intergenerational transmission of depression. *Journal of Consulting and Clinical Psychology, 79*(3), 353-363. https://doi.org/10.1037/a0023536

Harris, T. (2001). Recent developments in understanding the psychosocial aspects of depression. *British Medical Bulletin, 57*(1), 17-32. https://doi.org/10.1093/bmb/57.1.17

Hartwig, M. (2007). *Dictionary of critical realism.* Routledge.

Harwood, T. M., Beutler, L.E., & Charvat, M. (2010). Cognitive-behavioral therapy and psychotherapy integration. In K. Dobson (Ed.). *Handbook of cognitive-behavioral therapies* (3rd ed.), (pp. 94-130). Guilford Press.

Hautamaki, A., Hautamamki, L., Neuvonen, L., & Malinimi-Piispanen, S. (2010). Transmission of attachment across three generations. *European Journal of Developmental Psychology, 7*(5), 618-634. https://doi.org/10.1080/17405620902983519

Havinghurst, R. J. (1972). *Developmental tasks and education* (3rd ed.). David McKay.

Hawton, K., Salkovskis, P., Kirk, J., & Clark, D. (1989). *Cognitive behaviour therapy for psychiatric problems.* Oxford University Press.

Hayes, S. C. (2004). Acceptance and commitment therapy, relational frame theory, and the third wave of behavioral and cognitive therapies. *Behavior Therapy, 35,* 639-665. https://doi.org/10.1016/j.beth.2016.11.006

Hayes, S. C., Barnes-Holmes, D., & Roche, B. (Eds.). (2001). *Relational frame theory: A post-Skinnerian account of human language and cognition.* Kluwer Academic/Plenum Publishers.

Hayes, S. C., Strosahl, K. D., & Wilson, K. G. (1999). *Acceptance and commitment therapy: An experiential approach to behavior change.* Guilford Press.

Hazan, C., & Shaver, P. (1987). Romantic love conceptualized as an attachment process. *Journal of Personality and Social Psychology, 52*(3), 511-524. https://doi.org/10.1037/0022-36514.52.3.511

Hendry. L. B., & Kloep, M. (2012). *Adolescence and adulthood. Transitions and transformations.* Palgrave MacMillan.

Hingley, S. M. (1981). *Depression and sex roles: The interaction of psychological and social factors.* [Unpublished undergraduate dissertation]. University of Sheffield.

Hingley, S. M. (1983). *Sex role stereotypes and depression in women: The interaction of psychological and social factors.* [Unpublished master's dissertation]. University of Liverpool.

Hingley, S. M. (1995). Cognition, emotion and defence: Processes and mechanisms of change in a brief psychotherapy of depression. *Clinical Psychology and Psychotherapy, 2* (2), 122-133. https://doi.org/10.1002/cpp.5640020207

Hingley, S. M. (2001). Psychodynamic theory and narcissistically related personality problems: Support from case study research. *British Journal of Medical Psychology, 74,* 5-72. https://doi.org/10.1348/000711201160803

Hobson, R. E. (1985). *Forms of feeling. The heart of psychotherapy.* Tavistock Publications.

Hollanders, H. (2000). Eclecticism/Integration: Some key issues and research. In S. Palmer, & R. Woolfe (Eds.), *Integrative and eclectic counselling and psychotherapy* (pp. 31-55). Sage

Holmes, J. (1993). *John Bowlby and attachment theory.* Routledge.

Holmes, J. (1996). *Attachment, intimacy, autonomy: Using attachment theory in adult psychotherapy.* Jason Aronson.

Holmes, J. (2001). *The search for the secure base. Attachment theory and psychotherapy.* Routledge.

Holmes, J., & Slade, A. (2018). *Attachment in therapeutic practice.* Sage Publications.

Honderich, T. (Ed.). (1995). *The oxford companion to philosophy.* Oxford University Press.

Hopcroft, R. L., & Bradley, D. B. (2007). The sex difference in depression across 29 countries. *Social Forces, 85*(4), 1483-1507. https://doi.org/10.1353/sof.2007.0071

Horowtiz, M. J. (1994). States, schemas, and control: General theories for psychotherapy integration. *Clinical Psychology & Psychotherapy, 1,* 143-152.

Ingvarssonn, E.T., & Morris, E.K. (2004). Post-Skinnerian, post-Skinner, or neo-Skinnerian? Hayes, Barnes-Holmes, and Roche's relational frame theory: A post-Skinnerian account of human language and cognition. *The Psychology Record,* 54, 497-504.

Irons, C., & Beaumont, E. (2017). *The compassionate mind work book.* Robinson.

Ivanov-Smolensky, A. G. (1927). On methods of examining conditioned food reflexes in children and in mental disorders. *Brain, 50,* 138-141. https://doi.org/10.1093/brain/50.2.138

Iversen, I.H. (1992). Skinner's early research. From reflexology to operant conditioning. *American Psychologist, 47* (11), 1318-1328.

Jacobs, M. (1995). *D. W. Winnicott.* Sage Publications.

Jacobs, M. (2004). *Psychodynamic counselling in action.* Sage Publications.

Joseph, S. (2010). *Theories of counselling and psychotherapy. An introduction to the different approaches.* Palgrave Macmillan.

Jung, C. G. (2014). *The structure and dynamics of the psyche* (2nd ed.). Routledge. (Original work published 1960)

Kagan, C., Burton, M., Duckett, P., Lawthom, R., & Siddiquee, A. (2020). *Critical community psychology* (2nd ed.). Routledge.

Kahn, M. (1997). *Between therapist and client. The new relationship.* Owl Books.

Kanfer, F. H., & Goldstein, A. P. (1986) *Helping people change. A textbook of methods* (2nd ed.). Pergammon.

Kanter, J. W., Bush, A. M., & Rusch, L. C. (2009). *Behavioral activation.* Routledge.

Katz, S. J., Hammen, C. L., & Brennan, P. A. (2013). Maternal depression and intergenerational transmission of relational impairment. *Journal of family psychology, 27*(1), 86-95. https://doi.org/10.1037/a0031411

Kelly, G. A. (1963). *A theory of personality. The psychology of personal constructs.* W. W. Norton.

Kennerley, H., Kirk, J., & Westbrook, D. (2016). *An introduction to cognitive behaviour therapy. Skills & applications* (3rd ed.). Sage.

Kingerlee, R., Precious, D., Sullivan, L., & Barry, J. (2014). Engaging with the emotional lives of men. *The Psychologist, 27*(6), 418-421.

Kohlenberg, R. J., & Tsai, M. (1991). *Functional analytic psychotherapy. Creating intense and curative therapeutic relationships.* Plenum Press. https://doi.org/10.1007/978-0-387-70855-3

Kohut, H. (1977). *The restoration of the self.* International Universities Press.

Kohut, H. (1984). *How does analysis cure?* (A. Goldberg & P. E. Stepansky, Eds.). University of Chicago Press.

Kuehner, C. (2003). Gender differences in unipolar depression: An update of epidemiological findings and possible explanations. *Acta Psychiatrica Scandinavica, 108*(3), 163-174. https://doi.org/10.1034/j.1600-0447.2003.00204.x

Larkin, P. (1974). This be the verse. In *High Windows* (p. 30). Faber and Faber.

Lazarus, A. A. (1958). New methods in psychotherapy: A case study. *South African Medical Journal, 32*(26), 660-663.

Lazarus, A. A. (1997). *Brief but comprehensive psychotherapy. The multimodal way.* Springer Publishing.

Lazarus, A. A. (2005). Multimodal therapy. In J. C. Norcross & M. R. Goldfried (Eds.), *Handbook of psychotherapy integration* (2nd ed. pp. 105-120). Oxford University Press.

Lebow, J. (2002). Emergent issues in integrative and eclectic psychotherapies. In F. W. Kaslow & J. Lebow (Eds.), *Comprehensive handbook of psychotherapy, Vol. 4: Integrative/eclectic* (pp. 569-578). Wiley.

Leiper, R., & Maltby, M. (2004). *The psychodynamic approach to therapeutic change.* Sage Publications.

Lemma, A., Target, M., & Fonagy, P. (2011). *Brief dynamic interpersonal therapy. A clinician's guide.* Oxford University Press.

Levinson, D. J. (1978). *The seasons of a man's life.* Ballantine.

Levinson, D. J. (1986). A conception of adult development. *American Psychologist, 42,* 3-13. https://doi.org/10.1037/0003-066X.41.1.3

Levinson, D. J. (2011). *The seasons of a woman's life. A fascinating exploration of the events, thoughts, and life events that all women share.* Random House. (Original work published 1996)

Lewinsohn, P. (1974). A behavioral approach to depression. In R. J. Friedman & M. M. Katz (Eds.), *Psychology of depression: Contemporary theory and research.* Wiley.

Linehan, M. M. (1993). *Cognitive-behavioral treatment of borderline personality disorder.* Gilford Press.

McConnell, M., & Moss, E. (2011). Attachment across the lifespan: Factors that contribute to stability and change. *Australian Journal of Educational and Developmental Psychology, 11*, 60-77.

Magnavita, J. J. (2008). Toward unification of clinical science: The next wave in the evolution of psychotherapy? *Journal of Psychotherapy Integration, 18*(3), 264-291. https://doi.org/10.1037/a0013490

Magnavita, J. J., & Anchin, J. C. (2014). *Unifying psychotherapy: Principles, methods and evidence from clinical science.* Springer Publishing.

Mahler, M. S., Pine, F., & Bergman, A. (1975). *The psychological birth of the human infant.* Basic Books.

Mahoney. M.J., (2003). *Constructive psychotherapy: A practical guide.* Guilford Press.

Main, M., Kaplan, N., & Cassidy, (1985). Security in infancy, childhood and adulthood: A move to the level of representation. *Monographs of the Society for Research in Child Development, 50*(1-2), 66-104. https://doi.org/10.2307/3333827

Main, M., & Solomon, J. (1990). Procedures for identifying infants as disorganized/disoriented during the Ainsworth strange situation. In M. Greenberg, D. Cicchetti & E. M. Cummings (Eds.), *Attachment during the preschool years: Theory, research and intervention* (pp. 121-160). University of Chicago Press.

Malan, D. H. (1995). *Individual psychotherapy and the science of psychodynamics.* Butterworth-Heinemann.

Marcotte, D., & Safran, J. D. (2002). Cognitive-interpersonal psychotherapy. In F. W. Kaslow & J. Lebow (Eds.), *Comprehensive handbook of psychotherapy, Vol. 4: Integrative/eclectic* (pp. 273-293). Wiley.

Maroda, K. J. (1998). Enactment. When the patient's and analyst's pasts converge. *Psychoanalytic Psychology, 15*(4), 517-535. https://doi.org/10.1037/0736-9735.15.4.517

Martell, C. R., Dimidjian, S., & Herman-Dunn, R. (2010). *Behavioral activation for depression.* Guilford Press.

Martens, A., Goldenberg, J. L., & Greenberg, J. (2005). A terror management perspective on ageism. *Journal of Social Issues, 61*(2), 223-239. https://doi.org/10.1111/j.1540.4560.2005.00403.x

Maslow, A. H. (1943). A theory of human motivation. *Psychological Review, 50*(4), 370-396. https://doi.org/10.1037/h0054346

Mearns, D., & Thorne, B. (2000). *Person-centred therapy today. New frontiers in theory and practice.* Sage Publications.

Mearns, D., & Thorne, B. (with McLeod, J.). (2013). *Person-centred counselling in action* (4th ed.). Sage Publications.

Messer, S. B. (1986). Behavioral and psychoanalytic perspectives at therapeutic choice points. *American Psychologist, 41*(11), 1261-1272.

Meth, R. L., & Pasick, R. S. (1990). *Men in therapy. The challenge of change.* Guilford Press.

Miller, S., & Konorski, J. (1937). On two types of conditioned reflex. *Journal of General Psychology, 16,* 264-272. https://doi.org/10.1080/00221309.1937.9917950

Möller-Leimkühler, A. (2002). Barriers to help-seeking by men: A review of sociocultural and clinical literature with particular reference to depression. *Journal of Affective Disorders, 71*(1-3), 1-9. https://doi.org/10.1016/SO165-0327(01)00327-2

Mooney, K. A., & Padesky, C. (2000). Applying client creativity to recurrent problems: Constructing possibilities and tolerating doubt. *Journal of Cognitive Psychotherapy, 14*(2), 149-161. https://doi.org/10.1891/0889-8391.14.2.149

Moore, J. (2001). On distinguishing methodological from radical behaviorism. *European Journal of Behavior Analysis, 2,* 221-244. https://doi.org/10.1080/15021149.2001.11434196

Morrissey, J., & Tribe, R. (2001). Parallel process in supervision. *Counselling Psychology Quarterly, 14,* 103-110. https://doi.org/10.1080/09515070126329

Mowrer, O. H. (1951). Two-factor learning theory: summary and comment. *Psychological Review, 58*(5), 350-354. https://doi.org/10.1037/h0058956

Murphy, D., & Joseph, S. (2016). Client-centred therapy and post-traumatic growth. In P. Wilkins (Ed.), *Person-centred and experiential therapies. Contemporary approaches and issues in practice* (pp. 119-132). Sage Publications.

Murphy, K., & Gilbert, M. (2000). A systematic integrative relational model for counselling and psychotherapy. In S. Palmer & R. Woolfe (Eds.), *Integrative and eclectic counselling and psychotherapy* (pp. 93-109). Sage Publications.

National Collaborating Centre for Mental Health (2019). *Improving access to psychological therapies* (version 3).

Neimayer, R. A. (2009). *Constructivist psychotherapy.* Routledge.

Neimayer, R. A., & Mahoney, M. J. (1995). *Constructivism in psychotherapy.* American Psychological Association.

Nelson, T. D. (Ed.). (2017). *Ageism. Stereotyping and prejudice against older persons* (2nd ed.). MIT Press.

Nelson-Jones, R. (1982). *The theory and practice of counselling psychology.* Holt, Rineheart and Winston.

Nolen-Hoeksema, S. (2006). The etiology of gender differences in depression. In C. M. Mazure & G. P. Keita (Eds.), *Understanding depression in women: Applying empirical research to practice and policy* (pp. 9-43). American Psychological Association. https://doi.org/10.1037/11434-001

Norcross, J. C., & Goldfried, M. R. (Eds.). (2005). *Handbook of psychotherapy integration* (2nd ed.). Oxford University Press.

O'Brien, M., & Houston, G. (2000). *Integrative psychotherapy. A practitioner's guide* (2nd ed.). Sage Publications.

O'Donohue, W. (2013). *Clinical psychology and the philosophy of science.* Springer.

Oliver, J. M., & Baumgart, E. P. (1985). The Dysfunctional Attitudes Scale: Psychometric properties and relation to depression in an unselected adult population. *Cognitive Therapy and Research, 9,* 161-168. https://doi.org/10.1007/BF01204847

Owens, R. G., & Ashcroft, J. B. (1982). Functional analysis in applied psychology. *British Journal of Clinical Psychology, 21*(3), 181-189. https://doi.org/10.1111/j.2044-8260.1982.tb00550.x

Padesky, C. A. (1994). Schema change processes in cognitive therapy. *Clinical Psychology & Psychotherapy, 2*(5), 267-278. https://doi.org/10.1002/cpp.5640010502

Palmer, S. (2000). Multimodal therapy. In S. Palmer & R. Woolfe (Eds.), *Integrative and eclectic counselling and psychotherapy* (pp. 141-162). Sage Publications.

Parloff, M. B. (1986). Frank's "common elements" in psychotherapy: Nonspecific factors and placebos. *American Journal of Orthopsychiatry, 56*(4), 521-439. https://doi.org/10.1111/j.1939-0025.1986.tb03485.x

Pavlov, I. (1927). *Conditioned reflexes.* Oxford University Press.

Persons, J. (1989). *Cognitive therapy in practice: A case formulation approach.* W. W. Norton.

Phillipson, H. (1995). *The object relations technique.* Tavistock Publications.

Pietersma, H. (2000). *Phenomenological epistemology.* Oxford University Press.

Pilgrim, D. (2018). Paying the price of positivism. *Clinical Psychology Forum, 309,* 12-15.

Pilgrim, D. (2019). *Critical realism for psychologists.* Routledge.

Pocock, D. (2015). A philosophy of practice for systemic psychotherapy: The case for critical realism. *Journal of Family Therapy, 37*(2), 167-183. https://doi.org/10.1111/1467-6427.12027

Porges, S. W. (2011). *The polyvagal theory: Neurophysiological foundations of emotions, attachment, communication, and self-regulation.* W.W. Norton.

Power, M. (2010). *Emotion-focused cognitive therapy.* Wiley-Blackwell.

Power, M., & Brewin, C. R. (1997). *The transformation of meaning in psychological therapies. Integrating theory and practice.* Wiley.

Power, M., & Dalgleish, T. (2008). *Cognition and emotion. From order to disorder* (2nd ed.). Psychology Press.

Prochaska, J. O., & DiClemente, C. C. (1983). Stages and processes of self-change of smoking: Toward an integrative model of change. *Journal of Consulting and Clinical Psychology, 51*(3), 390-395. https://doi.org/10.1037/0022-006X.51.3.390

Prochaska, J. O., & DiClemente, C. C. (2005). The transtheoretical approach. In J. C. Norcross & M. R. Goldfried (Eds.), *Handbook of psychotherapy integration* (2nd ed., pp. 147-171). Oxford University Press.

Rafaeli, E., Bernstein, D. P., & Young, J. (2011). *Schema Therapy.* Routledge.

Rank, O. (1978). *Truth and reality.* W. W. Norton. (Original work published 1936)

Rogers, C. R. (1942). *Counseling and psychotherapy: Newer concepts in practice.* Houghton Mifflin.

Rogers, C. R. (1957). The necessary and sufficient conditions of therapeutic personality change. *Journal of Consulting and Clinical Psychology, 21* (3), 95-103. https://doi.org/10.1037/h0045357

Rogers, C. (1967). *A therapist's view of psychotherapy. On becoming a person.* Constable. (Original work published 1961)

Rogers, C. (1980). *A way of being.* Houghton Mifflin.

Rogers, C. (2003). *Client-centered therapy. Its current practice, implications and theory.* Constable. (Original work published 1951)

Rosenberg, A. (2012). *Philosophy of social science, A contemporary introduction* (3rd ed.). Routledge.

Rosenzweig, S. (2002). Some implicit common factors in diverse methods of psychotherapy. *Journal of Psychotherapy Integration, 12*(1), 5-9. (Original work published 1936) https://doi.org/10.1037/1053-0479.12.1.5

Roth, A., & Fonagy, P. (2006). *What works for whom?: A critical review of psychotherapy research.* Guilford Press.

Rutter, M. (1991) *Maternal deprivation reassessed* (2nd ed.). Penguin Press.

Ryle, A. (1975). Self-to-self, self-to-other: The world's shortest account of object relations. *New Psychiatry, 24,* 12-13.

Ryle, A. (1994a). Projective identification: A particular form of reciprocal role procedure. *British Journal of Medical Psychology, 67,* 107-114. https://doi.org/10.1111/j.2044-8341.1994.tb01776.x

Ryle, A. (1994b). Consciousness and psychotherapy. *British Journal of Medical Psychology, 67,* 115-123. https://doi.org/10.1111/j.2044-8341.1944.tb01777.x

Ryle, A. (Ed.). (1995a). *Cognitive analytic therapy. Developments in theory and practice.* Wiley.

Ryle, A. (1995b). Psychoanalysis, cognitive analytic psychotherapy, mind and self. *British Journal of Psychotherapy, 11*(4), 567-596. https://doi.org/10.1111/j.1752-0118.1995.tb00766.x

Ryle, A., & Kerr, I. B. (2020). *Introducing Cognitive Analytic Therapy. Principles and practice of a relational approach to mental health* (2nd ed.). Wiley.

Safran, J. D. (1998). *Widening the scope of cognitive therapy: The therapeutic relationship, emotion and the processes of change.* Jason Aronson.

Safran, J. D., & Ink, T. A. (1995). Psychotherapy integration: Implications for the treatment of depression. In E. E. Beckham & W. R. Leber (Eds.) *Handbook of Depression* (2nd ed., pp. 425-434). Guilford Press.

Sanders, P. (2013). The 'family' of person-centred and experiential therapies. In M. Cooper, M. O'Hara, P. F. Schmid & A. C. Bohart, (Eds.), *The handbook of person-centred psychotherapy & counselling* (2nd ed., pp. 46-65). Palgrave Macmillan.

Sanders, D., & Wills, F. (2005). *Cognitive therapy. An introduction* (2nd ed.). Sage Publications.

Scarvalone, P., Fox, M., & Safran, J. D. (2005). Interpersonal schemas: Clinical theory, research and implications. In M. W. Baldwin (Ed.), *Interpersonal cognition.*

Schore, A. N. (2012). *The science of the art of psychotherapy.* W. W. Norton.

Scott, M. M., Slavich, G. M., & Georgiades, K. (2014). The social environment and depression: The roles of life stress. In I. H. Gotlib & C. L. Hammen (Eds.), *Handbook of Depression,* (3rd ed., pp. 296-314). Guilford Press.

Segal, H. (2018). *Introduction to the work of Melanie Klein.* Routledge. (Original work published 1973)

Segal, Z. V., Williams, J. M. G., & Teasdale, J. D. (2002). *Mindfulness-based cognitive therapy for depression: A new approach to preventing relapse.* Guilford Press.

Seligman, M. E. P. (1975). *Learned helplessness. On depression, development and death.* Freeman.

Shean, G. D. (2013). Controversies in psychotherapy research: Epistemic differences in assumptions about human psychology. *American Journal of Psychotherapy, 67*(1), 73-87. https://doi.org/10.1176/appl.psychotherapy.2013.67.1.73

Sheftall, A. H., Schoppe-Sullivan, S. J., & Bridge, J. A. (2014). Insecure attachment and suicidal behaviour in adolescents. *Crisis: The Journal of Crisis Intervention and Suicide Prevention, 35*(6), 426-430. https://doi.org/10.1027/0227-5910/a000273

Shiraev, E. B., & Levy, D. A. (Eds). (2016). *Cross-cultural psychology. Critical thinking and contemporary applications* (6th ed.). Routledge.

Siegel, A. M. (1996). *Heinz Kohut and the psychology of the self.* Routledge.

Skinner, B. F. (1938). *The behavior of organisms: An experimental analysis.* Appleton-Century-Crofts.

Skinner, B. F. (1974). *About behaviorism.* Random House.

Smidt, S. (2018). *Introducing Trevarthen. A guide for practitioners and students in early years education.* Routledge.

Stern, D. N. (2018). *The interpersonal world of the infant. A view from psychoanalysis and developmental psychology.* Routledge. (Original work published 1984)

Stovall-McClough, K. C., & Dozier, M. (2016). Attachment states of mind and psychopathology in adulthood. In J. Cassidy & P. R. Shaver (Eds.), *Handbook of Attachment. Theory, research and clinical applications* (3rd ed., pp. 715-738). Guilford Press. https://doi.org/10.1002/imhj.21730

Stricker, G. (2010). *Psychotherapy integration.* American Psychological Association.

Striker, G., & Gold, J. (2002). An assimilative approach to integrative psychodynamic psychotherapy. In F. W. Kaslow & J. Lebow (Eds.), *Comprehensive handbook of psychotherapy, Vol. 4: Integrative/eclectic* (pp. 295-315). Wiley.

Sugarman, L. (2001). *Life-span development. Frameworks, accounts and strategies.* Psychology Press.

Sugarman, L. (2004). *Counselling and the life course.* Sage Publications.

Sullivan, H. S. (1953). *The interpersonal theory of psychiatry.* W. W. Norton.

Super, D. E. (1980). A life-span, life-space approach to career development. *Journal of Vocational Behaviour, 16,* 282-298. https://doi.org/10.1016/0001-8791(80)90056-1

Suttie, I. D. (1988). *The origins of love and hate.* Routledge. (Original work published 1935)

Swales, M. A., & Heard, H. L. (2009). *Dialectical behaviour therapy.* Routledge.

Symington, J., & Symington, N. (1996). *The clinical thinking of Wilfred Bion.* Routledge.

Taft, J. (1933). *The dynamics of therapy in a controlled relationship.* Macmillan. https://doi.org/10.1037/10602-000

Teasdale, J. D., & Barnard, P. J. (1993). *Affect, cognition and change.* Psychology Press.

Thomas-Anttila, K. (2015). Confidentiality and consent issues in psychotherapy case reports. The Wolf Man, Gloria and Jeremy. *British Journal of Psychotherapy, 31*(3), 360-375. https://doi.org/10.1111/bjp.12157

Thorndike, E. L. (1927). The law of effect. *The American Journal of Psychology, 39*(1/4), 212-222. https://doi.org/10.2307/1415413

Thorne, B. (2003). *Carl Rogers* (2nd ed.). Sage Publications.

Timulak, L., & Pascual-Leone, A. (2015). New developments for case conceptualization in emotion-focused therapy. *Clinical Psychology and Psychotherapy, 22,* 619-636. https://doi.org/10.1002/cpp.1922

Tolan, J. (2003). *Skills in person-centred counselling & psychotherapy.* Sage Publications.

Trevarthen, C. (2005). First things first: infants make good use of the sympathetic rhythm of imitation, without reason or language. *Journal of Child Psychotherapy,* 31(1), 91-113. https://doi.org/10.1080/00754170500079651

Trevarthen, C., & Aitken, K. J. (2001). Infant intersubjectivity: Research, theory, and clinical applications. *J. Child Psychology and Psychiatry,* 42(1), 3-48. https://doi.org/10.1111/1469-7610.00701

Tsai, M., Yard, S., & Kohlenberg, R. J. (2014). Functional analytic psychotherapy: A behavioral relational approach to treatment. *Psychotherapy, 51* (3), 364-371. https://doi.org/10.1037/a0036506

Vaillant, G. E. (1971). Theoretical hierarchy of adaptive ego mechanisms. A 30-year follow-up of 30 men selected for psychological health. *Archives of General Psychiatry,* 24, 107-118. https://doi.org/10.1001/archpsyc.1971.01750080011003

Wachtel, P. L. (1977). *Psychoanalysis and behavior therapy: Toward an integration.* Basic Books.

Wachtel, P. L. (1997). *Psychoanalysis, behavior therapy and the relational world.* American Psychological Association.

Wachtel, P. L. (2010). Psychotherapy integration and integrative psychotherapy: Process or product? *Journal of Psychotherapy Integration, 20* (4), 406-416. https://doi.org/10.1037/a0022032

Wachtel, P. L. (2014). *Cyclical psychodynamics and the contextual self. The inner world, the intimate world and the world of culture and society.* Routledge.

Wachtel, P. L., Kruk, J. C., & McKinney, M. K. (2005). Cyclical psychodynamics and integrative relational psychotherapy. In J. C. Norcross & M. R. Goldfried (Eds.), *Handbook of psychotherapy integration* (2nd ed., pp. 172-195). Oxford University Press.

Wallin, D.J. (2007). *Attachment in psychotherapy.* Guilford Press.

Wampold, B. E. (2019). *The basics of psychotherapy. An introduction to theory and practice* (2nd ed.). American Psychological Association. https://dx.doi.org/10.1037/0000117-000

Wampold, B. E., & Imel, Z. E. (2015). *The great psychotherapy debate. The evidence for what makes psychotherapy work* (2nd ed.). Routledge.

Warner, M. (2000). Person-centred therapy at the difficult edge: a developmentally based model of fragile and dissociated process. In D. Mearns & B. Thorne, *Person-centred therapy today. New frontiers in theory and practice* (pp. 144-171). Sage Publications.

Waters, E., Hamilton, C. E., & Weinfield, S. (2000). The stability of attachment security from infancy to adolescence and early adulthood. General introduction. *Child Development,* 71(3), 678-683. https://doi.org/10.1111/1467-8624.00175

Watson, J. B. (1924). *Behaviorism.* People's Institute.

Watson, J. B., & Raynor, R. (1920). Conditioned emotional reactions. *Journal of Experimental Psychology,* 3(1), 1-14. https://doi.org/10.1037/h0069608

Welch, I. D. (2003). *The therapeutic relationship: Listening and responding in a multicultural world*. Praeger/Greenwood.

West, M., & Sheldon, A. E. R. (1988). Classification of pathological attachment patterns in adults. *Journal of Personality Disorders, 2*(2), 153-159. https://doi.org/10.1521/pedi.1988.2.2.153

Westwell, G. (2016). Experiential therapy. In P. Wilkins (Ed.), *Person-centred and experiential therapies. Contemporary approaches and issues in practice* (pp. 64-88). Sage Publications.

Wilkins, P. (2016). *Person-centred and experiential therapies. Contemporary approaches and issues in practice*. Sage Publications.

Williams, J., Stephenson, D., & Keating, F. (2014). A tapestry of oppression. *The Psychologist, 27*(6), 406-409.

Williams, J. M. G., Watts, F. N., MacLeod, C., & Matthews, A. (1997). Nonconscious processing. In *Cognitive psychology and emotional disorders* (2nd ed., pp. 231-275). Wiley.

Winnicott, D. W. (1974). *Playing and reality*. Penguin Books. (Original work published 1971)

Winnicott, D. W. (1986). *Home is where we start from*. W. W. Norton.

Winnicott, D. W. (1990). *The maturational process and the facilitating environment*. Karnac Books. (Original work published 1965)

Wolpe, J. (1958). *Psychotherapy by reciprocal inhibition*. Stanford University Press.

Young, J. (1990). *Cognitive therapy for personality disorders: A schema focused approach*. Professional Resource Exchange.

Young, J., & Klosko, J. S. (1993). *Reinventing your life*. Dutton.

Young, J. E., Klosko, J. S., & Weishaar, M. S. (2003). *Schema therapy: A practitioners guide*. Guilford Press.

www.ingramcontent.com/pod-product-compliance
Lightning Source LLC
Chambersburg PA
CBHW050643270326
41927CB00012B/2859